T. Tsubokawa · A. Marmarou
C. Robertson · G. Teasdale (Eds.)

Neurochemical Monitoring in the Intensive Care Unit

Microdialysis, Jugular Venous Oximetry,
and Near-Infrared Spectroscopy

Proceedings of the 1st International Symposium on Neurochemical
Monitoring in the ICU held concurrently with the 5th Biannual
Conference of the Japanese Study Group of Cerebral Venous
Oximetry in Tokyo, Japan, May 20–21, 1994

With 82 Figures

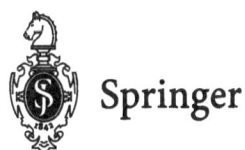 Springer

Takashi Tsubokawa, M.D., D.Sc.
Professor and Chairman, Department of Neurological Surgery
Nihon University School of Medicine
Tokyo, Japan

Anthony Marmarou, Ph.D.
Professor, Division of Neurosurgery
Medical College of Virginia, Virginia Commonwealth University
Richmond, Virginia, USA

Claudia Robertson, M.D.
Professor, Department of Neurosurgery
Baylor College of Medicine
Houston, Texas, USA

Graham Teasdale, M.D.
Professor and Chairman, Department of Neurosurgery
Southern General Hospital, University of Glasgow
Glasgow, Scotland
ISBN 978-4-431-68524-1   ISBN 978-4-431-68522-7 (eBook)
DOI 10.1007/978-4-431-68522-7

Printed on acid-free paper

Library of Congress Cataloging-in-Publication Data. Neurochemical monitoring in the inten-
sive care unit : microdialysis, jugular venous oximetry, and near-infrared spectroscopy /
T. Tsubokawa . . . [et al.] (eds.). p. cm. Includes bibliographical references and index.
                    1. Neurological intensive care—Congresses.   2. Patient monitoring—
Congresses. 3. Neurochemistry—Congresses.   4. Brain   microdialysis—Congresses. 5.
Oximetry—Congresses. 6. Near   infrared   spectroscopy—Congresses. I. Tsubokawa,
Takashi. RC350.N49N43 1995 616.8′0428—dc20   95-6883 CIP

Preface

Neurophysiological recording is the major neuromonitoring technique employed in ICU. In addition, continuous recording of intracranial pressure has proved to provide infomation useful for critical care of the patient with severe brain damage. It is, however, difficult to assess neurochemical and/or metabolic environments of the brain with these conventional neuromonitoring techniques. Information regarding these changes, if available on a real-time basis, is undoubtedly useful for patient care. Many important developments in bedside techniques to monitor these changes have been achieved during the last few years. It was the consensus of the editors that a symposium to exchange knowledge concerning recent advances in such techniques would be valuable.

With this background, the First International Symposium of Neurochemical Monitoring in ICU held May 20–21, 1994, in Tokyo, Japan. It was not the intention of the organizers that this symposium should survey the whole field of neuromonitoring in ICU. The symposium was thus focused on clinical application of microdialysis, jugular venous oximetry, and near-infrared spectroscopy, which currently appear to be the most promising techniques for monitoring neurochemical and metabolic changes in the brain in a clinical setting. We termed these techniques collectively as neurochemical monitoring, contrasting them with neurophysiological monitoring in ICU. The concept that has motivated this symposium was to provide an opportunity to exchange up-to-date summaries on issues currently debated for these techniques. This volume is based on the papers presented at the symposium.

The editors appreciate having received contributions from many active investigators in this field. These contributions were provided generously and promptly, despite the authors' other commitments. The editors also express sincere thanks to Dr. Yoichi Katayama, who agreed as the chair of the Japanese Study Group of Cerebral Venous Oximetry to hold the symposium concurrently with their Fifth Biannual Conference and served as a co-organizer of the symposium. The contribution of Dr. Atsuo Yoshino as secretary is also greatly appreciated.

Takashi Tsubokawa, M.D., D.Sc.

Proceedings of the First International Symposium on Neurochemical Monitoring in ICU held concurrently with the Fifth Biannual Conference of the Japanese Study Group of Cerebral Venous Oximetry in Tokyo, Japan, May 20–21, 1994.

Contents

Part 1

Basic Problems of Microdialysis Technique

Basic Problems in Clinical Application of Microdialysis Technique
YOICHI KATAYAMA 3
Glutamate Neurotoxicity as a Mechanism of Ischemic Brain Damage:
A Basic Study Using a New in Vivo Model
HIROSUKE FUJISAWA, HANS LANDOLT, ROSS BULLOCK 26
Delayed Neuronal Damage Following Focal Ischemic Injury in
Stroke-Prone Spontaneously Hypertensive Rats
TOSHIKI SHIROTANI, KATSUJI SHIMA, MIWAKO IWATA, HIDEYUKI KITA,
HIROO CHIGASAKI 34
Prolonged Stimulation-Induced Afterdischarges of Hippocampal CA1
Pyramidal Cells After Ischemia in Vivo
MAKOTO FURUICHI, SHUHEI MIYAZAKI, YOICHI KATAYAMA,
TAKASHI TSUBOKAWA 42
The Use of Microdialysis for Monitoring the Effect of the
Neuroprotective Drug CI-977 on Extracellular Excitatory Amino Acid
S. GALBRAITH, K.B. MACKAY, T.R. PATEL, J. McCULLOCH 47

Part 2

Clinical Application of Microdialysis Technique

Microdialysis for Neurochemical Monitoring in Human Brain Injury
LARS HILLERED, LENNART PERSSON 59
Patterns of Excitatory Amino Acid Release and Ionic Flux after
Severe Human Head Trauma
R. BULLOCK, A. ZAUNER, O. TSUJI, J.J. WOODWARD,
A.T. MARMAROU, H.F. YOUNG 64

Measurement of Excitatory Amino Acid Release in Glioma and
Contused Brain Tissue During Intracranial Surgery
    TATSURO KAWAMATA, YOICHI KATAYAMA, KOSAKU KINOSHITA,
    TAKASHI TSUBOKAWA   72
Measurement of Lactic Acid and Amino Acid in the Cerebral Cortex
of Head Injury Patients Using Microdialysis
    J. CLAY GOODMAN, DANIEL P. ROBERTSON, SHANKAR P. GOPINATH,
    RAJ K. NARAYAN, ROBERT G. GROSSMAN, RICHARD K. SIMPSON JR.,
    CLAUDIA S. ROBERTSON   78

Part 3

Clinical Impact of Jugular Bulb Oximetry

Benefits and Pitfalls of Jugular Bulb Venous Oxygen Saturation
Monitoring
    N. MARK DEARDEN   87
Continuous Monitoring of Jugular Venous Oxygen Saturation in
Neurosurgical ICU
    HIROYUKI YOKOTA, YASUHIRO YAMAMOTO, MATOAKI NAKABAYASHI,
    AKIRA FUSE, KUNIHIRO MASHIKO, HIROSHI HENMI, TOSHIBUMI OTSUKA,
    SHIRO KOBAYASHI, SHOZO NAKAZAWA   98
The Optimal Cerebral Perfusion Pressure Management of Patients
with Severe Brain Injury
    K.H. CHAN, S.C.P. NG   105
Bilateral Jugular Bulb Oximetry
    HIROSHI INAGAWA, YASUSEI OKADA, SOU SUZUKI, KAZUYUKI ONO,
    KAZUHIKO MAEKAWA   112
Causes and Treatment of Desaturation in SjO_2 Monitoring
    MOTOAKI NAKABAYASHI, HIROYUKI YOKOTA, AKIRA FUSE,
    HIDETAKA SATO, SHIGEKI KUSHIMOTO, KAZUYOSHI KATO,
    AKIRA KUROKAWA   120
Evaluation of Continuous Monitoring of Jugular Venous
Oxygen Saturation (SjO_2), Regional Cerebral Oxygen Saturation
(rSO_2) and EEG Power Spectrum for Intraoperative Cerebral
Ischemia
    YOSHIHIRO IKUTA, TATSUHUKO KANO, EIJI ABE, MARI SESHITA,
    KANEMITSU HIGASHI   127
Jugular Bulb Oxygen Saturation and Oxygen Consumption in Patients
Receiving Barbiturate Therapy
    KAZUMI IKEDA, NARIHIRO YOSHIMATSU, HIDETO KANEKO,
    MASATOSHI SUGI, TOHRU IIZUKA, YOSHIYUKI KAMEYAMA,
    NAGAO ISHII   134

Does the Transient Decrease in SvO_2 and SjO_2 During the Rewarming
Phase in a Cardiopulmonary Bypass (CPB) Merely Reflect a Recovery
of the Metabolic Rate?: A case Report
  H. OKAMOTO, K. IRITA, T. TANIYAMA, T. KAWASAKI, Y. KAI,
  S. TAKAHASHI 140
Jugular Bulb Oximetry in Patients with Cerebral Arteriovenous
Malformation
  TERUYASU HIRAYAMA, YOICHI KATAYAMA,
  TAKASHI TSUBOKAWA 146

Part 4

Jugular Bulb Oximetry in Head Injured Patients

$SjvO_2$ Monitoring in Head Injured Patients
  CLAUDIA S. ROBERTSON 153
Intraoperative Monitoring of Jugular Venous Oxygen Saturation in
Patients with Severe Head injury
  S.P. GOPINATH, A.M. RITTER, C.S. ROBERTSON 160
Multimodal Evaluation of Cerebral Oxygen Metabolism Disturbances in
Patients with Severe Head Injury
  TOSHIYUKI SHIOGAI, AKIO NOGUCHI, EISHI SATO, ISAMU SATO 164
Continuous Monitoring of Jugular Bulb Oxygen Saturation in the
Management of the Patients with Severe Closed Head Injury
  YASUFUMI MIZUTANI, TSUYOSHI KATABAMI, MASAHIKO UDZURA,
  TAKEKI OGAWA, HIROAKI SEKINO, YOSHIO TAGUCHI,
  IKUO YAMANAKA 172
CO_2-Reactivity and Autoregulation in Severe Head Injury: Bedside
Assessment by Relative Changes in AVDO2
  JUAN SAHUQUILLO, MARCELINO BAGUENA, LAURA CAMPOS,
  MONTSERRAT OIVE.. 180

Part 5

Characteristics of Near-Infrared Spectroscopy

Validation of a Noninvasive Measurement of Regional Hemoglobin
Oxygen Saturation
  VALERIE POLLARD, ERIC A. DEMELO, DONALD J. DEYO,
  REBECCA DALMEIDA, R. WIDMAN, DONALD S. PROUGH 193
Validation of Monitoring of Cerebral Oxygenation by Near Infrared
Spectroscopy (NIRS) in Comatose Patient
  A. UNTERBERG, A. ROSENTHAL, G.H. SCHNEIDER, K. KIENIG,
  W.R. LANKSCH 204

Near-Infrared Spectroscopy at the Sagittal Sinus Region: Comparison
with Jugular Buld Oxymetry
  HIDEHIKO KUSHI, TADASHI SHIBUYA, MOTOAKI FUJII,
  YOICHI KATAYAMA, TAKASHI TSUBOKAWA 211
Bilateral Simultaneous Monitoring of Regional Cerebrovascular Oxygen
Saturation Using Near-Infrared Spectroscopy
  ISSEI NARA, TOSHIYUKI SHIOGAI, NAHOKO TANAKA, MANABU TOKITSU,
  ISAMU SAITO 218
Effects of Hyperventilation and CO_2 Inhalation on Cerebral Oxygen
Metabolism of Moyamoya Disease Measured by Near Infrared
Spectroscopy
  KAORU SAKATANI, MASAFUMI OHTAKI, MASATAKA KASHIWASAKE,
  KAZUO HASHI 226

Index 235

List of Contributors

E. Abe
Department of Anesthesiology, Kumamoto University Hospital,
Kumamoto, Japan   127

M. Báguena
Department of Neurotraumatology Intensive Care Unit, Vall d'Hebron
University Hospital, Barcelona, Spain   180

R. Bullock
Division of Neurosurgery, Medical College of Virginia, Virginia, USA
                                                               26, 64

L. Campos
Department of Neurotraumatology Intensive Care Unit, Vall d'Hebron
University Hospital, Barcelona, Spain   180

K.H. Chan
Division of Neurosurgery, Department of Surgery, University of Hong
Kong, Hong Kong   105

H. Chigasaki
Department of Neurosurgery, National Defense Medical College,
Saitama, Japan   34

R. Dalmeida
Department of Anesthesia, The University of Texas Medical Branch in
Galveston, Texas, USA   193

M.N. Dearden
Department of Anaesthesia, Leeds General Infirmary, Leeds, UK   87

E.A. DeMelo
Department of Anesthesia, The University of Texas Medical Branch in
Galveston, Texas, USA   193

D.J. Deyo
Department of Anesthesia, The University of Texas Medical Branch in
Galveston, Texas, USA   193

J.C. Goodman
Department of Neurosurgery and Pathology, Baylor College of Medicine,
Houston, USA   78

M. Fujii
Department of Neurological Surgery, Nihon University School of
Medicine, Tokyo, Japan   211

H. Fujisawa
Department of Neurosurgery, Yamaguchi University School of Medicine,
Yamaguchi, Japan   26

M. Furuichi
Department of Neurological Surgery, Nihon University School of
Medicine, Tokyo, Japan   42

A. Fuse
Department of Emergency and Critical Care Medicine, Nihon Medical
School, Tokyo, Japan   98, 120

S. Galbraith
Wellcome Surgical Institute & Hugh Fraser Neuroscience Labs.,
University of Glasgow, Glasgow, UK   47

S.P. Gopinath
Department of Neurosurgery, Baylor College of Medicine, Houston,
USA   78, 160

R.G. Grossman
Department of Neurosurgery and Pathology, Baylor College of Medicine,
Houston, USA   78

K. Hashi
Department of Neurosurgery, Sapporo Medical University, Sapporo,
Japan   226

H. Henmi
Department of Emergency and Critical Care Medicine, Nihon Medical
School, Tokyo, Japan   98, 120

K. Higashi
Surgical Center, Kumamoto University Hospital, Kumamoto, Japan   127

L. Hillered
Department of Neurosurgery, Department of Clinical Chemistry, Uppsala
University Hospital, Uppsala, Sweden   59

T. Hirayama
Department of Neurological Surgery, Nihon University School of
Medicine, Tokyo, Japan   146

T. Iizuka
Department of Anesthesiology, Tokyo Medical College, Tokyo, Japan
                                                              134

K. Ikeda
Department of Anesthesiology, Tokyo Medical College, Tokyo, Japan
                                                              134

T. Ikeda
Department of Anesthesiology, Tokyo Medical College, Tokyo, Japan
                                                              134

Y. Ikuta
Surgical Center, Kumamoto University Hospital, Kumamoto, Japan   127

H. Inagawa
Department of Traumatology and Critical Care, Faculty of Medicine,
University of Tokyo, Tokyo, Japan   112

K. Irita
Department of Anesthesiology and Critical Care Medicine, Faculty of
Medicine, Kyushu University, Fukuoka, Japan   140

N. Ishii
Department of Anesthesiology, Tokyo Medical College, Tokyo, Japan
                                                              134

M. Iwata
Department of Neurosurgery, National Defense Medical College,
Saitama, Japan   34

Y. Kai
Department of Anesthesiology and Critical Care Medicine, Faculty of
Medicine, Kyushu University, Fukuoka, Japan   140

Y. Kameyama
Department of Anesthesiology, Tokyo Medical College, Tokyo, Japan
                                                              134

H. Kaneko
Department of Anesthesiology, Tokyo Medical College, Tokyo, Japan
                                                              134

T. Kano
Surgical Center, Kumamoto University Hospital, Kumamoto, Japan   127

M. Kashiwasake
Hamamatsu Photonics Tsukuba Laboratory, Ibaraki, Japan   226

T. Katabami
Department of Neurosurgery, St. Marianna University School of
Medicine, Yokohama, Japan   172

Y. Katayama
Department of Neurological Surgery, Nihon University School of
Medicine, Tokyo, Japan   3, 42, 72, 146, 211

K. Kato
Department of Emergency and Critical Care Medicine, Nihon Medical
School, Tokyo, Japan   120

T. Kawamata
Department of Neurological Surgery, Nihon University School of
Medicine, Tokyo, Japan   72

T. Kawasaki
Department of Anesthesiology and Critical Care Medicine, Faculty of
Medicine, Kyushu University, Fukuoka, Japan   140

K. Kiening
Department of Neurosurgery, Rudolf Virchow Medical Center, Free
University of Berlin, Berlin, Germany   204

K. Kinoshita
Department of Neurological Surgery, Nihon University School of
Medicine, Tokyo, Japan   72

H. Kita
Department of Neurosurgery, National Defense Medical College,
Saitama, Japan   34

S. Kobayashi
Department of Neurosurgery, Nihon Medical School, Tokyo, Japan   98

A. Kurokawa
Department of Emergency and Critical Care Medicine, Nihon Medical
School, Tokyo, Japan   120

H. Kushi
Department of Neurological Surgery, Nihon University School of
Medicine, Tokyo, Japan   211

S. Kushimoto
Department of Emergency and Critical Care Medicine, Nihon Medical
School, Tokyo, Japan   120

H. Landolt
Neurochirurgische Universitätsklinik, Kantonsspital, Basel, Switzerland
                                                                              26

W.R. Lanksch
Department of Neurosurgery, Rudolf Virchow Medical Center, Free
University of Berlin, Berlin, Germany   204

K.B. Mackay
Wellcome Surgical Institute & Hugh Fraser Neuroscience Labs.,
University of Glasgow, Glasgow, UK   47

K. Maekawa
Department of Traumatology and Critical Care, Faculty of Medicine,
University of Tokyo, Tokyo, Japan   112

A. T. Marmarou
Division of Neurosurgery, Medical College of Virginia, Virginia, USA 64

K. Mashiko
Department of Emergency and Critical Care Medicine, Nihon Medical
School, Tokyo, Japan   98

J. McCulloch
Wellcome Surgical Institute & Hugh Fraser Neuroscience Labs.,
University of Glasgow, Glasgow, UK   47

S. Miyazaki
Department of Neurological Surgery, Nihon University School of
Medicine, Tokyo, Japan   42

Y. Mizutani
Department of Neurosurgery, St. Marianna University School of
Medicine, Yokohama, Japan   172

M. Nakabayashi
Department of Emergency and Critical Care Medicine, Nihon Medical
School, Tokyo, Japan   98, 120

S. Nakazawa
Department of Neurosurgery, Nihon Medical School, Tokyo, Japan   98

I. Nara
Department of Neurosurgery, Kyorin University School of Medicine,
Tokyo, Japan   218

R.K. Narayan
Department of Neurosurgery and Pathology, Baylor College of Medicine,
Houston, USA   78

S.C.P. Ng
Division of Neurosurgery, Department of Surgery, University of Hong
Kong, Hong Kong   105

A. Noguchi
Department of Neurosurgery, Kyorin University School of Medicine, Tokyo, Japan   164

T. Ogawa
Department of Neurosurgery, St. Marianna University School of Medicine, Yokohama, Japan   172

M. Ohtaki
Department of Neurosurgery, Sapporo Medical University, Sapporo, Japan   226

Y. Okada
Department of Traumatology and Critical Care, Faculty of Medicine, University of Tokyo, Tokyo, Japan   112

H. Okamoto
Department of Anesthesiology and Critical Care Medicine, Faculty of Medicine, Kyushu University, Fukuoka, Japan   140

M. Olivé
Department of Anesthesiology, Vall d'Hebron University Hospital, Barcelona, Spain   180

K. Ono
Department of Traumatology and Critical Care, Faculty of Medicine, University of Tokyo, Tokyo, Japan   112

T. Otsuka
Department of Emergency and Critical Care Medicine, Nihon Medical School, Tokyo, Japan   98, 120

T.R. Patel
Wellcome Surgical Institute & Hugh Fraser Neuroscience Labs., University of Glasgow, Glasgow, UK   47

L. Persson
Department of Neurosurgery, Uppsala University Hospital, Uppsala, Sweden   59

V. Pollard
Department of Anesthesia, The University of Texas Medical Branch in Galveston, Texas, USA   193

D.S. Prough
Department of Anesthesia, The University of Texas Medical Branch in Galveston, Texas, USA   193

A. M. Ritter
Department of Neurosurgery, Baylor College of Medicine, Houston, USA   160

C.S. Robertson
Department of Neurosurgery, Baylor College of Medicine, Houston,
USA   78, 153, 160

D.P. Robertson
Department of Neurosurgery and Pathology, Baylor College of Medicine,
Houston, USA   78

A. Rosenthal
Department of Neurosurgery, Rudolf Virchow Medical Center, Free
University of Berlin, Berlin, Germany   204

J. Sahuquillo
Department of Neurosurgery, Vall d'Hebron University Hospital,
Barcelona, Spain   180

I. Saito
Department of Neurosurgery, Kyorin University School of Medicine,
Tokyo, Japan   164, 218

K. Sakatani
Department of Neurosurgery, Sapporo Medical University, Sapporo,
Japan   226

E. Sato
Department of Neurosurgery, Kyorin University School of Medicine,
Tokyo, Japan   164

H. Sato
Department of Emergency and Critical Care Medicine, Nihon Medical
School, Tokyo, Japan   120

G.H. Schneider
Department of Neurosurgery, Rudolf Virchow Medical Center, Free
University of Berlin, Berlin, Germany   204

H. Sekino
Division of Neurosurgery, The Second Department of Surgery, St.
Marianna University School of Medicine, Yokohama, Japan   172

M. Seshita
Department of Anesthesiology, Kumamoto University Hospital,
Kumamoto, Japan   127

T. Shibuya
Department of Neurological Surgery, Nihon University School of
Medicine, Tokyo, Japan   211

K. Shima
Department of Neurosurgery, National Defense Medical College,
Saitama, Japan   34

T. Shiogai
Department of Neurosurgery, Kyorin University School of Medicine,
Tokyo, Japan   164, 218

T. Shirotani
Department of Neurosurgery, National Defense Medical College,
Saitama, Japan   34

R.K. Simpson
Department of Neurosurgery and Pathology, Baylor College of Medicine,
Houston, USA   78

M. Sugi
Department of Anesthesiology, Tokyo Medical College, Tokyo, Japan
                                    134

S. Suzuki
Department of Traumatology and Critical Care, Faculty of Medicine,
University of Tokyo, Tokyo, Japan   112

Y. Taguchi
Division of Neurosurgery, The Second Department of Surgery, St.
Marianna University School of Medicine, Yokohama, Japan   172

S. Takahashi
Department of Anesthesiology and Critical Care Medicine, Faculty of
Medicine, Kyushu University, Fukuoka, Japan   140

N. Tanaka
Department of Neurosurgery, Kyorin University School of Medicine,
Tokyo, Japan   218

T. Taniyama
Intensive Care Unit, Faculty of Medicine, Kyushu University, Fukuoka,
Japan   140

M. Tokitsu
Department of Neurosurgery, Kyorin University School of Medicine,
Tokyo, Japan   218

T. Tsubokawa
Department of Neurological Surgery, Nihon University School of
Medicine, Tokyo, Japan   42, 72, 146, 211

O. Tsuji
Division of Neurosurgery, Medical College of Virginia, Virginia, USA   64

M. Udzura
Department of Neurosurgery, St. Marianna University School of
Medicine, Yokohama, Japan   172

A. Unterberg
Department of Neurosurgery, Rudolf Virchow Medical Center, Free
University of Berlin, Berlin, Germany   204

R. Widman
Somanetics Corp., Missouri, USA   193

J. J. Woodward
Division of Neurosurgery, Medical College of Virginia, Virginia, USA 64

Y. Yamamoto
Department of Emergency and Critical Care Medicine, Nihon Medical
School, Chiba, Japan   98

I. Yamanaka
Department of Critical Care Medicine, St. Marianna University School of
Medicine, Yokohama, Japan   172

H. Yokota
Department of Emergency and Critical Care Medicine, Nihon Medical
School, Chiba, Japan   98, 120

N. Yoshimatsu
Department of Anesthesiology, Tokyo Medical College, Tokyo, Japan
                                                                        134

H.F. Young
Division of Neurosurgery, Medical College of Virginia, Virginia, USA 64

A. Zauner
Division of Neurosurgery, Medical College of Virginia, Virginia, USA 64

Part 1

Basic Problems of Microdialysis Technique

Basic Problems in Clinical Application of Microdialysis Technique

Yoichi Katayama

Introduction

There are three major advantages in using the microdialysis technique [1,2] for investigating neurochemical processes in the central nervous system (CNS). First, this technique enables various neurochemical changes to be monitored simultaneously. Second, this technique provides a means of examining the mechanisms of the neurochemical changes by modifying various neurochemical environments in situ via the dialysis probe. Finally and most importantly, the changes detected by this technique represent those occurring in the extracellular space (ECS), which permits neuro-chemical changes in the ECS to be distinguished from those in the intracel-lular space (ICS). These advantages have provided valuable data for elucidating the neurochemical processes in a variety of diseases, including ischemic [3–7] and traumatic brain injuries [8–10]. Based on such data, a major advance has been made in understanding pathological processes within the CNS during the last decade [e.g., 11,12].

There are, however, several possibilities for misinterpretation of the data obtained from the diseased CNS. To avoid such misinterpretation, it is probably most important to note that the information provided by the microdialysis technique sensitively reflects the biochemical properties of the cellular membrane separating the ECS and ICS, which are not always the same volume. For example, dialysate concentration of a given substance is dependent on the ECS volume, which is maintained by cellular membrane function. During cerebral ischemia or anoxia, an abrupt change in cellular membrane function develops [13]. Similar changes can be induced by various forms of traumatic brain injury [14–17]. Because these changes cause ionic fluxes and water movement through the cellular membrane into the cells,

Department of Neurological Surgery, Nihon University School of Medicine, 30-1, Oyaguch, Kamimachi, Itabashi-ku, Tokyo 173, Japan, and Division of Neurosurgery, UCLA School of Medicine, University of California at Los Angeles, California 90024, U.S.A.

cellular swelling develops concomitantly with ionic shifts [18–21]. Accordingly, possible changes in function of the cellular membrane should always be taken into consideration before any conclusions are drawn from the data obtained by this technique.

This chapter discusses how these changes in cellular membrane function influence the data obtained by the microdialysis technique. Such properties of microdialysis can, on the other hand, be viewed as another advantage for detecting alterations in cellular membrane function in the diseased CNS. This chapter also reviews the data obtained from experimental models of ischemic and traumatic brain injury to delineate the unique value of microdialysis for investigating the mechanisms of the changes in cellular membrane function.

Methodological Problems

Methodological problems associated with the microdialysis technique have been the subject of numerous publications [e.g., 22–27]. These difficulties are not repeated here. A discussion is given of the methodological aspects that are important to note for maximizing the unique capability of the technique of detecting changes in cellular membrane function. As mentioned, these aspects must of course also be borne in mind in any experiments using the microdialysis technique to study the diseased CNS.

Depletion of Substances from the Extracellular Space

The microdialysis technique involves insertion of a dialysis probe into the cerebral tissue, which causes a kind of focal traumatic brain injury. To exclude such initial effects of probe insertion, a certain period of time must be allowed to elapse before conducting the actual experiment. The duration of the time required for stabilization of the baseline data is highly variable depending on the substance of interest. Broadly speaking, the longer the duration for stabilization of the baseline data, the better the experimental data obtained appear to be. When the duration of dialysis is too long, however, there may be an *unphysiological stabilization* that is sometimes critical for the data analysis. There have been no extensive studies of how much of the period required for baseline data stabilization results from the initial effects of probe insertion and how much from unphysiological stabilization.

The dialysis process is basically a removal of substances located within the ECS. With the microdialysis techique, the brain tissue is dialyzed for a certain period of time by the perfusate. This will inevitably lead to a slow but continuous removal of the substance of interest from the ECS, and could potentially produce an unphysiologically lowered level of many substances.

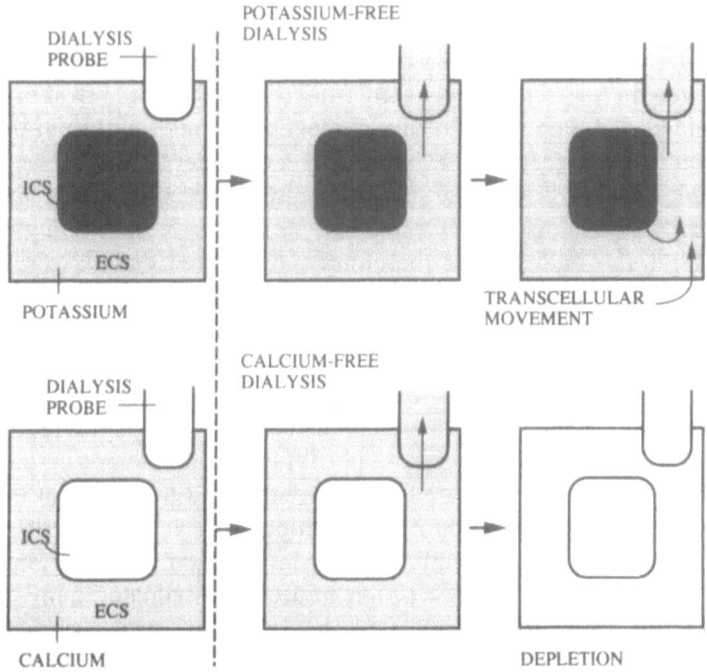

FIG. 1. Effects of K⁺-free (*upper panel*) and Ca²⁺-free dialysis (*lower panel*). Following initiation of K⁺-free dialysis (*dashed line*), $[K^+]_d$ remains at approximately the same level for a considerable period of time because K^+ is replenished continuously by the *transcellular movement* of K^+. In contrast, $[Ca^{2+}]_d$ decreases rapidly following initiation of the Ca²⁺-free dialysis (*dashed line*), and Ca^{2+} can be depleted by Ca²⁺-free dialysis. *ECS*, extracellular space; *ICS*, intracellular space. *Darker tone* indicates higher concentrations of K^+ (*upper*) or Ca^{2+} (*lower*)

The best example of such a problem is provided by the outcome of Ca²⁺-free dialysis (Fig. 1) [28]. Following initiation of the Ca²⁺-free dialysis, the dialysate concentration of Ca^{2+} ($[Ca^{2+}]_d$) decreases rapidly from the higher values because of the previous Ca²⁺-containing perfusate, and $[Ca^{2+}]_d$ continues to decrease. The baseline $[Ca^{2+}]_d$ is often decreased to less than half within 40 min following initiation of the Ca²⁺-free dialysis. Employing ⁴⁵Ca autoradiography, we have confirmed extensive Ca^{2+} depletion within a brain area of approximately 2–3 mm in diameter when Ca²⁺-free dialysis is continued for more than 30 min (unpublished observations).

In contrast to Ca^{2+}, extracellular concentration of K^+ ($[K^+]_e$) is quite resistant to removal by microdialysis (see Fig. 1) [28]. Following the initiation of K⁺-free dialysis, the dialysate concentration of K^+ ($[K^+]_d$) decreases rapidly from the higher values because of the previous K⁺-containing perfusate, but a stationary level of $[K^+]_d$ is obtained within 5 min. Although a very slow progressive decrease does occur thereafter, the $[K^+]_d$ remains at approximately the same level for a considerable period of time. The presence of a slight but significant decrease in the baseline $[K^+]_d$ becomes apparent only when the K^+-free dialysis is continued for 60 min.

If K^+-free dialysis removes K^+ only from the ECS, the removal of 0.2 mM at 5 μl/min as dialysate would result in a loss of 1.0 nmol/min from the ECS, which could deplete all the K^+ in 3.3 μl ECS after 10 min. The lack of remarkable changes in baseline $[K^+]_d$ actually observed indicates that K^+ is replenished continuously by *transcellular movement* of K^+ during K^+-free dialysis [29]. It would appear therefore that K^+-free dialysis can provide reasonable information regarding alterations in $[K^+]_e$ and associated neurochemical changes, such as those observed during cerebral ischemia, in short-term experiments.

The foregoing two examples clearly demonstrate the critical role of the transcellular movement of substances in determining the period required for stabilization of the baseline data. The diffusion parameters of each substance [29], which may be altered by the volume and tortuosity of the ECS, must also be taken into account. In addition, passive movements of substances across the cellular membrane may be changed under certain pathological conditions. Some of these problems are discussed later in this chapter. Active uptake from and release into the ECS obviously represent other determinants of the data obtained with this technique. Although most experiments are designed to measure or modify these functions [e.g., 1–10], and no detailed analysis may be called for, it should be remembered that these are always determinants of the stabilization of the baseline data.

Cellular Swelling and Shrinkage of the Extracellular Space

When rapid cellular swelling occurs, water moves from the ECS into the cells and causes shrinkage of the ECS, that is, a decrease in water volume in the ECS. If the substance of interest does not move from the ECS into the cells and is left behind, the concentration of the substance in the ECS will increase and the data yielded by the microdialysis technique will thereby be influenced.

The occurrence of cellular swelling and resultant shrinkage of the ECS during cerebral ischemia, anoxia, or spreading depression has been repeatedly demonstrated in in vitro [30,31] as well as in vivo [20,21,32,33] studies by various methods. The cellular swelling and ECS shrinkage can be detected as an increase in concentration of ECS markers, such as tetraethylammonium, tetraethyltrismethylammonium, and choline, which do not move from the ECS into the cells [20,32]. These markers are introduced into the ECS by a superfusion technique, and changes in their ECS concentration are monitored by employing electrodes sensitive to ammonium ions [20,32].

Cellular swelling during cerebral ischemia can be detected by microdialysis based on similar principles [34]. ^{14}C-labeled sucrose is preperfused into the ECS through the dialysis probe. This substance has been widely employed in in vitro studies as an ECS marker. Changes in the ECS concentration of ^{14}C-labeled sucrose ($[^{14}C\text{-labeled sucrose}]_e$) are then determined from the dialysate with perfusate without ^{14}C-labeled sucrose. Following termination of the ^{14}C-labeled sucrose perfusion, $[^{14}C\text{-labeled sucrose}]_d$ decreases rapidly during initial period of a few minutes and decreases slowly thereafter. Autoradiograms have demonstrated that an area approximately 1.5 mm distant from the probe is perfused by the ^{14}C-labeled sucrose.

A sudden and marked increase in $[^{14}C\text{-labeled sucrose}]_d$ is observed at 1–3 min after the induction of cerebral ischemia [34]. The value of $[^{14}C\text{-labeled sucrose}]_d$ usually remains elevated for 2–4 min and decreases thereafter (see following). Because sucrose is not taken up by either the cells or capillaries, the absolute amount of ^{14}C-labeled sucrose in the ECS must be unchanged. The observed increase therefore represents a relative decrease in water volume in the ECS resulting from movement of water into the cells, that is, cellular swelling (Fig. 2). The increase in $[^{14}C\text{-labeled sucrose}]_e$ is

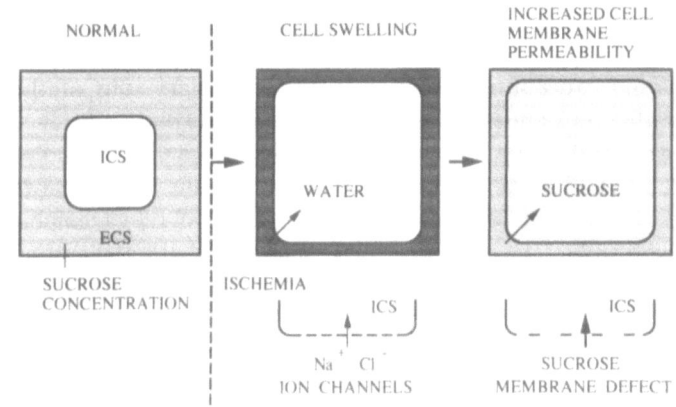

FIG. 2. Detection of cellular swelling (*middle*) and an increase in cellular membrane permeability (*right*) after ischemia induction (*dashed line*). ^{14}C-labeled sucrose was preperfused into the ECS through the dialysis probe as an ECS marker. A sudden and marked increase in $[^{14}C\text{-labeled sucrose}]_d$ is observed at 1–3 min after the induction of cerebral ischemia. $[^{14}C\text{-labeled sucrose}]_d$ usually remains elevated for 2–4 min. Because sucrose is not taken up by either the cells or capillaries, the absolute amount of ^{14}C-labeled sucrose in the ECS must remain unchanged. The increase therefore represents a relative decrease in water volume in the ECS resulting from movement of water into the cells, that is, cellular swelling. The increase in $[^{14}C\text{-labeled sucrose}]_e$ is concomitant with an abrupt increase in $[K^+]_e$, indicating that the increase in $[^{14}C\text{-labeled sucrose}]_e$ represents cellular swelling induced by massive ionic shifts across the cellular membrane. The value of $[^{14}C\text{-labeled sucrose}]_d$, however, declines rapidly after this initial increase. This fall in $[^{14}C\text{-labeled sucrose}]_d$ could result from penetration of the ^{14}C-labeled sucrose into the cells. Membrane defects may be produced at this period of ischemia so that ^{14}C-labeled sucrose can enter the cells. *ECS*, extracellular space; *ICS*, intracellular space. *Darker tone* indicates higher concentrations of sucrose

concomitant with an abrupt increase in $[K^+]_e$, indicating that the increase in $[^{14}C\text{-labeled sucrose}]_e$ represents cellular swelling induced by massive ionic shifts across the cellular membrane.

The increase in $[^{14}C\text{-labeled sucrose}]_d$ (approximately 1.4 fold) is generally smaller than the increase in ECS marker concentration detected by other methods [20]. This difference may be partly the result of the continuous background decrease in $[^{14}C\text{-labeled sucrose}]_d$ following termination of the ^{14}C-labeled sucrose perfusion [34]. Another reason for the smaller increase in $[^{14}C\text{-labeled sucrose}]_d$ could be a decreased recovery rate of the dialysis system in vivo during cerebral ischemia [28] (see following). In addition, it is possible that the smaller response of $[^{14}C\text{-labeled sucrose}]_d$ is caused by sucrose administration into the ECS, which may prevent cellular swelling to a certain degree. In any experiment, therefore, possible changes in ECS volume should be taken into consideration when interpreting the data obtained by the microdialysis technique. This is clearly the case in ischemic [34] and traumatic [35,36] brain injuries.

Changes in Effective Surface Area and Recovery Efficiency

It is a routine procedure to determine the recovery rate of the dialysis system for the substances of interest before the experiment. It should be noted, however, that the recovery rate in vivo is smaller than the recovery rate in vitro [27,28]. For example, the recovery rate of the dialysis system for K^+ in vivo as determined from $[K^+]_d$ and $[K^+]_e$, each measured by microdialysis and a K^+-sensitive electrode ($[K^+]_d/[K^+]_e$), is always far smaller than the recovery rate in vitro [28]. This may reflect the smaller effective surface area of the dialysis system in vivo [27].

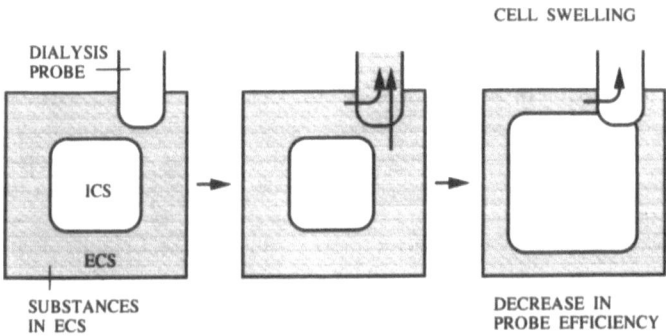

FIG. 3. Decrease in recovery efficiency during ischemia. Following ischemia induction (*middle* to *right*), the recovery rate of the dialysis system in vivo drops dramatically. This may be accounted for by a decrease in the effective surface area of the dialysis system in vivo, presumably caused by cellular swelling and shrinkage of the ECS volume (*right*). *ECS*, extracellular space; *ICS*, intracellular space

Furthermore, the ratio of the recovery rate in vivo to that in vitro is not constant in the diseased CNS. Following ischemia induction, this ratio drops dramatically in association with elevation of $[K^+]_e$ during ischemia [28]. This may be accounted for by a decrease in the effective surface area of the dialysis system in vivo, presumably caused by cellular swelling and shrinkage of the ECS volume (Fig. 3) [34]. The decrease in the recovery rate in vivo can also be viewed as reflecting changes in the diffusion parameters [29] within the ECS. The effect of the shrunken ECS after the onset of cellular swelling would be to retard diffusion in general. Substances cannot therefore be replenished from areas adjacent to the site of dialysis, and the substances available for dialysis will become depleted rapidly. The smaller response of the ECS marker concentration, as detected by microdialysis (see earlier), may be partly the result of the decreased recovery efficiency following the onset of cellular swelling.

Without knowing the dynamic changes in effective surface area and recovery efficiency of the dialysis system in vivo, microdialysis can provide only a qualitative measure of the changes in concentration of any substance in the ECS in the diseased CNS.

Increase in Permeability and Breakdown of the Cellular Membrane

The ECS concentration of a given substance is dependent on the equilibrium across the ECS, ICS, and blood vessels. The permeability of the cellular membrane separating the ECS and ICS to a given substance is therefore a critical determinant of its ECS concentration. During cerebral ischemia, the ECS concentration of ^{14}C-labeled sucrose, which has been preperfused through the dialysis probe, increases suddenly, as was mentioned earlier. The value of [^{14}C-labeled sucrose]$_d$, however, declines rapidly after this initial increase [37]. Similar findings have been reported with trimethylammonium and choline employed as an ECS marker [20]. This decrease in ECS marker concentration could result from either reexpansion of the ECS or penetration of the ECS marker into the cells. The latter possibility seems the more likely (see Fig. 2), because no reexpansion has been detected by other methods [18].

Such a rapid decrease in ECS marker concentration is not clearly observed when ECS markers of much larger molecular size, such as ^{3}H-labeled inulin, are used [37]. Although the data regarding this phenomenon are not yet conclusive, it can be speculated that defects are starting to be produced in the cellular membrane at this period of ischemia so that ECS markers of smaller molecular size can enter the cells through the membrane defects (see Fig. 2). Similar observations, although over a different time course, have been reported in in vitro studies [30,31]. In support of this idea, liberation of free fatty acid, an indicator of membrane breakdown, has been demonstrated to commence at such an early period of ischemia in vivo [38,39]. Our data also support this earlier finding (see following).

In addition to passive movements of substances across the cellular membrane, active uptake from and release into the ECS are also determinants of the ECS concentration. Because the ECS concentration of any substance sensitively reflects the biochemical properties of the cellular membrane separating the ECS and ICS, the possible contribution of the ECS and ICS to the data obtained by microdialysis should always be borne in mind.

Changes in Cerebrovascular Permeability

Another determinant of the ECS concentration of any substance is the capability of this substance to cross the capillary wall. Because the micro-dialysis technique involves insertion of a dialysis probe into the cerebral tissue, there is concern that this procedure might disrupt the normal cerebrovascular permeability through a kind of focal traumatic brain injury [23,25]. Changes in cerebrovascular permeability following experimental traumatic brain injury have been described previously employing various intravascular tracers [40].

An altered cerebrovascular permeability can be detected by the micro-dialysis technique from the appearance of an intravascular tracer in the ECS [3,23,25]. For such a purpose, it is desirable that the intravascular tracer remains in the ECS after its entrance from the capillary into the ECS. If the intravascular tracer is taken up by the cells, detection of the tracer entering the ECS will also be dependent on the rate of uptake by the cells. As mentioned earlier, sucrose in the ECS is not taken up by the cells or capillaries for the most part. An increased cerebrovascular permeability can therefore be detected as the appearance of ^{14}C-labeled sucrose in the ECS after intravascular administration of ^{14}C-labeled sucrose [41].

Only a very low radioactivity is evident in the dialysate as baseline data, suggesting that insertion of the dialysis probe into the cerebral tissue does not cause any marked disruption of the normal cerebrovascular permeability [3,23,41]. Immediately after traumatic brain injury [41], however, a clear increase in $[^{14}$C-labeled sucrose$]_d$ is observed. Because the dialysis probe was temporarily withdrawn at the moment of injury and repositioned in the same place immediately after the injury, destruction of the moving brain tissue with the dialysis probe at the moment of injury was not the cause of this increase. In addition, these observations indicate that repositioning of the dialysis probe causes minimal changes in the cerebrovascular permeability.

Because the fluid percussion produces a transient cellular swelling [35,36], the increase in $[^{14}$C-labeled sucrose$]_d$ immediately after fluid percussion could have been amplified by a decrease in ECS volume. $[^{14}$C-labeled sucrose$]_d$ does not return to the baseline level, however, after the period of cellular swelling [41]. This indicates that a certain amount of sucrose has entered the ECS after the fluid percussion. In contrast, no change in radioactivity is detected in the dialysate after irreversible ischemia. It should be remembered that substances originating in the blood can appear in the dialysate. This is dependent on passive as well as active movements of the substances across the capillary wall, and also across the cellular membrane separating the ECS and ICS.

Experimental Procedures

There are several advantages in employing microdialysis technique for investigation of the neurochemical environments of the CNS. They can be classified into two aspects: evaluation and modification of the neurochemical environments.

Detection of Changes in Neurochemical Environments

The microdialysis technique can measure various neurochemical changes occurring within the ECS simultaneously. For example, microdialysis can identify the timing of the abrupt K^+ flux during cerebral ischemia [28]. It is then possible to evaluate various neurochemical changes, such as the excitatory amino acids (EAA) release and lactate accumulation, in relation to the abrupt K^+ flux, employing the same dialysate fractions. However, as mentioned earlier, the data yielded by microdialysis are influenced directly or indirectly by various changes in cellular membrane function. For this reason, the results should be interpreted in conjunction with possible changes in cellular membrane function. Moreover, the data obtained by this technique themselves frequently reveal changes in cellular membrane function in the diseased CNS. For example, massive, changes in $[K^+]_d$ are likely to be a result of changes in the ion permeability of the cellular membrane. Cellular swelling detected as an increase in the ECS concentration of ^{14}C-labeled sucrose preperfused into the ECS represents another example of the consequence of an altered cellular membrane function. Thus, the microdialysis technique can provide a unique opportunity to detect functional changes of the cellular membrane in the diseased CNS.

We usually place a pair of microdialysis probes at symmetrical sites of the brain bilaterally.The probes are initially perfused with Ringer solution. The temperature of the perfusate is adjusted to 37°C, and the temperature is maintained using a chamber filled with water at 37°C into which the whole length of the inlet tubing is placed. Dialysate fractions are usually collected at 1-min intervals, except in some experiments in which the fractions are collected at 2-min intervals. The total volume of the outlet tube and the probe is adjusted to 5.0 µl. The second 1-min dialysate fraction collected after the induction of ischemia or trauma thus corresponds to the initial postischemic fraction.

Modification of Neurochemical Environments

In addition to measurement of neurochemical changes in the ECS and functional changes in the cellular membrane, various modifications of the neurochemical environments can be made when employing dialysis probes. Modifications can be produced by the removal of certain bioactive substances from the ECS by dialysis. For example, we have demonstrated that Ca^{2+}-free dialysis can efficiently remove Ca^{2+} from the ECS (see earlier). Furthermore, the neurochemical processes can be manipulated experimentally through the administration of various agents in situ via the dialysis probes.

The effects of such modification can be evaluated not only by measurement with microdialysis but also by applying various morphological techniques. For example, we have demonstrated that perfusion of EAA antagonist through the dialysis probe can attenuate the increase in local glucose utilization rate induced by traumatic brain injury as demonstrated by [^{14}C]deoxyglucose autoradiography and by selective death of hippocampal pyramidal cells induced by transient forebrain ischemia (see following). We perform experimental modification of the neurochemical environment through one of the two probes placed bilaterally (test probe). Dialysis with the other probe serves as the control (control probe). The effects of such experimental modification can then be evaluated by making comparisons between the control and test probes and examining the statistics for paired data.

Experimental Applications

As examples of data from experiments utilizing above-mentioned techniques, data obtained with experimental models of cerebral ischemia and trauma in our laboratories are herein briefly summarized. We have employed decapitation as a model of permanent cerebral ischemia, bilateral occlusion of the carotid arteries with hypotension as a model of transient cerebral ischemia (10 min), and fluid-percussion brain injury as a model of cerebral trauma. The fluid percussion is applied at the vertex at the level of injury, which causes loss of righting response for 5–15 min without overt morphological damage of the cerebral parenchyma.

Ionic Fluxes

The abrupt increase in $[K^+]_e$ occurring during cerebral ischemia can be detected by microdialysis with K^+-free perfusate [28]. Similarly, the increase in $[K^+]_e$ following traumatic brain injury can be demonstrated by microdialysis [9,35]. A large increase in $[K^+]_d$ occurred for 2–5 min immediately after fluid-percussion injury of the rat. The abrupt and large increase in $[K^+]_e$ during cerebral ischemia begins when $[K^+]_e$ reaches a level of

$6-10\,\text{m}M$ [13]. Neurotransmitter release and a sudden K^+ flux through ligand-gated ion channels of neuronal cells have been postulated to be responsible for this phenomenon [42-44]. If the Ca^{2+}-dependent exocytotic release of neurotransmitters is responsible for the abrupt increase in $[K^+]_e$, inhibition of Ca^{2+} entry into the nerve terminals [45,46] would be expected to alter the time course of the changes in $[K^+]_e$ during cerebral ischemia. In support of this hypothesis, the abrupt, large increase in $[K^+]_d$ following the induction of ischemia is significantly delayed by dialysis with Ca^{2+}-free perfusate containing Co^{2+} or Mg^{2+}, which blocks Ca^{2+} entry [28]. The increase in $[K^+]_e$ after concussive levels of fluid-percussion brain injury is also partially Ca^{2+} dependent [9], suggesting involvement of Ca^{2+}-dependent exocytotic release of neurotransmitters.

Release of Excitatory Amino Acids

Employing brain microdialysis, the ECS concentration of glutamate ($[Glu]_e$) has been demonstrated to increase during cerebral ischemia [3-5,7,47,48]. (See chapters entitled "Effect of CI-977 on Glutamate Release Following Cerebral Ischemia in the Cat" and "Measurements of Lactic Acid and Amino Acids in the Cerebral Cortex of Head-Injured Patients" in this volume.) It is well documented that glutamate at a sufficient concentration is neurotoxic [49-52]. The increase in $[Glu]_e$ has therefore been proposed to be a causative factor in the development of ischemic neuronal death. In addition, glutamate induces massive ionic fluxes across the plasma membrane [49-51]. For this reason, the elevation of $[Glu]_e$ has been suggested to play an important role in producing rapid ionic fluxes during cerebral ischemia or anoxia. The elevation of the dialysate concentration of glutamate ($[Glu]_d$) during cerebral ischemia begins concomitantly with the large increase in $[K^+]_d$ [7,47], suggesting that the elevation of $[Glu]_d$ is the result of glutamate release from the nerve terminal depolarized by the elevated $[K^+]_e$ through Ca^{2+}-dependent exocytosis. Consistent with this inference, the earlier rapid increase in $[Glu]_d$ during cerebral ischemia is markedly attenuated by Ca^{2+}-free perfusate containing Co^{2+} [7,46]. An increase in $[Clu]_d$ simultaneous with the increase in $[K^+]_e$ is also seen following concussive levels of fluid-percussion brain injury [9]. Because this sudden increase in $[K^+]_e$ is also partially Ca^{2+} dependent [9], exocytotic release of glutamate from the nerve terminals depolarized by the elevated $[K^+]_e$ may account for part of the $[Glu]_d$ increase.

Excitatory Amino Acid-Coupled Ion Channels

The ionic fluxes observed after ischemic and traumatic brain insults are too rapid to be accounted for by failure of the energy-dependent ion pump activity alone. Sudden changes in the ion permeability of the cellular membranes have therefore been postulated to occur presumably through indiscriminate release of neurotransmitters. EAAs are the most likely

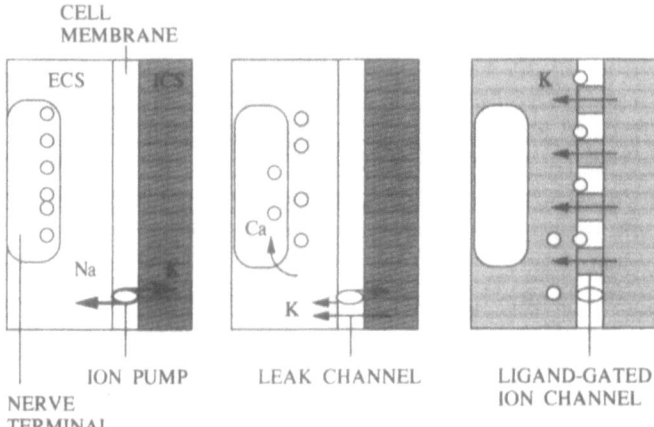

FIG. 4. Possible mechanisms of massive ionic (e.g., K^+) shifts during ischemia. After ischemia induction, the energy-dependent ion pump fails to restore leaked K^+ completely so that $[K^+]_e$ slowly increases. Elevation of $[K^+]_e$ to a certain level causes depolarization of nerve terminals. This depolarization of the nerve terminals results in Ca^{2+}-dependent exocytotic release of excitatory amino acids (EAAs) (*middle*). Further flux of K^+ together with other ions occurs through EAA-coupled ion channels (*right*). It appears therefore that the sudden and rapid increase in $[K^+]_e$ observed during cerebral ischemia represents the result of a malignant cycle beween the K^+ flux and EAA release. *ECS*, extracellular space; *ICS*, intracellular space. *Open circles*, EAA neurotransmitter; *darker tone* indicates a higher concentration of K^+

neurotransmitter that could produce such marked ionic shifts [49–52]. Consistent with this hypothesis, the abrupt increase in $[K^+]_d$ following ischemia induction is significantly delayed by the broad-spectrum EAA antagonist, kynurenic acid (KYN) [53–55], administered in situ through microdialysis [56]. The delay in latency induced by KYN was comparable to the previously mentioned delay induced by Ca^{2+}-free dialysis with Co^{2+} or Mg^{2+}. Systemically administered EAA antagonists have been reported to inhibit spreading cortical depression [57–61], but they fail to delay [58,59] and may even accelerate [61] sudden ionic shifts during cerebral ischemia or anoxia. Denervation of glutamatergic afferents has, however, been reported to delay ionic changes in the hippocampus during cerebral ischemia [62]. The disparity in results from systemically administered EAA antagonists may reflect the difference in the efficiency of elimination of the effect of EAAs. Together with the role of elevated $[K^+]_e$ in the Ca^{2+} dependent exocytotic release of EAAs, it appears that the sudden and rapid increase in $[K^+]_e$ occurring during cerebral ischemia represents a result of a malignant cycle beween the K^+ flux and EAA release (Fig. 4). The increase in $[K^+]_d$ after concussive levels of fluid-percussion brain injury is also inhibited by KYN administered in situ through microdialysis [9]. This finding suggests that indiscriminate release of EAAs and the EAA-receptor-coupled ion channels may also play a vital role in the production of the massive ionic fluxes induced by traumatic brain injury.

Cellular Swelling

As mentioned previously, the microdialysis technique can identify the timing of development of cellular swelling in vivo. EAAs cause large fluxes of Na^+, K^+, Ca^{2+}, and Cl^- across the cellular membrane in vitro, which have been shown to generate cellular swelling [18,20,34]. Among the various EAA antagonists, KYN attenuates such cellular swelling in vitro most effectively [63]. It would not be surprising therefore if ionic fluxes through EAA-coupled ion channels are also responsible for the cellular swelling during cerebral ischemia in vivo. As expected, KYN administered in situ through microdialysis inhibits both the cellular swelling and the massive ionic fluxes occurring simultaneously [34]. This implies that pathological processes quite similar to the EAA-mediated ionic fluxes and cellular swelling which are seen in vitro may underlie the early cellular swelling during cerebral ischemia in vivo. Transient cellular swelling is also observed after concussive levels of fluid-percussion brain injury [36,41]. Such cellular swelling is again inhibited by KYN administered in situ through the dialysis probe [36]. Although ionic shifts are not the sole cause of the cellular swelling occuring during cerebral ischemia, these findings indicate that Ca^{2+}-dependent exocytotic release of EAAs may play a major role in producing cellular swelling during the early period after ischemia induction and traumatic brain injury. This conclusion apparently accounts for the reported effect of KYN in reducing the brain edema and neuronal damage induced by ischemia or anoxia [64–68].

Increased Glucose Utilization

The energy metabolism of the brain increases during the period soon after traumatic brain injury [69–74]. A diffuse increase in glucose utilization is observed by ^{14}C-labeled deoxyglucose autoradiography following fluid percussion (Fig. 5) [74]. Sudden ionic perturbation across the cell membrane discussed previously. Because the major component of the ionic fluxes across the cellular membrane, such as those observed in spreading depression, strongly activate the energy-dependent ion pump for restoration of ionic homeostasis [75–81]. The observed increase in glucose utilization after traumatic brain injury may thus be caused by the ionic fluxes after fluid-percussion brain injury appears to be mediated by EAA-coupled ion channels, KYN would attenuate the increase in glucose utilization rate. Consistent with this hypothesis, the increase is clearly inhibited in areas perfused with KYN through microdialysis (Fig. 5) [82]. Removal of EAA-mediated afferents also prevents the increase in glucose utilization rate following fluid-percussion brain injury [83]. An increase in glucose utiliza-

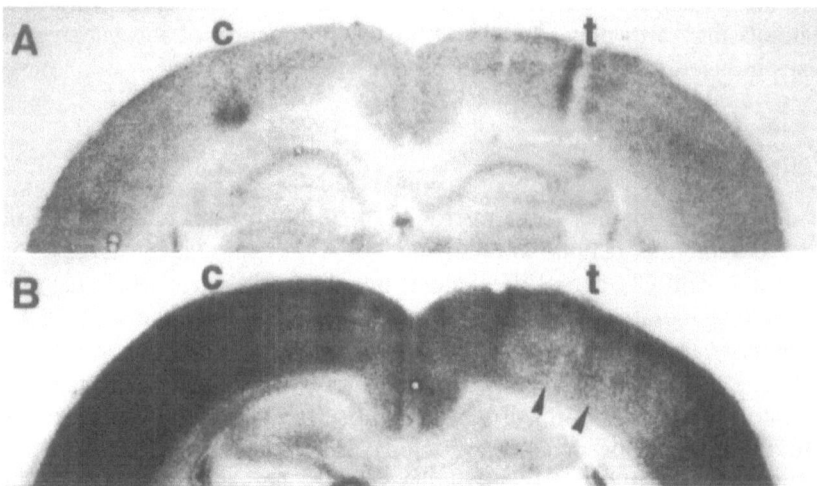

FIG. 5A,B. Representative examples of changes in local glucose utilization rate as evaluated by ^{14}C-labeled deoxyglucose autoradiography. **A** Sham injury. **B** Fluid-percussion injury. The control probe (*c*) perfused without kynurenic acid (KYN) and test (*t*) probe perfused with KYN were placed bilaterally in the cortex. The increase in ^{14}C-labeled deoxyglucose uptake in **B** is inhibited in the area perfused by KYN (*t*), but not in the area perfused without KYN (*c*)

tion rate and its inhibition by EAA antagonists have also been demonstrated in other models of traumatic brain injury [84,85].

Lactate Accumulation

Lactate accumulation has been suggested to be one of the most important factors affecting cell viability under pathological conditions such as ischemia [86–91]. The dialysate concentration of lactate ([lactate]$_d$) increases dramatically, beginning at a few minutes after ischemia induction [68]. The increase in [lactate]$_d$ is clearly delayed by KYN administered in situ through microdialysis at doses that delay the anoxic depolarization [68]. This finding indicates that the early increase in lactate is caused by the anoxic depolarization. A sudden change in ionic gradients across the plasma membrane strongly activates the energy-dependent ion pumps and increases adenosine triphosphate (ATP) hydrolysis for activating energy-dependent ion pumps, thereby stimulating lactate formation [75–81,92,93]. During a single passage of cortical spreading depression, which causes quite similar ionic events, almost parallel decreases in glucose content and pH in addition to elevation of the lactate concentration have been reported [75–81,94–97]. Such data suggest that the sudden ionic shifts during cerebral ischemia may be mediated at their commencement by EAA-coupled ion channels, rather than merely be a result of depletion of energy that terminates ion-pump activity. The value of $[\text{lactate}]_d$ also increases after concussive levels of fluid-percussion brain injury for 15–20 min [98,99]. The increase in $[\text{lactate}]_d$ can be inhibited by KYN administered in situ through micro-dialysis [99]. Furthermore, inhibition of the energy-dependent ion pump by oubain administered in situ through the dialysis probe can clearly attenuate the increase in $[\text{lactate}]_d$ [99]. These findings suggest that the lactate accumulation after traumatic brain injury is also partially caused by strong activation of the energy-dependent ion pump for the restoration of ionic homeostasis.

Free Fatty Acid Liberation

The tissue levels of free fatty acids increase rapidly after induction of cerebral ischemia [38,39]. This early and rapid increase in free fatty acids is an unique characteristic of adult brain, which is not seen in the neonate or in other organs. A rapid increase in free fatty acid levels, superimposed on a continued slow increase, is observed beginning at 1–2 min after ischemia induction [100]. The early and rapid increase in free fatty acids was profoundly inhibited by KYN administered in situ through a microdialysis, suggesting that EAAs are critically involved in the early phase of free fatty acid liberation [100]. Because the development of anoxic depolarization can be delayed for several minutes by KYN administered with the same pro-cedure, the observed inhibition of early free fatty acid liberation may be attributable to the delay in developing massive ionic shifts and resultant neurotransmitter release, which may activate phospholipase A_2 and C through a mechanism coupled to Ca^{2+} entry and a guanosine triphosphate-binding protein.

Changes in Synaptic Efficacy

It has been demonstrated that Schaffer collateral/CA1 response of the rat is potentiated [101] and a prolonged afterdischarge to repetitive stimulation with relatively low frequency is seen [102] beginning at 6–8 h after transient cerebral ischemia in vivo. The long-term potentiation has been shown to be attenuated at the same time [103]. Following ischemia in vivo, similar but not identical changes occurs after fluid-percussion brain injury [104]. The postischemic potentiation (PIP) was not affected by 2-amino-5-phosphonovalerate (APV), a N-methyl-D-aspartate- (NMDA-) coupled ion channel antagonist, administered via microdialysis at 7 h post ischemia. The prolonged afterdischarges in response to repetitive stimulation were, however, reversed to short-duration afterdischarges by the same procedure, leaving the response to single stimulation unaffected. These findings suggest that during the reperfusion period the Ca^{2+} influx to CA1 pyramidal cells can be greatly increased through NMDA receptor-coupled ion channels if appropriately timed multiple synaptic input bombards these cells.

Neuronal Cell Death

Transient cerebral ischemia causes selective death of hippocampal CA1 pyramidal cells after a period of 2–3 days [105–108]. The death of these cells can be selectively inhibited in an area perfused by KYN via micro-dialysis at doses that delay the occurrence of anoxic depolarization [68]. Although the beneficial effects of EAA antagonists, such as KYN [65–68], have been attributed mainly to inhibition of Ca^{2+} fluxes through EAA-receptor coupled ion channels, it is thought that inhibition of early occurrence of lactate accumulation, free fatty acid liberation, and other consequences of anoxic depolarization may also contribute to the mechanisms whereby KYN is able to attenuate ischemic neuronal damage. The effects of in situ administration of other drugs can also be tested by microdialysis [48]. While similar damage of hippocampal neurons occurs following traumatic brain injury [109–111], effects of in situ administration of drugs have not been tested.

Conclusion

Changes in cellular membrane function in response to neurotransmitter release are characteristically unique to neuronal cells as compared to any other kinds of cells within the body [112]. The microdialysis technique is useful for revealing such changes in cellular membrane function, rather than merely detecting changes in concentration of substances in the ECS. Although the interpretation of the data from clinical application of the microdialysis technique would be more complicated than those from experimental models, this technique would provide a deeper insight into the pathological processes involved.

Acknowledgments. The data reviewed in this chapter are from experiments conducted in collaboration with Drs. T. Tamura, T. Kawamata, A. Yoshino, T. Kano, T. Maeda and T. Tsubokawa (Department of Neurological Surgery, Nihon University, Tokyo), and Drs. D.A. Hovda and D.P. Becker (Department of Neurosurgery, University of California at Los Angeles, Los Angeles). These investigations were supported by grants from the U.S. National Institutes of Health (NS27544) and a research grant for cardiovascular disease (2A-2) from the Ministry of Health and Welfare of Japan.

References

1. Delgado JMR, Defeudis FV, Roth RH, Ryugo DK, Mitruka BM (1971) Dialytrode for long term intercerebral perfusion in awake monkeys. Arch Int Pharmacodyn Ther 198:9–12

2. Ungerstedt U, Herrera-Manschitz M, Jungnelius U, Stahle L, Tossman U, Zetterstrom T (1982) Dopamine synaptic mechanisms reflected in studies combining behavioral recordings and brain dialysis. Adv Dopamine Res 17:219–231

3. Benveniste H, Drejer J, Schousboe A, Diemer NH (1984) Elevation of the extracellular concentrations of glutamate and aspartate in rat hippocampus during transient cerebral ischemia monitored by intracerebral microdialysis. J Neurochem 43:1369–1374

4. Hagberg H, Lehmenn A, Sandberg M, Nystrom B, Jacobson I, Hamberger A (1985) Ischemia-induced shift of inhibitory and excitatory amino acids from intra- to extracellular compartments. J Cereb Blood Flow Metab 5:413–419

5. Globus MY-T, Busto R, Dietrich WD, Martinez E, Valdes I, Ginsberg MD (1988) Effect of ischemia on the in vivo release of striatal dopamine, glutamate and γ-aminobutyric acid studied by intracerebral microdialysis. J Neurochem 51:1455–1464

6. Hillered L, Hallstrom A, Segersvard S, Persson L, Ungerstedt U (1989) Dynamics of extracellular metabolites in the striatum after middle cerebral artery occlusion in the rat monitored by intracerebral microdialysis. J Cereb Blood Flow Metab 9:607–616

7. Katayama Y, Kawamata T, Tamura T, Becker DP, Tsubokawa T (1991) Calcium-dependent glutamate release concomitant with massive potassium flux during cerebral ischemia in vivo. Brain Res 558:136–140

8. Faden AI, Demediuk P, Panter SS, Vink R (1989) The role of excitatory amino acids and NMDA receptors in traumatic brain injury. Science 244:798–800

9. Katayama Y, Becker DP, Tamura T, Hovda D (1990) Massive increase in extracellular potassium and indiscriminative glutamate release after concussive brain injury. J Neurosurg 73:889–900

10. Bullock R, Butcher SP, Chen M-H, Kendall L, McCulloch J (1991) Correlation of the extracellular glutamate concentration with extent of blood flow reduction after subdural haematoma in the rat. J Neurosurg 74:794–802

11. Hayes RL (1991) Central nervous system trauma: neurotransmitter-mediated mechanisms of traumatic brain injury: acetylcholine and excitatory amino acids. J Neurotrauma 9(suppl 1):s157–s164

12. Bullock R, Fujisawa H (1992) The role of glutamate antagonists for the treatment of CNS injury. J Neurotrauma 9:s443–s462

13. Hansen AJ (1977) Extracellular potassium concentration in juvenile and adult rat brain cortex during anoxia. Acta Physiol Scand 99:412–420

14. Takahashi H, Manaka S, Sano K (1981) Changes in extracellular potassium concentration in cortex and brain stem during the acute phase of experimental closed head injury. J Neurosurg 55:708–717

15. Tsubokawa T (1983) Cerebral circulation and metabolism in concussion. Neurol Surg (Tokyo) 11:563–573

16. Hubschmann OR, Kornhauser D (1983) Effects of intraparenchymal hemorrhage on extracellular cortical potassium in experimental head trauma. J Neurosurg 59:289–293

17. Nilsson P, Hillered L, Olsson Y, Sheardown MJ, Hansen AJ (1993) Regional changes in interstitial K^+ and Ca^{2+} levels following cortical compression contusion trauma in rats. J Cereb Blood Flow Metab 13:183–192

18. Van Harreveld A, Ochs S (1956) Cerebral impedance changes after circulatory arrest. Am J Physiol 187:180–192

19. Maknight AD, Leaf A (1977) Regulation of cellular volume. Physiol Rev 57:510–573

20. Hansen AJ, Olsen CE (1980) Brain extracellular space during spreading depression and ischemia. Acta Physiol Scand 108:355–365

21. Hansen AJ (1985) Effect of anoxia on ion distribution in the brain. Physiol Rev 165:101–148

22. Imperat A, DiChiara G (1984) Trans-striatal dialysis coupled to reverse phase high performance liquid chromatography with electrochemical detection: a new method for the study of the in vivo release of endogenous dopamine and metabolites. J Neurosci 4:966–977

23. Tossman U, Ungerstedt U (1986) Microdialysis in the study of extracellular levels of amino acids in the rat brain. Acta Physiol Scand 128:9–14

24. Damsma G, Westernink BHX, Imperato A, Rollema H, DeVries JB, Horn AS (1987) Automated brain dialysis of acetylcholine in freely moving rats: detection of basal acetylcholine. Life Sci 41:873–876

25. Benveniste H, Drejer J, Schousboe A, Diemer NH (1987) Regional cerebral glucose phosphorylation and blood flow after insertion of a microdialysis fiber through the dorsal hippocampus in the rat. J Neurochem 49:729–734

26. Westerink BHC, Damsma G, Rollema H, De Vries JB, Horn AS (1987) Scope and limitation of in vivo brain dialysis: a comparison of its application to various neurotransmitter systems. Life Sci 41:1763–1776

27. Alexander GM, Grothusen JR, Schwartzman RJ (1988) Flow-dependent changes in the effective surface area of microdialysis probes. Life Sci 43:595–601

28. Katayama Y, Tamura T, Becker DP, Tsubokawa T (1991) Calcium-dependent component of massive increase in extracellular potassium during cerebral ischemia as demonstrated by microdialysis in vivo. Brain Res 567:57–63

29. Nicholson C, Phillips JM, Gardner-Medwin AR (1979) Diffusion from a iontophoretic point source in the rat brain. Role of tortuosity and volume fraction. Brain Res 169:580–584

30. Parks JM, Shay J, Ames A III (1976) Cell volume and permeability of oxygen- and glucose-deprived retina in vitro. Arch Neurol 33:709–714

31. Ames A III, Nesbett FB (1983) Pathophysiology of ischemic cell death: II. Changes in plasma membrane permeability and cell volume. Stroke 14:227–233

32. Phillips JM, Nicholson C (1979) Anion permeability in spreading depression investigated with ion-sensitive microelectrodes. Brain Res 173:567–571

33. Katayama Y, Becker DP, Tamura T, Tsubokawa T (1990) Cellular swelling during cerebral ischemia demonstrated by microdialysis in vivo: preliminary data indicating the role of excitatory amino acids. Acta Neurochir (Suppl) 51:183–185

34. Katayama Y, Tamura T, Becker DP, Tsubokawa T (1992) Early cellular swelling during cerebral ischemia in vivo is mediated by excitatory amino acids released from nerve terminal. Brain Res 577:121–126

35. Katayama Y, Cheung MK, Alves A, Becker DP (1989) Ion fluxes and cell swelling after experimental traumatic brain injury: the role of excitatory amino

acids. In: Hoff JT, Betz AL (eds) Intracranial pressure, vol 7. Springer, Berlin Heidelberg New York, pp 584–588

36. Katayama Y, Becker DP, Tamura T, Ikezaki K (1990) Early cellular swelling in experimental traumatic brain injury: a phenomenon mediated by excitatory amino acids. Acta Neurochir (Suppl) 51:271–273

37. Katayama Y, Tamura T, Becker DP, Tsubpkawa T (1991) Detection of cellular swelling and subsequent increase in plasma membrane permeability during cerebral ischemia in vivo using microdialysis. J Cereb Blood Flow Metab 11:s479

38. Aveldano MI, Bazan NG (1975) Rapid production of diacylglycerols enriched in arachidonate and stearate during early brain ischemia. J Neurochem 25:919–920

39. Yasuda H, Kishiro K, Izumi N, Nakanishi M (1985) Biphasic liberation of arachidonic and stearic acids during cerebral ischemia, J Neurochem 45:168–172

40. Povlishock JT, Becker DP, Sullivan HG, Miller JD (1978) Vascular permeability alterations to horseradish peroxidase in experimental brain injury. Brain Res 153:223–239

41. Katayama Y, Becker DP, Tamura T (1992) Changes in cerebrovascular permeability and excitatory amino acid-mediated cellular swelling in experimental concussive brain injury. In: Averzaat CJJ, van Eijndhoven JHM, Mass AIR, Tans JTJ (eds) Intracranial pressure, vol 8. Springer, Berlin Heidelberg New York, pp 484–487

42. Van Harreveld A (1978) Two mechanisms for spreading depression in chicken retina. J Neurobiol 9:419–431

43. Nicholson C, Kraig RP (1981) The behavior of extracellular ions during spreading depression. In: Zeuthen T (ed) The application of ion electrodes. Elsevier/North-Holland, Amsterdam New York, pp 217–238

44. Moghaddam B, Schenk JO, Stewart WB, Hansen AJ (1987) Temporal relationship between neurotransmitter release and ion flux during spreading depression and anoxia. Can J Physiol Pharmacol 54:1105–1110

45. Martins-Ferreira H, DeOliveira Castro G, Struchiner CJ, Rodrigues PS (1974) Circulating spreading depression in isolated chick retina. J Neurophysiol 37:778–784

46. Drejer J, Benveniste H, Diemer NH, Schousboe A (1985) Cellular origin of ischemia-induced glutamate release from brain tissue in vivo and in vitro. J Neurochem 45:145–151

47. Scheller D, Heister U, Peters U, Hoeller M (1989) Glutamate and asparate are released concomitantly with the terminal DC-negativation after global cerebral ischemia. J Cereb Blood Flow Metab 9:s372

48. Kano T, Katayama Y, Kawamata T, Tsubokawa T (1994) Propentofylline administered by microdialysis attenuates ischemia-induced hippocampal damage but not excitatory amino acid release in gerbils. Brain Res 641:149–154

49. Olney JW, Price MT, Samson L, Lambuyere J (1986) The role of specific ions in glutamate neurotoxicity. Neurosci Lett 65:65–71

50. Choi DW (1987) Ionic dependence of glutamate neurotoxicity. J Neurosci 7:369–379

51. Mayer ML, Westbrook GL (1987) Cellular mechanisms underlying excitotoxicity. Trends Neurosci 10:59–61

52. Rothman SM, Olney JW (1987) Excitotoxicity and the NMDA receptor Trends Neurosci 10:299-302
53. Perkins MN, Stone TW (1982) An iontophoretic investigation of the actions of convulsant kynurenines and their interaction with the endogenous excitant quinolinic acid. Brain Res 247:184-187
54. Ganong AH, Lanthorn TH, Cotman CW (1983) Kynurenic acid inhibits synaptic and acidic amino acid-induced responses in the rat hippocampus and spinal cord. Brain Res 273:170-174
55. Ganong AH, Cotman CW (1986) Kynurenic acid and quinolinic acid act at N-methyl-D-aspartate receptors in the rat hippocampus. J Pharmacol Exp Ther 236:293-299
56. Katayama Y, Tamura T, Becker DP, Tsubokawa T (1992) Inhibition of rapid potassium flux during cerebral ischemia in vivo with excitatory amino acid antagonist. Brain Res 568:294-298
57. Gorelova NA, Koroleva VI, Amemori T, Pavlik V, Bures J (1987) Ketamine blockade of cortical spreading depression in rats. Electroencephalogr Clin Neurophysiol 66:440-447
58. Hernandez-Caceres J, Macias-Gonzalez R, Brozek G, Bures J (1987) Systemic ketamine blocks spreading depression but does not delay the onset of terminal anoxic depolarization in rats. Brain Res 437:360-364
59. Hansen JA, Lauritzen M, Wieloch T (1988) MK-801 inhibits spreading depression but not anoxic depolarization. In: Lehman J, Turski L (eds) Recent advances in excitatory amino acid research. Liss, New York
60. Marrannes R, Willems R, De Prins E, Wauquier A (1988) Evidence for a role of the N-methyl-D-aspartate (NMDA) receptor in cortical spreading depression in the rat. Brain Res 457:226-240
61. Marrannes R, De Prins E, Willems R, Wauquier A (1988) NMDA antagonists inhibit cortical spreading depression but accelerate the onset of neuronal depolarization induced by asphyxia. In: Somjen G (ed) Mechanisms of cerebral hypoxia and stroke. Plenum, New York, pp 303-304
62. Benveniste H, Jorgensen MB, Lundbaek JA, Hansen AJ (1989) Ionic changes in the normal and denervated hippocampus during ischemia. J Cereb Blood Flow Metab 9:s46
63. Choi DW, Koh J-Y, Peters S (1988) Pharmacology of glutamate neurotoxicity in cortical cell culture: attenuation by NMDA antagonist. J Neurosci 8:185-196
64. Simon RP, Young RSK, Stout S, Cheung J (1986) Inhibition of excitatory neurotransmission with kynurenate reduces brain edema in neonatal anoxia. Neurosci Lett 71:361-364
65. Simon RP, Swan JH, Griffith T, Meldrum BS (1984) Blockade of methyl-D-aspartate receptors may protect against ischemic damage in the brain. Science 226:850-852
66. Germano IM, Pitts LH, Meldrum BS, Bartkowski HM, Simon RP (1987) Kynurenate inhibition of cell excitation decreases stroke size and deficits. Ann Neurol 22:730-734
67. Gill R, Woodruff GN (1990) The neuroprotective actions of kynurenic acid and MK-801 in gerbils are synergistic and not related to hypothermia. Eur J Pharmacol 176:143-149
68. Katayama Y, Kawamata T, Kano T, Tsubokawa T (1992) Excitatory amino acid antagonist administered via microdialysis attenuates lactate accumulation

during cerebral ischemia and subsequent hippocampal damage. Brain Res 584:329–333

69. Nelson SR, Lowry OH, Passonneau JV (1966) Changes in energy reserves in mouse brain associated with compressive head injury. In: Careness WF, Walker AW (eds) Head injury. Lippincott, Philadelphia, pp 444–447

70. Nilsson B, Nordstrom CH (1977) Experimental head injury in the rat. Part 3: Cerebral blood flow and oxygen consumption after concussive impact acceleration. J Neurosurg 47:262–273

71. Nilsson B, Nordstrom CH (1977) Rate of cerebral energy consumption in concussive head injury in the rat. J Neurosurg 47:274–281

72. Nilsson B, Ponten U (1977) Experimental head injury in the rat. Part 2: Regional brain energy metabolism in concussive trauma. J Neurosurg 47:252–261

73. Duckrow RB, LaManna JC, Rosenthal M, Levasseur JE, Patterson JL Jr (1981) Oxidative metabolism activity of cerebral cortex after fluid-percussion head injury in the cat. J Neurosurg 54:607–614

74. Yoshino A, Hovda DA, Kawamata T, Katayama Y, Becker DP (1991) Dynamic changes in local cerebral glucose utilization following fluid-percussion injury: evidence of a hyper- and subsequent hypometabolic state. Brain Res 561:106–119

75. Tschirgi RD, Kazutoyo I, Taylor JL, Walker RM, Sonnenschein RR (1957) Changes in cortical pH and blood flow accompanying spreading cortical depression and convulsion. Am J Physiol 190:557–562

76. Krivanek J (1961) Some metabolic changes accompanying Leao's spreading cortical depression in the rat. J Neurochem 6:183–189

77. Rosenthal M, Somjen G (1973) Spreading depression sustained potential shifts and metabolic activity of cerebral cortex in cats. J Neurophysiol 36:739–745

78. Mayevsky A, Chance B (1974) Repetitive patterns of metabolic changes during cortical spreading depression of the awake rat. Brain Res 65:529–533

79. LaManna JC, Rosenthal M (1975) Effect of ouabain and phenobarbital on oxidative metabolic activity associated with spreading cortical depression in cats. Brain Res 88:145–149

80. Shinohara M, Dollinger B, Brown G, Rapoport S, Sokoloff L (1979) Changes in local cerebral glucose utilization during and following recovery from spreading depression. Science 203:188–190

81. Gjedde A, Hansen AJ, Quistorff B (1981) Blood brain glucose transfer in spreading depression. J Neurochem 37:807–812

82. Kawamata T, Katayama Y, Hovda DA, Yoshino A, Becker DP (1992) Administration of excitatory amino acid antagonists via microdialysis attenuates the increase in glucose utilization seen following concussive brain injury. J Cereb Blood Flow Metab 12:12–24

83. Yoshino A, Hovda DA, Katayama Y, Kawamata T, Becker DP (1992) Hippocampal CA3 lesion prevents the post-concussive metabolic derangement in CA1. J Cereb Blood Flow Metab 12:996–1006

84. Kuroda Y, Inglis FM, Miller JD, McCullocj J, Graham DI, Bullock R (1992) Transient glucose hypermetabolism after acute subdural hematoma in the rat. J Neurosurg 76:471–477

85. Inglis F, Kuroda Y, Bullock R (1992) Glucose hypermetabolism after subdural hematoma is ameliorated by a competitive NMDA antagonist. J Neurotrauma 9:73–74

86. Myers RE (1979) A unitary theory of causation of anoxic and hypoxic brain pathology. Adv Neurol 26:195–217
87. Ginsberg MD, Welsh FA, Budd WW (1980) Deleterious effect of glucose pretreatment on recovery from diffuse cerebral ischemia in the cat. Stroke 11:347–354
88. Welsh FA, Ginsberg MD, Rieder W, Budd WW (1980) Deleterious effect of glucose pretreatment on recovery from diffuse cerebral ischemia in the cat. Stroke 11:355–363
89. Kalimo H, Rehncrona S, Soderfelt B, Olsson Y, Siesjo BK (1981) Brain lactic acidosis and ischemic cell damage. 2. Histopathology. J Cereb Blood Flow Metab 1:313–327
90. Pulsinelli WA, Waldman S, Rawlinson D, Plum F (1982) Moderate hyperglycemia auguments ischemic brain damage. A neuropathologic study in the rat. Neurology 32:1239–1246
91. Marmarou A (1992) Intracellular acidosis in human and experimental brain injury. J Neurotrauma 9(suppl):s551–s562
92. Howse DC, Duffy TE (1975) Control of the redox state of the pyridine nucleotides in the rat cerebral cortex. Effect of electroshock-induced seizures. J Neurochem 24:935–940
93. Paschen W, Djuricic B, Mies G, Schmidt-Kastner R, Linn F (1987) Lactate and pH in the brain. Association and dissociation in different pathophysiological states. J Neurochem 48:154–159
94. Somjen GG (1984) Acidification of interstitial fluid in hippocampal formation caused by seizures and by spreading depression. Brain Res 311:186–188
95. Mutch WAC, Hansen AJ (1984) Extracellular pH changes during spreading depression and cerebral ischemia. Mechanisms of brain pH regulation. J Cereb Blood Flow Metab 4:17–27
96. Csiba L, Paschen W, Mies G (1985) Regional changes in tissue pH and glucose content during cortical spreading depression in rat brain. Brain Res 336:167–170
97. Harris RJ, Richards PG, Symon L, Habib A-HA, Rosenstein J (1987) pH, K^+, and PO_2 of the extracellular space during ischemia of primate cerebral cortex. J Cereb Blood Flow Metab 7:599–604
98. Hovda DA, Becker DP, Katayama Y (1991) Central nervous system trauma: secondary injury and acidosis. J Neurotrauma 9(suppl 1):s47–s70
99. Kawamata T, Katayama Y, Hovda DA, Yoshino A, Becker DP (to be published) Lactate accumulation following concussive brain injury. The role of ionic fluxes induced by excitatory amino acids. Brain Res
100. Katayama Y, Kawamata T, Maeda T, Tsubokawa T (1994) Inhibition of early phase of free fatty acid liberation during cerebral ischemia by excitatory amino acid antagonist administered by microdialysis. Brain Res 635:331–334
101. Miyazaki S, Katayama Y, Furuichi M, Kinoshita K, Kawamata T, Tsubokawa T (1993) Post-ischemic potentiation of Schaffer collateral/CA1 pyramidal cell response of the rat hippocampus in vivo: involvement of N-methyl-D-aspartate receptors. Brain Res 611:155–159
102. Miyazaki S, Katayama Y, Furuichi M, Kano T, Tsubokawa T (1994) N-Methyl-D-aspartate receptor-mediated, prolonged afterdischarges of CA1 pyramidal cells following transient cerebral ischemia in the rat hippocampus in vivo. Brain Res 657:325–329

103. Miyazaki S, Katayama Y, Furuichi M, Kinoshita K, Kawamata T, Tsubokawa T (1993) Impairment of hippocampal long-term potentiation following transient cerebral ischemia in rats. Effects of bifemelane, a potent inhibitor of ischemia-induced acetylcholine release. Neurol Res 15:249–251

104. Miyazaki S, Katayama Y, Lyeth BG, Jenkins LW, DeWitt DS, Goldberg SJ, Newlon PG, Hayes RL (1992) Enduring suppression of hippocampal long-term potentiation following traumatic brain injury in rat. Brain Res 585:335–339

105. Kirino T (1982) Delayed neuronal death in the gerbil hippocampus following ischemia. Brain Res 239:57–69

106. Pulsinelli WA, Brierley JB, Plum F (1982) Temporal profile of neuronal damage in a model of transient forebrain ischemia. Ann Neurol 11:491–498

107. Katayama Y, Tsubokawa T, Koshinaga M, Miyazaki S (1991) Temporal pattern of survival and dendritic growth of fetal hippocampal cells transplanted into ischemic lesions of the adult rat hippocampus. Brain Res 562:352–355

108. Kano T, Katayama Y, Miyazaki S, Kinoshita K, Kawamata K, Tsubokawa T (1933) Effects of indeloxazine on hippocampal CA1 pyramidal cell damage following transient cerebral ischemia in the gerbil. Neuropharmacology 32: 307–310

109. Jenkins LW, Moszynski K, Lyeth BG, et al (1989) Increased vulnerability of the mildly traumatized rat brain to cerebral ischemia: the use of controlled secondary ischemia as a research tool to identify common or different mechanisms contributing to mechanical and ischemic brain injury. Brain Res 477:211–224

110. Kotapka MJ, Gennarelli TA, Graham DI, et al (1991) Selective vulnerability of hippocampal neurons in acceleration-induced experimental head injury. J Neurotrauma 8:247

111. Smith DH, Okiyama K, Thomas MJ, et al (1991) Evaluation of memory dysfunction following experimental brain injury using the Morris water maze. J Neurotrauma 8:259–269

112. Siesjo BK, Wieloch T (1985) Molecular mechanisms of ischemic brain damage: calcium-related events. In: Plum F, Pulsinelli W (eds) Cerebrovascular diseases. Raven, New York, pp 187–197

Glutamate Neurotoxicity As a Mechanism of Ischemic Brain Damage: A Basic Study Using a New In Vivo Model

Hirosuke Fujisawa[1], Hans Landolt[2], and Ross Bullock[3]

Introduction

Ischemic brain damage is seen as a common feature in many pathological conditions such as ischemic stroke, subarachnoid hemorrhage, head injury, and prolonged seizures [1]. A number of animal studies have shown that there is a marked increase in the extracellular concentrations of glutamate under such conditions [2–7]. The neuroprotective effects of glutamate antagonists have also been demonstrated in the animal models of ischemia and head injury [1,8], and thus it has been suggested that these conditions share a common injury mechanism, that is, glutamate neurotoxicity.

Under normal conditions, glutamate in the extracellular space is kept at 1 micromolar (μM) [9]. Glutamate concentrations in the presynaptic cytoplasm and vesicles are as high as $10\,mM$ and $100\,mM$, respectively [9]. It has been demonstrated using brain microdialysis that extracellular concentrations of glutamate increase to several times the control levels during experimental cerebral ischemia and head injury [2,3,6,10] and subarachnoid hemorrhage in human [11], while the concentrations remain within the micromolar range ($20–1000\,\mu M$). There is still a question as to whether these concentrations of glutamate are really neurotoxic or whether they are merely an epiphenomenon. Choi et al. [12], has demonstrated using a neuronal cell culture that brief exposure to $100\,\mu M$ glutamate causes cell death. Is this also true in vivo? To answer this question, we have devised a new in vivo model of "pure" glutamate neurotoxicity in which predetermined concentrations of glutamate are infused into the normal rat brain via a microdialysis probe.

[1] Department of Neurosurgery, Yamaguchi University School of Medicine, 1144 Kogushi, Ube, Yamaguchi 755, Japan
[2] Chefarzt Neurochirurgische Universitätsklinik, Kantonsspital Aarau, Buchserstr. 1, 5001 Aarau, Schweiz
[3] Division of Neurosurgery, Medical College of Virginia, Virginia Commonwealth University, Box 980631, Richmond, Virginia, 23298 U.S.A.

Materials and Methods

General Preparation

Adult male Sprague-Dawley rats were used for this study. All experiments were performed under general anesthesia after tracheostomy using 0.5%–1% halothane and a 2:1 nitrous oxide:oxygen mixture. The animals were ventilated to normocarbia and normoxia. Body temperature was controlled at $37° \pm 0.5°C$ by means of a rectal thermometer and a heater system. The animals were mounted in a stereotactic frame, and a burr hole was made at the right parietal skull. The microdialysis probe (CMA/12, membrane length, 3 mm; outside diameter, 0.5 mm; Carnegie Medicine, Stockholm, Sweden) was angled at 15° to the sagittal plane and lowered 3.5 mm into the cortex through the burr hole after the dura-arachnoid had been incised (stereotactic coordinates: anteroposterior, 0.0 mm; lateral, 4.0 mm).

Glutamate Perfusion

Glutamate solutions were made up in mock cerebrospinal fluid (NaCl 135 mM, KCl 1 mM, KH_2PO_4 2 mM, $CaCl_2$ 1.2 mM, $MgCl_2$ 1 mM, pH 7.4) by adding 0.01 M, 0.1 M, 0.5 M, or 1 M monosodium glutamate. The 0.01 M and 0.1 M glutamate solutions were corrected to a sodium level of 135 mM. A 1 M NaCl solution was chosen as control.

For the autoradiographic study of glutamate diffusion, 2.5 µCi of ^{14}C-labeled glutamate was added to 5 ml of 0.01 M, 0.1 M, 0.5 M, and 1 M of "cold" glutamate solution to make the "hot" glutamate solutions. After 90 min of stabilization, a glutamate solution was perfused for 90 min at a flow rate of 1.5 µl/min.

Histological Examination

The animals were perfusion fixed with FAM fixative (40% formaldehyde, glacial acetic acid, absolute methanol, 1:1:8) 2.5 h after glutamate or control perfusion. The head was removed and immersion fixed in FAM for a further 24 h. After the brain had been removed from the skull, the forebrain was embedded in paraffin wax and 7-µm-thick coronal sections were cut at 200-µm intervals. The sections were stained with hematoxylin and eosin (H&E) and examined by light microscopy. For the electron microscopic study, Karnovsky's fixative (2% formaldehyde, 2% glutaraldehyde in 0.1 M phosphate buffer) was used.

Quantitative Histology

Serial H&E-stained cryostat sections were selected for study. After the removal of the probe, the animals were killed by decapitation. The brains were then removed and frozen in isopentane chilled with dry ice to −45°C.

The frozen brains were cut into 20-µm coronal sections, each 200 µm apart, in a cryostat. The sections were mounted on glass slides and stained with H&E. The areas of the glutamate-induced lesion were readily distinguished from the intact brain as areas of pallor and were measured on an image analyzer. The volume of damage was calculated by summing the damaged areas and multiplying by the interval thickness between sections.

Autoradiographic Study of ^{14}C Glutamate Diffusion

The "hot" glutamate solutions $(0.01\,M, 0.1\,M, 0.5\,M,$ and $1\,M)$ were perfused in the probe to investigate the diffusion characteristics of glutamate in the brain. After perfusion of the glutamate solutions for 90 min, the rat was killed by decapitation. The removed brain was frozen at $-45°C$ and cut into 20-µm coronal sections. The sections were mounted on glass cover slips and were used to expose X-ray film for 3 weeks to obtain the autoradiogram.

The Effects of Glutamate Antagonists

The effects of the glutamate antagonists (+)-5-methyl-10,11-dihydro-5H-dibenzo(a,d)cyclohepten-5,10-imine maleate (MK-801) and 2,3-dihydroxy-6-nitro-7-sulfamoyl-benzo(F)-quinoxaline (NBQX) on lesion size were investigated. In this experiment, glutamate $(0.5\,M)$ was perfused in the microdialysis probe and the brains were processed in the same way as for quantitative histology. NBQX was injected intravenously 30 min before and after the start of glutamate perfusion, and MK-801 30 min before the glutamate perfusion. A 5.5% glucose solution was used as control. Volumes of damage were compared using H&E-stained frozen coronal sections.

Results

In all the experiments adequate oxygenation, normocarbia, and normothermia were maintained throughout the procedure, and there were no significant differences between control and glutamate perfusion groups in these conditions.

Histological Findings

Macroscopically, glutamate-induced damage was seen in $0.1\,M, 0.5\,M,$ and $1\,M$ glutamate perfusion groups as an area of pallor staining (Fig. 1). In some animals, a hemorrhagic probe track was observed. The area of pallor staining was produced in the cortex and striatum, and extended in anterior and posterior directions. In the $1\,M$ NaCl-perfused control group and $0.01\,M$ glutamate perfusion group, pallor of staining was observed just around the probe track, and no difference could be detected between these two groups.

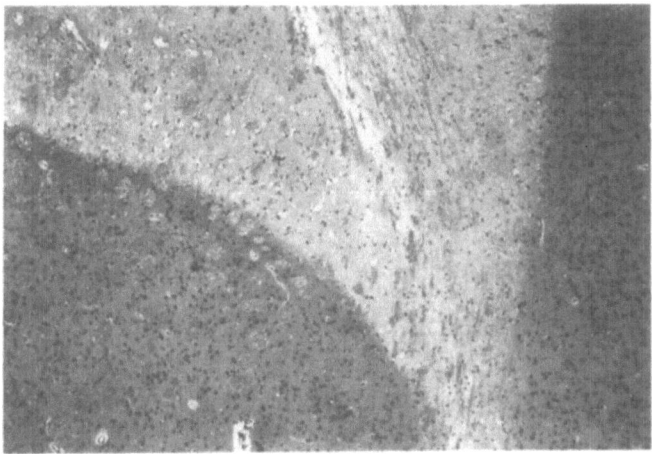

Fig. 1. Hematoxylin and eosin-stained brain section show the glutamate-induced lesion as an area of pallor staining. Histopathological features in the lesion were similar to those of acute ischemia

The histopathological features of the $0.1\,M$, $0.5\,M$, and $1\,M$ glutamate perfusion groups were similar in nature and quite similar to those of acute ischemia. Within the core of the lesion, there were shrinkage of neurons and neuropil, triangulation of the nucleus, and swelling of perineuronal astrocytes. There was a perilesional zone between the lesion core and the intact brain. In this zone, neurons demonstrated pyknosis and shrinkage to a lesser extent than in the lesion core. Beyond this zone, no histological abnormalities were found.

Electron microscopy also revealed remarkable changes. Neurons were electron dense and shrunken, and showed an irregular profile. Nucleus and cytoplasmic structures were severely damaged. Astrocytes and neurites were markedly swollen, observed as massive vacuolations. Neurons were indented by these vacuolations.

Volume of Glutamate-Induced Brain Damage

The volume of the glutamate-induced damage increased in relation to the increasing concentrations of glutamate. The volume of damage of the $0.1\,M$, $0.5\,M$, and $1\,M$ glutamate perfusion groups was significantly larger than that of the control group (Fig. 2).

^{14}C Glutamate Diffusion

The glutamate diffusion area was seen as a "cloud" formed by ^{14}C radioactivity on the autoradiogram. In the cloud of each glutamate perfusion group, ^{14}C concentration was high in the center and decreased gradually toward the

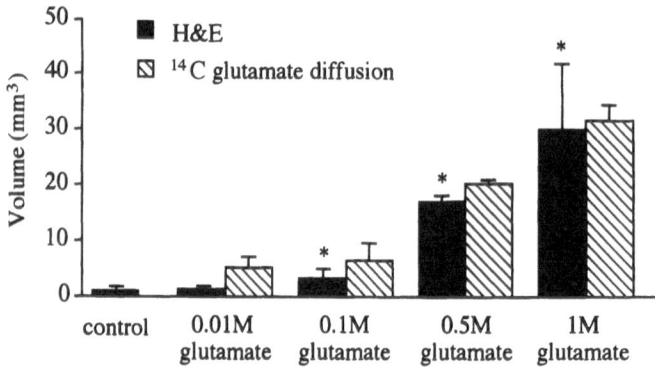

FIG. 2. Volume of glutamate-induced damage and ^{14}C glutamate diffusion (mean ± standard error of mean). *, Significantly different from control; $P < .05$; H&E, hematoxylin and eosin-stained cryostat section

periphery. The diffusion area increased in size as glutamate concentration was increased. The shapes of the clouds corresponded well to those of the histological lesions. However, the area of diffusion was larger than that of the corresponding histologic lesions, and this was marked in the lower level (0.01 M and 0.1 M) glutamate perfusion groups (Fig. 2).

The Effects of Glutamate Antagonists on Lesion Volume

Both NBQX and MK-801 significantly reduced the volume of glutamate-induced damage. The magnitude of the reduction was largely similar for each drug (30% from control).

Discussion

Using the newly devised reproducible model of glutamate neurotoxicity, we have demonstrated that ischemic brain damage can be produced by glutamate alone. Because ischemia is not a component of this model, the role of glutamate in cell injury mechanisms can be explored in vivo, uncomplicated by reduced tissue blood flow and oxygen delivery and compromised energy generation [13]. Van Harreveld and Fifkova [14] demonstrated that 150 mM glutamate was necessary to produce a lesion when applied electrophoretically to the normal cortex. However, their lesion was small, only 300 μm in diameter. In our model, glutamate is delivered through the microdialysis probe, leading to a continuous efflux of glutamate into the extracellular space. This may be why we produced a much larger lesion than that shown by van Harreveld and Fifkova [14].

We have demonstrated that the glutamate-induced lesions increase in size in a dose-dependent manner. In 0.1 M, 0.5 M, and 1 M glutamate perfusion groups, there were significant differences from the control group. In a separate in vitro study in which the diffusion rate of glutamate through the microdialysis probe was measured, the glutamate diffusion rate was found to be about 20%–30%. Taking this diffusion rate into account, $0.1\,M$ ($100\,mM$) glutamate perfused within the dialysis probe corresponds to an extracellular glutamate concentration of 20–$30\,mM$. Thus, the neurotoxic level of glutamate in the normal rat brain is thought to be about 20–$30\,mM$.

Our autoradiographic study of glutamate diffusion in the brain using ^{14}C-labeled glutamate has shown that the diffusion area increases in size as glutamate concentration is increased and that the shape of the diffusion corresponds to that of the histologic lesions. However, the diffusion areas were larger than the histologic lesion, particularly in the lower ($0.01\,M$ and $0.1\,M$) glutamate perfusion groups. The ^{14}C concentration was high in the center of the diffusion clouds and decreased gradually toward the periphery. It is likely that in the lower glutamate perfusion groups the glutamate concentration in the most peripheral areas was too low to exceed the capacity of the glutamate uptake mechanisms. The approximate glutamate concentrations in the ^{14}C diffusion clouds can be calculated by ^{14}C radioactivity measured optically with a calibrated gray scale on the autoradiogram. When $1\,M$ and $0.1\,M$ of "hot" glutamate was perfused, the calculated glutamate concentration in the zone that corresponded to the histologic lesion was $59\,mM$ and $56\,mM$, respectively. It should be noted, however, that these values may reflect both intra- and extracellular concentrations of glutamate because glutamate could be taken up and metabolized in astrocytes or neurons.

Two different glutamate antagonists, NBQX and MK-801, significantly reduced the volume of glutamate-induced brain damage. It has been demonstrated that antagonists of the N-methyl-D-aspartate (NMDA) and α-amino-3-hydroxy-5-methyl-4-isoxazolepropionic acid (AMPA) receptors can reduce excitotoxic damage to neurons in culture and ameliorate neuronal necrosis in vivo after cerebral ischemia [15,16]. The result, that the necrosis occurring after glutamate perfusion can be attenuated by agents acting at the NMDA (MK-801) or AMPA (NBQX) receptors, provides pharmacological validation of this model [13].

There is a discrepancy between the extracellular glutamate concentrations under pathological circumstances and the toxic levels in the normal rat brain demonstrated in our study. There are some possible explanations for this discrepancy. First, under the pathological circumstances, glutamate uptake into both astrocytes and neurons is inhibited by failure of energy substrate delivery and cessation of aerobic metabolism. It is well known that glutamate uptake, particularly by astrocytes, strongly regulates glutamate neurotoxicity. Rosenberg et al. [17], have shown that the potency of glutamate neurotoxicity in the astrocyte-poor culture is approximately 34 times that in the astrocyte-rich culture.

In addition to inhibition of glutamate uptake, other synergistic mechanisms are likely to operate to potentiate glutamate neurotoxicity. During pathological conditions such as ischemia, multiple neurochemical and vascular mechanisms are disturbed in addition to elevation in the extracellular glutamate and inhibition of glutamate uptake. Increased calcium ion influx to the cytoplasm leads to formation of a number of substances (for example, arachidonic acids, free radicals, protein kinase C, calpain I, or phospholipase A_2, etc.). These may multiply the effect of glutamate [18]. Furthermore, it has been shown in cell culture studies that changes in the ionic concentration (sodium, potassium) of the culture medium determine glutamate neurotoxicity [19]. Ionic changes are prominent after acute ischemia and head injury, and these changes may be other candidates for potentiating glutamate neurotoxicity.

The new in vivo model of glutamate neurotoxicity that we have described here can provide insight into one of the critical events in cell death caused by cerebral ischemia. A further understanding of this process in vivo may offer us more opportunity for therapeutic intervention.

References

1. McCullock J, Bullock R, Teasdale GM (1991) Excitatory amino acids antagonists: opportunities for the treatment of ischaemic brain damage in man. In: Excitatory amino acids antagonists. Meldrum BS (ed) Blackwell, Oxford London, pp 287–326
2. Benveniste H, Drejer J, Schousboe A, Diemer NH (1984) Elevation of the extracellular concentrations of glutamate and aspartate in rat hippocampus during transient cerebral ischemia monitored by intracerebral microdialysis. J Neurochem 43:1369–1374
3. Butcher SP, Bullock R, Graham DI, McCulloch J (1990) Correlation between amino acid release and neuropathologic outcome in rat brain following middle cerebral artery occlusion. Stroke 21:1727–1733
4. Collins RC, Olney JW (1982) Focal cortical seizures cause distant thalamic lesions. Science 218:177–179
5. Faden AI, Demediuk P, Panter SS, Vink R (1988) The role of excitatory amino acids and NMDA receptors in traumatic brain injury. Science 244:798–800
6. Katayama Y, Becker DP, Tamura T, Hovda DA (1990) Massive increases in extracellular potassium and the indiscriminate release of glutamate following concussive brain injury. J Neurosurg 73:889–900
7. Meldrum BS (1984) Amino acid neurotransmitters and new approaches to anticonvulsant drug action. Epilepsia 25 S2:S140–S149
8. Bullock R, Fujisawa H (1992) The role of glutamate antagonists for the treatment of CNS injury. J Neurotrauma 9:S443–S461
9. Nicholls D, Attwell D (1990) The release and uptake of excitatory amino acids. Trends Pharmacol Sci 11:462–468
10. Bullock R, Butcher SP, Chen MH, Kendall L, McCulloch J (1991) Correlation of the extracellular glutamate concentration with extent of blood flow reduction after subdural hematoma in the rat. J Neurosurg 74:794–802
11. Persson L, Hillered L (1992) Chemical monitoring of neurosurgical intensive care patients using intracerebral microdialysis. J Neurosurg 76:72–80
12. Choi DW, Maulucci-Gedde M, Kriegstein AR (1987) Glutamate neurotoxicity in cortical cell culture. J Neurosci 7:357–368

13. Fujisawa H, Dawson D, Browne SE, MacKay KB, Bullock R, McCulloch J (1993) Pharmacological modification of glutamate neurotoxicity in vivo. Brain Res 629:73–78

14. Van Harreveld A, Fifkova E (1971) Light- and electron-microscopic changes in central nervous tissue after electrophoretic injection of glutamate. Exp Mol Pathol 15:61–81

15. Gill R, Nordholm L, Lodge D (1992) The neuroprotective actions of 2,3-dihydroxy-6-nitro-7-sulfamoyl-benzo(F)quinoxaline (NBQX) in a rat focal ischaemic model. Brain Res 580:35–43

16. Park CK, Nehls DG, Graham DI, Teasdale GM, McCulloch J (1988) The glutamate antagonist MK-801 reduces focal ischemic brain damage in the rat. Ann Neurol 24:543–541

17. Rosenberg PA, Amin S, Leitner M (1992) Glutamate uptake disguises neurotoxic potency of glutamate agonists in cerebral cortex in dissociated cell culture. J Neurosci 12:56–61

18. Choi DW (1990) Cerebral hypoxia: some new approaches and unanswered questions. J Neurosci 10:2493–2501

19. Choi DW (1987) Ionic dependence of glutamate neurotoxicity. J Neurosci 7:369–379

Delayed Neuronal Damage Following Focal Ischemic Injury in Stroke-Prone Spontaneously Hypertensive Rats

TOSHIKI SHIROTANI, KATSUJI SHIMA, MIWAKO IWATA, HIDEYUKI KITA, AND HIROO CHIGASAKI

Introduction

The striatum is highly vulnerable to ischemia. It also is innervated richly by both the corticostriatal glutamatergic pathway and nigrostriatal dopaminergic projections, which have been shown to interact with each other [1]. Excitatory amino acids, such as glutamate, may contribute to ischemic cell death by causing an intracellular overload of Ca^{2+} [2]. It has been suggested that dopamine contributes to ischemic cell death by producing oxygen radicals [3] or by potentiating the excitotoxic effects of glutamate [4].

Coyle [5,6] demonstrated that distal occlusion to the striate branches of the middle cerebral artery (MCA) resulted in a reproducible focal infarction in stroke-prone spontaneously hypertensive rats, but not in normotensive rats. The infarct produced by this procedure was limited to the ipsilateral cerebral cortex and did not extend to the basal ganglia. The objective of the present study was twofold: first, to identify delayed neuronal damage in the focal ischemic injury of stroke-prone spontaneously hypertensive rats, and, second, to clarify the relationship between the glutamate release and calcium accumulation to be coincident with the development of delayed neuronal damage. The time course and distribution of calcium accumulation after occlusion of the MCA were investigated using ^{45}Ca autoradiography. Changes in neurotransmitters in the striatum were studied using intracerebral microdialysis. Microdialysis probes were inserted in the lateral or medial parts of the striatum to allow a comparison between each part.

Materials and Methods

Experimental Model

Male stroke-prone spontaneously hypertensive rats, 11–14 weeks of age and weighing 250–300 g, were used for all experiments. Following intubation,

Department of Neurosurgery, National Defense Medical College, 3-2, Namiki, Tokorozawa, Saitama 359, Japan

the animals were ventilated artificially with a mixture of 70% N_2, 30% O_2, and 1%–1.5% halothane. Body temperature was kept at 37°C using a heating lamp controlled by a rectal thermometer during surgical preparation. Under an operating microscope, the right MCA was exposed through a 2- to 3-mm burrhole craniectomy. The MCA was occluded with a microbipolar coagulation and divided. The occlusion was distal to the striate branches of the MCA and 0.7–1 mm dorsal to the rhinal fissure. After recovery, the animals were returned to their cages at the ambient temperature (22°–25°C) until decapitation.

Experiment 1: Time Course and Distribution of ^{45}Ca Accumulation

Experiments were performed as described previously [7,8]. Briefly, following 4 h, 24 h, 3 days, 7 days, and 14 dyas of MCA occlusion, animals ($n = 3$) for each group) were injected intravenously with $^{45}CaCl_2$ (3.7 MBq/100 g body weight; New England Nuclear, Boston, MA, U.S.A.). Rats were decapitated 5 h after the injection. Brains were removed and autoradiographed.

Experiment 2: Effect of MK-801 on ^{45}Ca Accumulation

The compound (+)-5-methyl-10,11-dihydro-5H-dibenzo(a,d) cyclohepten-5,10-imine maleate (MK-801) (0.5, 1.0, 5, 10 mg/kg; $n = 5$ for each group) was injected as an iv bolus at 15 min before MCA occlusion. Twenty minutes after MCA occlusion, rats were allowed to move freely within their cage. Seven days later, they were injected intravenously with $^{45}CaCl_2$, and autoradiographs were obtained. Five animals in the control group were injected with nomal saline, and autoradiographs were obtained 7 days after MCA occlusion. The volumes of ^{45}Ca accumulation were calculated by multiplying each sum of ^{45}Ca accumulated areas on each section of autoradiograph by the distance between sections.

Experiment 3: Microdialysis Study

The microdialysis probe (outer diameter, 0.22 mm; membrane length, 3 mm; molecular weight cutoff, 50,000; BDP-I-8-03, EICOM, Kyoto, Japan) was inserted into eigher the medial ($n = 14$) or lateral ($n = 14$) part of the right striatum. The corrdinates were 0.5 mm anterior, 3 mm lateral to the bregma, and 3.5 mm ventral from the brain surface in the medial side group, and 0.5 mm anterior, 4.5 mm lateral to the bregma and 2.8 mm ventral from the brain surface in the lateral side group. The dialysis probe was continually perfused at 2 μl/min with Ringer solution (NaCl, 148 mM; $CaCl_2$, 2.2 mM; KCl, 4.0 mM). After a 3-h period for stabilization of the baseline, the right MCA was occluded. The dialysate samples were collected every 20 min until 2 h after MCA occlusion. Glutamate (Glu) in the dialysate sample was analyzed in seven rats from each group. Dopamine (DA) in the sample was analyzed in the remaining rats. The dialysate content of DA was determined by high-performance liquid chromatography (HPLC) with an electrochemical detector (ECD-100, EICOM). The dialysate content of Glu was analyzed by HPLC with electrochemical detection and precolumn derivatization.

Statistical Analysis

Data are expressed as mean ± SD. Dunnett's tests or Student's t tests were used for the statistical analysis. Probability values less than 0.05 ($P < .05$) were considered significant.

Results

Time Course and Distribution of ^{45}Ca Accumulation

Autoradiograms of rat brains following MCA occlusion were studied in coronal sections (Fig. 1). ^{45}Ca accumulation was detected only in the cortex and corpus callosum at 4 h and 24 h postischemia, and extended to the pyramidal tract, thalamus, and lateral portion of the striatum by 3 days. After 7–14 days, the regional ^{45}Ca becomame more prominent. Regional distribution of calcium 7 days after MCA occlusion is also shown schematically in Fig. 1.

Effect of MK-801 on ^{45}Ca Accumulated Volume

Significant decreases of ^{45}Ca accumulation in the cortex, striatum, and thalamus were observed in MK-801-injected animals. The amount of neuroprotection afforded by MK-801 was dose related except for the highest dose (10 mg/kg) (Fig. 2).

Changes of Striatal Glu and DA after MCA Occlusion

The time course of change in Glu and DA is illustrated in Fig. 3. Following MCA occlusion, a threefold transient increase was observed in the lateral part of the striatum. The levels returned to baseline values 60 min after MCA occlusion. This increase of Glu was not observed in the medial part. DA in the lateral part increased with a twofold peak value. This release persisted for 2 h after MCA occlusion.

Discussion

In this study using ^{45}Ca autoradiography, ^{45}Ca accumulation was observed in the cerebral cortex supplied by the occluded MCA, in the corpus callosum, ipsilateral pyramidal tract, and ventral posterior nucleus of the thalamus,

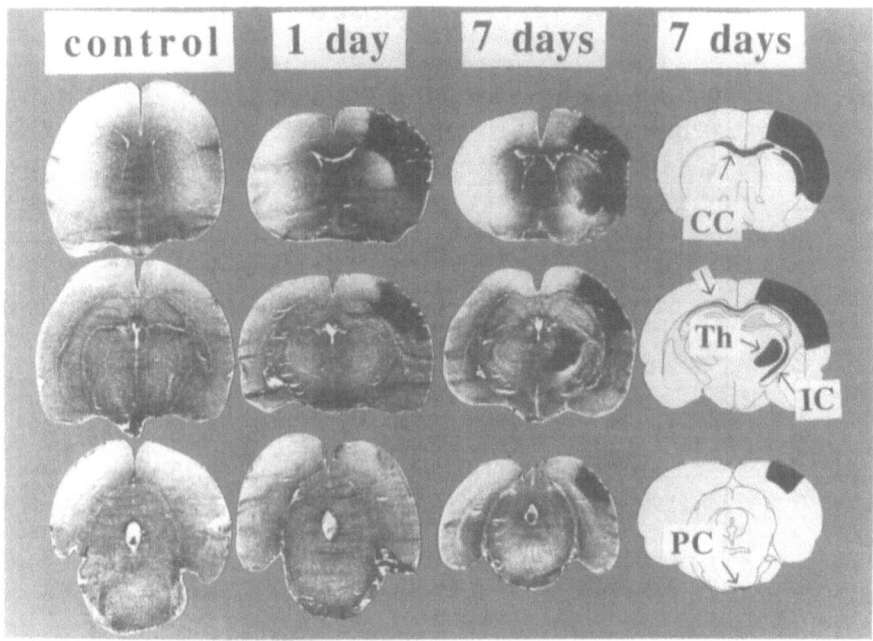

FIG. 1. ⁴⁵Ca autoradiographs of rat brains studied 4 h, 24 h, 3 days, and 7 days after middle cerebral artery (MCA) occlusion, and schematic diagram of accumulation of ⁴⁵Ca 7 days following MCA occlusion. Controls were obtained 3 days after sham operation. Autoradiographs show coronal sections at the level of striatum (*top*), thalamus (*middle*), and pons (*bottom*). ⁴⁵Ca accumulated in the cerebral cortex supplied by occluded MCA, the corpus callosum, the ipsilateral pyramidal tract, ventral posterior nucleus of the thalamus, and the lateral portion of the striatum not supplied by the occluded MCA. Corpus callosum, CC; thalamus, Th; internal capsule, IC; cerebral peduncle, PC

and also in the lateral portion of the striatum, which is not supplied by the occluded MCA. We speculate that ⁴⁵Ca had accumulated in the irreversibly damaged neuronal body and degenerating axons, as found by Benveniste et al. [9]. In the thalamus, ⁴⁵Ca accumulation was limited to the ventral posterior nucleus, which has fiber connections in anatomic proximity to the postcentral gyrus of the cerebral cortex. Damage in this area may be caused by retrograde degeneration resulting from thalamo cortical fiber damage caused by the precedent ischemic insult to the postcentral gyrus [10]. Furthermore, damage in the pyramidal tract and corpus callosum may be caused by anterograde degeneration resulting from ischemic injury in the cerebral cortex.

MK-801 is a noncompetitive *N*-methyl-D-aspartate (NMDA) receptor antagonist acting at the associated phencyclidine site [11]. In MK-801-injected animals, neuronal damaged volumes in the striatum were significantly

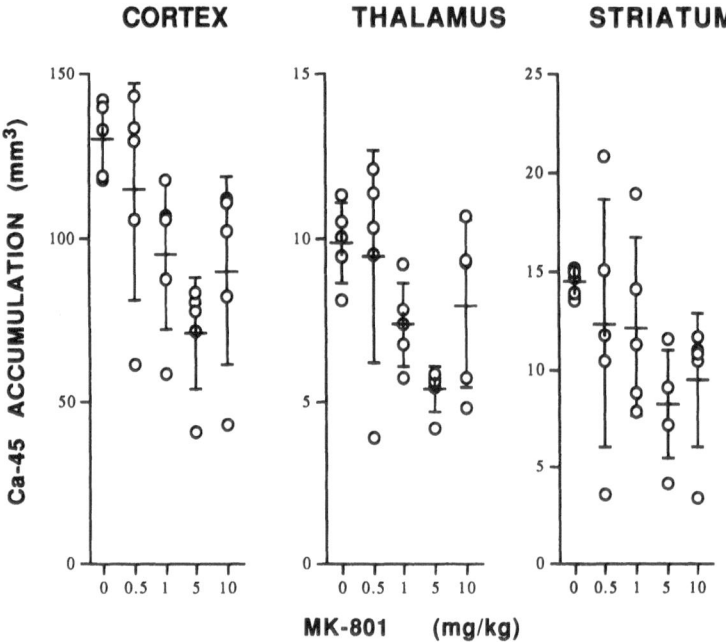

FIG. 2. The volumes of accumulation of ^{45}Ca in the cortex, striatum, and thalamus for the different doses of MK-801- and saline-treated animals. Data are presented as means ± SD (n = 5 in each group). *, $P < .05$; **, $P < .01$, as saline-treated animals (Dunnett's test)

decreased as well as in the cortex and thalamus, which suggests that glutamate plays a role in the neuronal damage in the striatum. McGeorge and Faull [12], while studying the organization of the corticostriate projection in the rat brain, demonstrated that the sensory and motor areas project topographically onto the dorsolateral striatum. These corticostriatal neurons use the excitatory amino acids glutamate or aspartate as neurotransmitters [13,14].

The results of our microdialysis study suggest that focal cortical ischemia is associated with different neurotransmitter changes in the medial and lateral parts of the striatum. Significant increases in the extracellular concentrations of Glu and DA were observed only in the lateral part of the striatum, which was not affected by ischemia following MCA occlusion. Glu attained its peak level after 20 min of ischemia and then rapidly declined to baseline. Sensory and motor areas were affected by ischemia in our study, suggesting that neuronal depolarization might occur in the cerebral cortex, causing a release of Glu stored in vesicles. Accordingly, spiky Glu release could be detected only in the lateral part of the striatum. DA release could be mediated via an NMDA-type glutamate receptor [15]. Massive release of these neurotransmitters may occur at the axon terminals of the striatum [14] inducing neuronal damage [16,17]. On the other hand, the lateral portion of

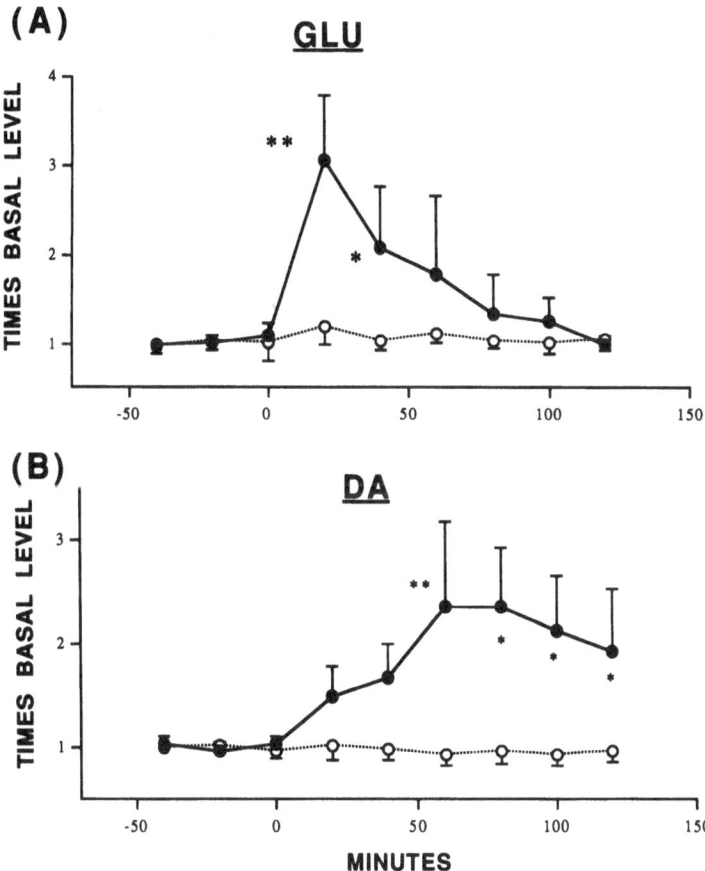

(A)

GLU

(B)

DA

Fig. 3. Changes in the concentration of glutamate (*GLU*) and dopamine (*DA*) in microdialysates from the medial (*open circles*) or lateral (*closed circles*) part of the striatum of seven rats subjected to MCA occlusion in relation to basal level. Values were the means and SD. GLU and DA were significantly elevated after MCA occlusion only in the lateral part. *, $P < .05$; **, $P < .01$, versus preischemic value (Dunnett's test)

the striatum is adjacent to the ischemic regions, and brain edema induced by ischemia may contribute to the changes observed in this segment [18].

Conclusions

A distal middle cerebral artery (MCA) occlusion model in stroke-prone spontaneously hypertensive rats using the ^{45}Ca autoradiographic technique demonstrated delayed ^{45}Ca accumulation in the corpus callosum, the ipsilateral pyramidal tract, the ventral posterior nucleus of the thalamus, and the lateral part of the striatum not affected by occluded MCA. Also, results from the intracerebral microdialysis study suggest that neurotransmitter changes in the lateral part of the striatum differ from those in the medial part of the striatum following MCA occlusion in stroke-prone spontaneously hypertensive rats. The delayed neuronal damage that occurred in the lateral part of the striatum in this model may have been caused by massive Glu release, which accompanied the DA release. Intracerebral microdialysis studies may produce different results if the microdialysis probes are not inserted into exactly the same place.

References

1. Cheramy A, Romo R, Godeheu G, Baruch P, Glowinski J (1986) In vivo presynaptic control of dopamine release in the cat caudate nucleus: II. Facilitatory or inhibitory influence of L-glutamate. Neuroscience 19:1081–1090
2. Choi DW (1987) Ionic dependence of glutamate neurotoxicity. J Neurosci 7: 369–379
3. Damsma G, Boisvert DP, Mudrick LA, Wenkstern D, Fibiger HC (1990) Effect of transient forebrain ischemia and pargyline on extracellular concentrations of dopamine, serotonin, and their metabolites in the rat striatum as determined by in vivo microdialysis. J Neurochem 54:801–808
4. Globus MY-T, Busto R, Dietrich WD, Martinez E, Valdes I, Ginsberg MD (1988) Intra-ischemic extracellular release of dopamine and glutamate is associated with striatal vulnerability to ischemia. Neurosci Lett 91:36–40
5. Coyle P (1982) Middle cerebral artery occlusion in the young rat. Stroke 13: 855–859
6. Coyle P, Jokelainen PT (1983) Differential outcome to middle cerebral artery occlusion in spontaneously hypertensive stroke-prone rats (SHRSP) and Wistar Kyoto (WKY) rats. Stroke 14:605–611
7. Dienel GA (1984) Regional accumulation of calcium in postischemic rat brain. J Neurochem 43:913–925
8. Shirotani T, Shima K, Iwata M, Kita H, Chigasaki H (1994) Calcium accumulation following middle cerebral artery occlusion in stroke-prone spontaneously hypertensive rats. J Cereb Blood Flow Metab 14:831–836
9. Benveniste H, Huttemeier PC, Johansen FF, Diemer NH (1989) Calcium 45 accumulation in the dentate hilus: possible effect of NMDA receptors blockers. In: Hartmann A, Kuschinsky W (eds) Cerebral ischemia and calcium. Springer, Berlin Heidelberg, pp 266–273
10. Nagasawa H, Kogure K (1990) Exo-focal postischemic neuronal death in the rat brain. Brain Res 524:196–202
11. Johnson RL, Koerner JF (1988) Excitatory amino acid neurotransmission. J Med Chem 31:2057–2066
12. McGeorge AJ, Faull RLM (1989) The organization of the projection from the cerebral cortex to the striatum in the rat. Neuroscience 29:503–537
13. Hassler R, Haug P, Nitsch C, Kim JS, Paik K (1982) Effect of motor and premotor cortex ablation on concentrations of amino acid, monoamines, and acetylcholine and on the ultrastructure in rat striatum. A confirmation of glutamate as the specific cortico-striatal transmitter. J Neurochem 38:1087–1098

14. Perschak H, Cuenod M (1990) In vivo release of endogenous glutamate and aspartate in the rat striatum during stimulation of the cortex. Neuroscience 35:283–287

15. Leviel V, Gobert A, Guibert B (1990) The glutamate-mediated release of dopamine in the rat striatum: further characterization of the dual excitatory-inhibitory function. Neuroscience 39:305–312

16. Rothman SM, Olney JW (1987) Glutamate and the pathophysiology of hypoxic-ischemic brain damage. Ann Neurol 19:105–111

17. Choi DW, Maulucci-Gedde M, Kriegstein AR (1987) Glutamate neurotoxicity in cortical cell curture. J Neurosci 7:357–368

18. Nordborg C, Sokrab TEO, Johansson BB (1991) The relationship between plasma protein extravasation and remote tissue changes after experimental brain infarction. Acta Neuropathol (Berl) 82:118–126

Prolonged Stimulation-Induced Afterdischarges of Hippocampal CA1 Pyramidal Cells After Ischemia In Vivo

Makoto Furuichi, Shuhei Miyazaki, Yoichi Katayama, and
Takashi Tsubokawa

Introduction

Transient cerebral ischemia causes selective death of hippocampal CA1 pyramidal cells after a period of 3–5 days [1]. We previously demonstrated that Schaffer collateral/CA1 responses of the rat are potentiated beginning at 6–8 h after transient cerebral ischemia in vivo [2]. The present study examined whether the utilization of N-methyl-D-aspartate (NMDA) receptor-coupled ion channels is increased or not during the period in which post-ischemic potentiation (PIP) of Schaffer collateral/CA1 responses is observed.

Material and Methods

Male Wistar rats (250–300 g, $n = 21$) were used for the experiments. To induce transient cerebral ischemia, the systemic blood pressure was repidly reduced to 30–50 mmHg through withdrawal of blood from the femoral artery, the anesthesia was discontinued, and the common carotid arteries were occluded with thread loops bilaterally. Occlusion of the carotid arteries was terminated at 12 min after the occurence of flat electroencephalograms, and the previously withdrawn blood was injected into the femoral artery. Sham controls were subjected to an identical experimental procedure except for the induction of ischemia. Craniectomy was then performed so that recording micropipets, a stimulation electrode, and microdialysis probe could be inserted into the hippocampus. A microdialysis probe was carefully positioned in the hippocampus. The recording micropipet was placed at the depth where synaptic responses to stimulation of Schaffer collaterals were best recorded.

The stimulus intensity–response relationship (input-output curve) was determined for a population excitatory postsynaptic potential (EPSP) and a

Department of Neurological Surgery, Nihon University School of Medicine, 30-1, Oyaguchi Kamimachi, Itabashi-ku, Tokyo 173, Japan population spike (PS) of Schaffer collateral/CA1 responses. The initial slope of EPSP was measured. The microdialysis probe was perfused with Ringer solution (adjusted to pH 7.4) at a rate of $5.0\,\mu l/min$ for 30 min, beginning at 7 h after reperfusion. A competitive antagonist of NMDA receptor, 2-amino-5-phosphonovalerate (APV, $0.1\,mM$), was administered via the perfusate for microdialysis. The input-output curves of the EPSP slope were compared before and after perfusion of APV, employing the paired t test. The synaptic responses to repetitive stimulation of Schaffer collaterals were then recorded. Only the data obtained with the first repetitive stimulation were analyzed to exclude the effect of long-term changes in synaptic responses induced by preceding repetitive stimulation. The responses to repetitive stimulation were compared between animals treated differently, employing the unpaired t test.

Results

In agreement with our previous study, the input-output curves of the EPSP slope of Schaffer collateral/CA1 responses were shifted to the left at 6 h postischemia ($n = 6$) as compared to those in the sham controls ($P < .01$, unpaired t test; $n = 7$). The EPSP slope in the postischemia animals ($n = 4$) as well as the sham controls ($n = 4$) was not significantly altered by $0.1\,mM$ APV administered in situ via microdialysis (paired t test).

We next examined the effect of APV on the synaptic responses to repetitive stimulation. A prolonged repetitive stimulation at high frequency produces NMDA receptor-mediated afterdischarges (ADs) even in normal animals. To maximize the opportunity to detect a possible increase in the utilization of NMDA receptor-coupled ion channels, the effect of NMDA antagonist was examined on ADs induced by brief repetitive stimulation at a low frequency (5 Hz, 6 s) that do not normally involve NMDA receptors. In the sham controls, the stimulation intensity was adjusted to levels that caused 95% maximal EPSP when applied as a single stimulus. Because the maximal synaptic response to single stimulation was slightly greater in the postischemia animals because of the PIP, the stimulation intensity in the postischemia animals was adjusted to levels that caused 85% maximal EPSP. The PS amplitude recorded at this intensity level in the postischemia animals was widely variable but often lower than the PS amplitude recorded in the sham controls (Table 1). The EPSP slope was comparable to the EPSP slope recorded in the sham controls (Table 1).

During repetitive stimulation, the synaptic responses to each stimulus demonstrated an initial augmentation followed by a decline and subsequent reaugmentation. The temporal changes in synaptic responses during repetitive stimulation were identical in the sham controls and postischemia animals (Fig. 1). In the sham controls, short-duration ADs were observed following the termination of repetitive stimulation, which continued for 1.0–6.4 s (mean $\pm$ SD = 4.49 $\pm$ 4.26 s; $n = 7$; see Table 1 and Fig. 1). The period of

TABLE 1. Duration of afterdischarges induced by repetitive stimulation and the effect of in situ administration of APV through microdialysis

Animal group	Microdialysis	n	PS amplitude in response to single stimulation (mV)[a]	EPSP slope in response to single stimulation (mV/ms)[a]	Duration of afterdischarges after repetitive stimulation (sec)
Sham	Vehicle	7	6.06 ± 1.03	0.79 ± 0.12	4.49 ± 4.26
	0.1 mM APV	4	5.91 ± 1.18	0.73 ± 0.21	2.13 ± 1.65
Ischemia	Vehicle	6	4.40 ± 4.12	0.75 ± 0.29	26.33 ± 12.63*
	0.1 mM APV	4	4.30 ± 3.81	0.64 ± 0.05	7.13 ± 1.44 **

Mean ± SD; APV, 2-amino-5-phosphonovalerate; PS, population spike; EPSP, excitatory postsynaptic potential.
[a] The stimulation intensity was adjusted to the level that caused comparable EPSPs in the sham controls (95% maximal EPSP) and postischemia animals (85% maximal EPSP).
* $P < .001$, as compared to sham/vehicle (unpaired t test).
** $P < .02$, as compared to ischemia/vehicle (unpaired t test).

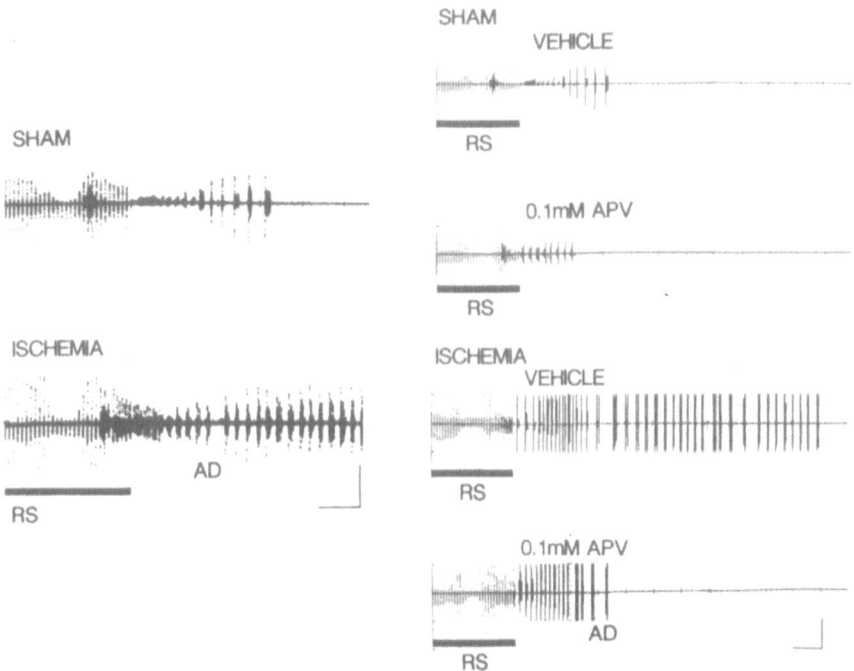

FIG. 1. *left*; Temporal changes in synaptic responses during repetitive stimulation (*RS*; 5 Hz, 6 s) in the sham controls (*SHAM*) and postischemia animals (*ISCHEMIA*). Scales: 2 s, 4 mV. *right*; afterdischarge (*AD*) induced by repetitive stimulation (*RS*; 5 Hz, 6 s) in the sham controls (*SHAM*) and in the postischemia animals (*ISCHEMIA*) perfused with vehicle (*VEHICLE*) alone (*upper trace*) and those perfused with 0.1 mM 2-amino-5-phosphonovalerate (*APV*) (*lower trace*). Scales: 2 s, 4 mV

the short-duration ADs in the sham controls was minimally affected by 0.1 mM APV (2.13 ± 1.65 s; $n = 4$; see Table 1 and Fig. 1). In clear contrast, it was found that the postischemia animals demonstrated ADs with a markedly long duration in the range of 14.0–44.0 s (26.33 ± 12.63 s; $n = 6$; see Table 1 and Fig. 1), which was evidently longer than the period of the short-duration ADs observed in the sham controls ($P < .001$, unpaired t test). The prolonged ADs did not appear to be attributable to potentiation of synaptic responses to each stimulus, because the PS amplitudes and EPSP slopes in response to single stimulation, and the temporal changes in synaptic responses during repetitive stimulation, were not larger than those recorded in the sham controls at the stimulation intensities examined. These prolonged ADs in the postischemia animals were reversed by microdialysis with 0.1 mM APV to short-duration ADs (7.13 ± 1.44 s; $n = 4$; $P < .02$, unpaired t test; see Table 1 and Fig. 1), which were similar to those observed in the sham controls. Because the synaptic responses to single stimulation in the postischemia animals were unaffected by APV, an NMDA receptor-mediated component does not appear to be involved in the PIP.

Conclusion

This investigation has provided evidence to indicate that NMDA receptor-coupled ion channels can be utilized more easily in the reperfusion period than under normal conditions. This finding is consistent with the data reported by Andiné et al. [3] in which an NMDA-mediated increase in Ca^{2+} uptake in response to repetitive stimulation was demonstrated during the reperfusion period. These data suggest that, during the reperfusion period, Ca^{2+} influx into the CA1 pyramidal cells can be greatly enhanced through NMDA receptor-coupled ion channels if appropriately timed multiple synaptic inputs bombard these cells. Such enhancement of the Ca^{2+} influx may facilitate delayed death of CA1 pyramidal cells.

References

1. Pulsinelli WA, Brierley JB, Plum F (1982) Temporal profile of neuronal damage in a model of transient forebrain ischemia. Ann Neurol 11:491–498
2. Miyazaki S, Katayama Y, Furuichi M, Kinoshita K, Kawamata T, Tsubokawa T (1993) Post-ischemic potentiation of Schaffer collateral/CA1 pyramidal cell responses of the rat hippocampus in vivo: involvement of N-methyl-D-aspartate receptors. Brain Res 611:155–159
3. Andiné P, Jacobson I, Hagberg H (1988) Calcium uptake evoked by electrical stimulation is enhanced postischemically and precedes delayed neuronal death in CA1 of rat hippocampus: involvement of N-methyl-D-asparate receptors. J Cereb Blood Flow Metab 8:799–807

The Use of Microdialysis for Monitoring the Effect of the Neuroprotective Drug CI-977 on Extracellular Excitatory Amino Acids

S. Galbraith, K.B. Mackay, T.R. Patel, and J. McCulloch

Introduction

The excitatory amino acid glutamate is now accepted as an important cause of brain damage in animals following ischemia [1,2]. Its effects can be ameliorated by various neuroprotective drugs that either block the post-synaptic N-methyl-D-aspartate (NMDA) and α-amino-3-hydroxy-5-methyl-4-isoxazole propionate (AMPA) receptors or which putatively inhibit the presynaptic release of glutamate [3]. In man, ischemia is a cause of brain damage, not only in stroke but also in head injury; as many as 85% of patients who die following a head injury have evidence of hypoxic ischemic brain damage [4,5]. The use of neuroprotective drugs in these conditions could be beneficial, and there are currently several clinical studies under way.

To properly assess the value of these drugs, it is important to limit their use to patients in whom glutamate is elevated and to monitor closely the effect of drug intervention. The best method of doing this would be by microdialysis, and preliminary studies have been reported [6,7]. Before developing this technique further in patients, however, we have studied microdialysis in the laboratory to examine its consistency in reflecting changes in excitatory amino acids resulting from pathology and its ability to monitor alterations following intervention with neuroprotective drugs.

The most widely studied neuroprotective drugs at the present time are the NMDA antagonists. They are effective in reducing experimental ischemic injury in animal models, but there is concern about their side effects in humans [8–10]. In animals, neuronal vacuolation and swelling and behavioral changes have been reported [11,12]. It is therefore prudent to examine also drugs that may reduce the amount of glutamate in the extracellular space. One such drug is the opioid agonist CI-977 (enadoline). It is neuroprotective in focal cerebral ischemia in rats and cats, but its clinical development is hindered by the uncertainty as to its precise mode of action [13].

Wellcome Surgical Institute & Hugh Fraser Neuroscience Labs., University of Glasgow, Garscube Estate, Bearsden Road, Glasgow G61 1QH, United Kingdom

We have therefore used this study into the usefulness of microdialysis to investigate further the mechanism of the neuroprotective action of CI-977.

Methods

Surgical Preparation

The investigations were carried out in nine cats weighing between 2.3 and 3.5 kg. The cats were anesthetized initially with saffan (9 mg · kg^{-1}, iv total steroids), intubated, and connected to a positive pressure ventilator delivering nitrous oxide (70%) and oxygen (30%) in an open circuit. Catheters were inserted into one femoral vein (for the administration of drugs) and two femoral arteries (for continuous monitoring of mean arterial blood pressure (MABP), repeated sampling of arterial blood, and controlled withdrawal of arterial blood for induction of hypotension). Anesthesia was maintained throughout the course of the investigation with a nitrous oxide/oxygen mixture (70% : 30%) containing 1%–1.5% halothane, to maintain sufficient anesthesia in each animal as determined by loss of the corneal reflex.

Microdialysis Probe/Hydrogen Electrode Implantation

The parietal skull was exposed and, using an operating microscope, craniectomies 7–10 mm in diameter were made with a saline-cooled dental drill above the right and left suprasylvian gyri. A microdialysis probe (CMA 10: membrane length 1 mm, outside diameter 0.5 mm; Carnegie Medicine, Stockholm, Sweden) and an electrode (etched platinum/iridium wire: diameter 250 μm, Teflon coated to 1 mm of the tip; Clark Electromedical, Reading, England) were assembled with a tip-to-tip distance of 1 mm. The dura was opened, and two probe/electrode assemblies were implanted stereotactically into the left suprasylvian gyrus, in the affected post-middle cerebral artery (MCA) occlusion penumbral region at a depth of 1.5 mm. A further probe/electrode was inserted into the right suprasylvian gyrus at a depth of 1.5 mm. Following placement, craniectomies were sealed with cyanoacrylate glue, and assemblies fixed in place with dental cement.

Dialysate Collection

Microdialysis probes were perfused continuously with Krebs–Ringer bicarbonate solution (NaCl 122 mM, KCl 3 mM, CaCl$_2$ 1.2 mM, MgSO$_4$ 1.21 mM KH$_2$PO$_4$, 0.4 mM, NaHCO$_3$ 25 mM, pH 7.4) at a constant flow rate of 2 μl · min^{-1} using a microinfusion pump (CMA/100; Carnegie Medicine). The probes were then left for a stabilization period of approximately 2 h, during which time any dialysate samples collected were discarded.

After the stabilization period, dialysates were collected in 20-min fractions for a total volume of 40 μl. Two baseline samples were collected and CI-977 or vehicle was administered 30 min before MCA occlusion. A further fraction was collected over the subsequent 20 min, and the left MCA was permanently occluded. Thereafter, MABP was reduced in 10–15 mmHg decrements by withdrawal of arterial blood. Dialysate samples were taken when MABP had stabilized at each decrement (approximately 10–15 min). This procedure was repeated to a minimum MABP of 40 mmHg.

Measurement of Cerebral Blood Flow

The platinum electrodes were used to measure cortical cerebral blood flow (CBF) by means of the hydrogen clearance technique. The CBF was calculated using the initial slope index method. Data were collected over a 1-min period, 1 min after the hydrogen gas mixture had been removed. The first minute of the clearance curve was discarded to avoid artifacts caused by recirculating hydrogen. CBF values were determined simultaneously with the collection of each sample of dialysate.

Induction of Focal Ischaemia

The cat's head was placed in a stereotactic frame (Kopf, Clark Electromedical), the left MCA occluded via a transorbital approach, and the left orbit exenterated. The optic foramen was enlarged with a saline-cooled dental drill, and the posterolateral and superior walls of the orbit removed to expose the dura mater overlying the MCA from the origin of the artery to its bifurcation. The dura was incised and the MCA exposed. The trunk of the MCA, all collateral vessels, and all visible branches of the lenticulostriate arteries were coagulated with bipolar diathermy, and the main trunk transected with microscissors to assure completeness of the vascular occlusion. Further ischemia was produced by systemic hemorrhagic hypertension.

Physiological Variables

Regular samples of arterial blood were taken throughout the experiment for determination of respiratory blood gas status (238 pH/Blood Gas System, Ciba Corning, Halstead, England) and plasma glucose concentration (Glucose Analyser 2, Beckman, Bucks, England). Animals were maintained normothermic throughout by a thermostatically controlled heating blanket. A thermistor probe was also inserted periosteally, overlying the parietal cortex, via a scalp incision ipsilateral to the MCA to be occluded.

Dosing Regimen

CI-977 ($0.3 \text{ mg} \cdot \text{kg}^{-1}$) dissolved in isotonic saline was administered as a slow (3-min) iv injection 30 min before occlusion of the MCA. A constant iv infusion of CI-977 ($0.15 \text{ mg} \cdot \text{kg}^{-1} \cdot \text{h}^{-1}$) was initiated immediately and maintained thereafter until death. Control animals received a bolus injection of isotonic saline $(0.1 \, mg \cdot kg^{-1}$ iv) 30 min before MCA occlusion. An iv infusion of saline $(0.15 \, ml \cdot min^{-1})$ was initiated immediately thereafter and maintained until death. Control animals were treated contemporaneously and randomized with the drug-treated animals. This is the same dosing regimen employed in the neuroprotection study in the cat in which it was shown to produce stable plasma levels of CI-977 $(\sim 200 \, ng \cdot ml^{-1})$ [13].

Determination of Microdialysate Amino Acid Content

Dialysate amino acids were detected fluorometrically following precolumn derivatization with orthophthaldialdehyde according to the method of Lindroth and Mopper (1979) [14]. Analysis of microdialysate fractions was carried out by Dr. P.K. Hitchott (Parke-Davis, Cambridge, UK).

Statistical Analysis

All data are presented as mean $\pm$ SE of the mean (SEM). Comparisons between groups were made using the two-tailed Student's t test. Intergroup comparisons were made using a paired t test. A significance level of $P < .05$ was chosen.

Results

Physiological Variables

There were no significant differences between the vehicle-treated control group and CI-977-treated group in respiratory blood gases (po_2, pco_2, pH), temperature (rectal or periosteal), plasma glucose concentration, and hematocrit at MCA occlusion and during the subsequent 3 h postocclusion period.

The bolus administration of CI-977 30 min before the induction of ischemia produced a significant reduction in MABP of approximately 27% of control values (but only within the initial 5-min postinjection period (control, 90 $\pm$ 6 mmHg; CI-977, 66 $\pm$ 3 mmHg; $P < .05$, Student's unpaired t test). The hypotension was transient, and there was no difference in MABP between the two groups at the start of dialysate collection and concomitant CBF measurement 20 min before MCA occlusion (control, 89 $\pm$ 4 mmHg; CI-977, 81 $\pm$ 5 mmHg).

Cerebral Blood Flow

CI-977 had no significant effect on the level of CBF in the suprasylvian gyrus during the control period before occlusion of the MCA in either the ipsilateral or contralateral hemisphere (Fig. 1). Following the induction of

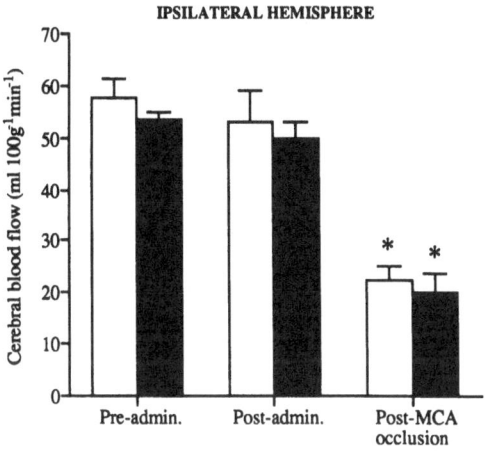

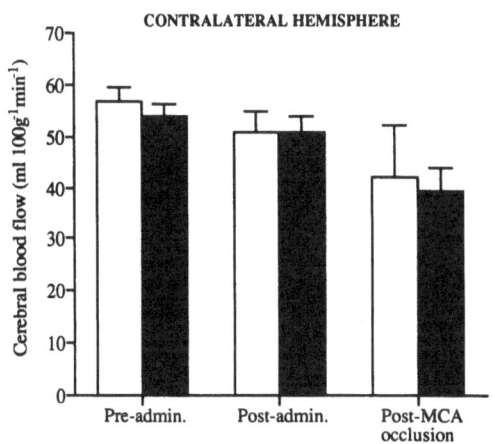

FIG. 1. The effect of CI-977 administration (*admin.*) on the level of cerebral blood flow in the ipsilateral (*upper half*) and contralateral (*lower half*) hemispheres immediately before and immediately after permanent middle cerebral artery (*MCA*) occlusion. Data are presented as mean ± SEM, and represent 4–15 measurements in cerebral blood flow (CBF) in five vehicle-treated controls and four CI-977-treated animals. *Asterisk indicates P* < .05 (paired *t*-test) relative to preischemic CBF level. *White bars*, control; *black bars* CI-977

ischemia, there was a significant reduction (approximately 50%) in cortical CBF in the ischemic hemisphere in both the vehicle-treated and drug-treated groups (*P* < .05, Student's paired *t* test) (Fig. 1). There was a minimal, nonsignificant reduction (approximately 18%) in CBF in the nonischemic hemisphere of both groups (Fig. 1). CI-977 did not alter significantly the level of postischemic CBF in either the ipsilateral or contralateral hemisphere (Fig. 1).

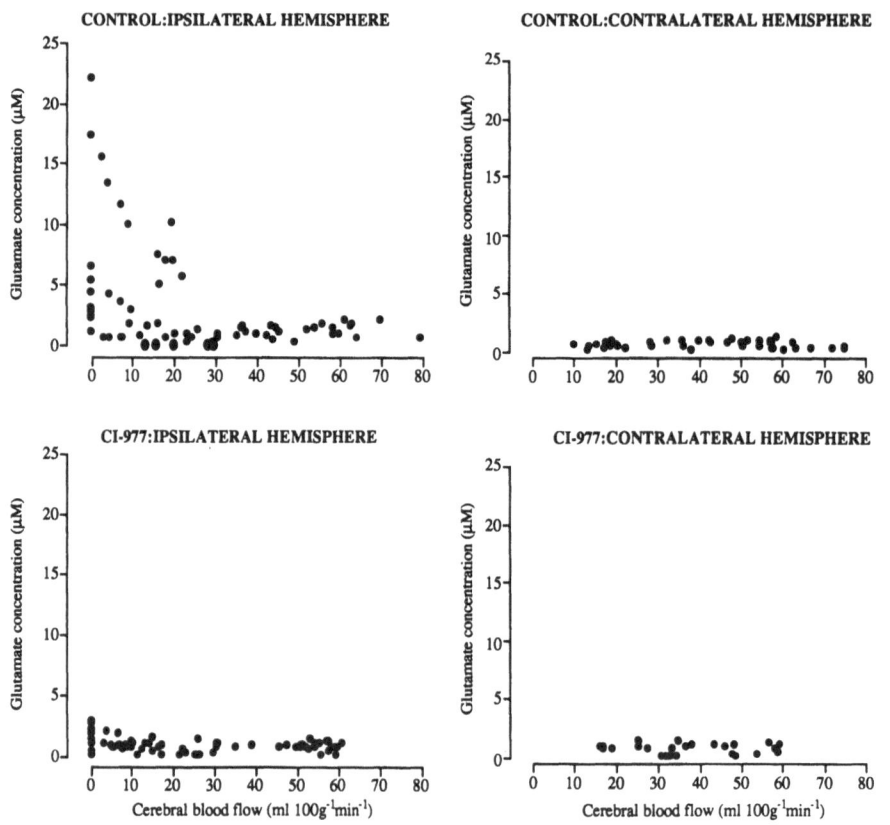

FIG. 2. Scatterplots of the relationships between CBF and the extracellular concentration of glutamate in the ipsilateral hemisphere before and after MCA occlusion in vehicle-treated control (*n* = 5) (*upper half*) and CI-977-treated (*n* = 4) (*lower half*) animals. Each data point represents all values obtained throughout the course of the investigation

FIG. 3. Scatterplots of the relationships between CBF and the extracellular concentration of glutamate in the contralateral hemisphere pre- and post-MCA occlusion in vehicle-treated control (*n* = 5) (*upper half*) and CI-977-treated (*n* = 3; one probe malfunctioned) (*lower half*) animals. Each data point represents all values obtained throughout the course of the investigation

Amino Acid Levels in Dialysate

At normal control CBF values, there was no difference in the concentration of glutamate in either the ipsilateral or contralateral hemisphere (Fig. 2). After the induction of ischemia, there was a marked increase in glutamate levels in the ipsilateral hemisphere when CBF fell to a threshold value of approximately $20 \, \text{ml} \cdot 100 \, \text{g}^{-1} \cdot \text{min}^{-1}$ in vehicle-treated control animals (Fig. 2). In the ischemic hemisphere in the CI-977-treated group, there was no such threshold (see Fig. 2). In the hemisphere contralateral to MCA

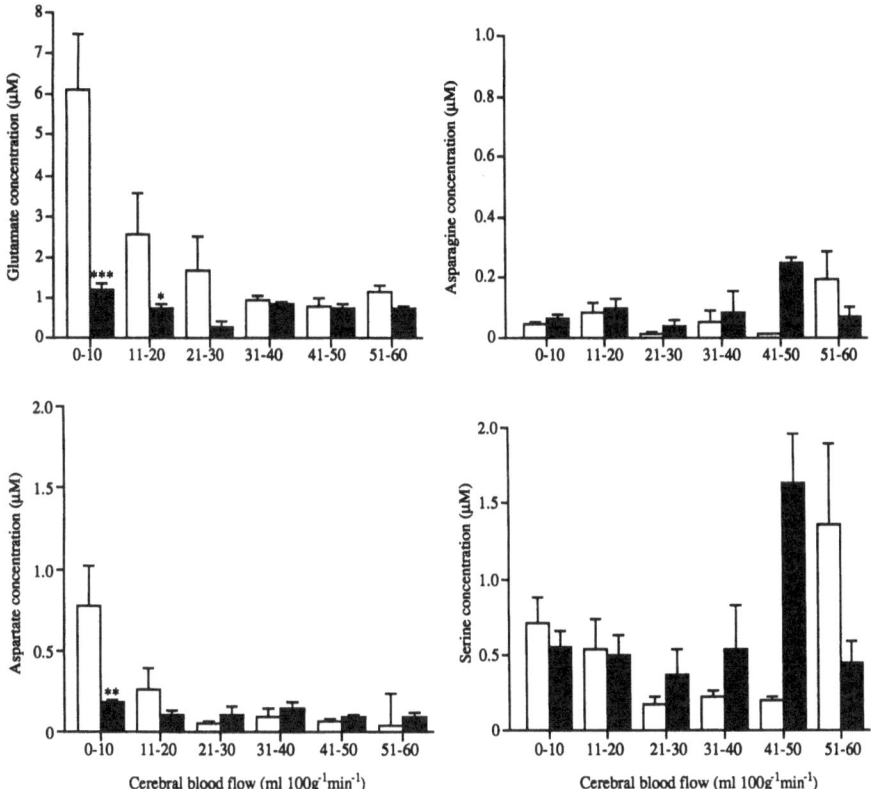

4

5

FIG. 4. The effect of pretreatment with CI-977 on the extracellular concentrations of glutamate (*upper half*) and aspartate (*lower half*) in the ipsilateral hemisphere before and after permanent MCA occlusion. Data are presented as mean ± SEM, and represent 3–26 determinations in five vehicle-treated control (*white bars*) and four CI-977-treated (*black bars*) animals. $*P < .05$; $**P < .01$; $***P < .01$ (Student's two-tailed t-test)

FIG. 5. The effect of pretreatment with CI-977 on the extracellular concentrations of asparagine '(*upper half*) and serine (*lower half*) in the ipsilateral hemisphere before and after permanent MCA occlusion. Data are presented as mean ± SEM, and represent 3–26 determinations in five vehicle-treated control (*white bars*) and four CI-977-treated (*black bars*) animals

occlusion, there was no increase in glutamate levels after the induction of ischemia in either vehicle-treated controls or CI-977-treated groups (Fig. 3). Similarly, there was no elevation in the levels of any of the other 11 amino acids examined in the contralateral hemisphere in either group after the onset of ischemia.

Glutamate was elevated in the ipsilateral hemisphere in vehicle-treated control animals when CBF fell to less than $30 \, ml \cdot 100 \, g^{-1} \cdot min^{-1}$ (Fig. 4). This increase was attenuated significantly by CI-977 at CBF of less than $20 \, ml \cdot 100 \, g^{-1} \cdot min^{-1}$ (Fig. 4). There was no difference between the two groups in the time elapsed after MCA occlusion for CBF values to fall to less than $30\,\text{ml} \cdot 100\,\text{g}^{-1} \cdot \text{min}^{-1}$, where increases in glutamate levels were observed (CBF bin $0.10\,\text{ml} \cdot 100\,\text{g}^{-1} \cdot \text{min}^{-1}$: control $123 \pm 10\,\text{min}$ ($n = 23$), CI-977 $124 \pm 11\,\text{min}$ ($n = 35$); CBF bin $1\text{–}20\,\text{ml} \cdot 100\,\text{g}^{-1} \cdot \text{min}^{-1}$: control $83 \pm 21\,\text{min}$ ($n = 11$), CI-977 $78 \pm 17\,\text{min}$ ($n = 14$); CBF bin $2\text{–}30\,\text{ml} \cdot 100\,\text{g}^{-1} \cdot \text{min}^{-1}$: control $57 \pm 10\,\text{min}$ ($n = 13$), CI-977 51 ± 18 ($n = 11$)). The extracellular concentration of the excitatory amino acid L-aspartate was also markedly increased at low flow levels (see Fig. 4). Administration of CI-977 significantly reduced this elevation such that the levels of asparatate did not increase over basal levels in the drug-treated group (Fig. 4). There was no obvious significant alteration in the glutamate-to-aspartate ratio in either circumstance.

There was no significant effect of CI-977 on the ischemia-induced release of the structural amino acids asparagine and serine (Fig. 5). The CBF bin $0\text{–}10\,\text{ml} \cdot 100\,\text{g}^{-1} \cdot \text{min}^{-1}$ was selected for comparison between control and CI-977-treated animals because in this CBF bin the response is robust with n typically 20–25. In contrast, the CBF bin $40\text{–}50\,\text{ml} \cdot 100\,\text{g}^{-1} \cdot \text{min}^{-1}$, where there is an apparent increase after CI-977, is not a robust response, with n approximately 3–4, arising as a consequence of the design of the study. Thus, in such a small group one large value will make a huge impact on the mean of the data in that CBF bin.

Discussion

Microdialysis is now being used clinically to determine the levels of extracellular amino acids. It is however demanding on resources, and its role is not yet clearly established. We have shown in experimental focal ischemia that microdialysis is a robust technique for measuring the extracellular levels of amino acids. Microdialysis gives a consistency of values both within and between animals. It is sensitive to alterations in excitatory amino acid level whether these changes result from pathology or modification by neuroprotective drugs. It will therefore be a useful clinical tool for the further development of such drugs.

The recovery rate of the substrate in the dialysate requires further consideration. Is any correction required, and if so, what? In experimental animals, it is possible as in our study to estáblish a baseline and relate changes to this. It was therefore unnecessary for us to introduce a correction. This is not possible clinically, especially when comparisons are made between patients. It will therefore be necessary to agree on a standard correction. This has previously been considered in this volume. Also, there is controversy related to the composition of the perfusate, particularly in relation to calcium and glucose, and this too was discussed previously (Katayama Y, Basic Problems in Clinical Apprication of Microdialysis Technique).

Extracellular glutamate begins to rise in the ischemic penumbra of the cat at CBF levels of about $30\,\text{ml} \cdot 100\,\text{g}^{-1} \cdot \text{min}^{-1}$. This is in keeping with previous findings [15,16]. The rise in glutamate is blocked by pretreatment with the opioid agonist CI-977.

This release of glutamate and its prevention by CI-977 is specific and unlikely to be the result of widespread neuronal damage. Glutamate is present in presynaptic terminals both in vesicles and in the general cytoplasmic pool. In the presynaptic vesicles, the ratio between glutamate and aspartate is approximately $10:1$, while in the cytoplasm it is less than $2:1$. The calcium-dependent release of vesicular glutamate is not accompanied by a parallel increase in aspartate; cell lysis or reversal of the electrogenic glutamate uptake mechanism produces marked increases in both glutamate and aspartate [17]. CI-977 is thought to act via the opioid receptor site specifically on the calcium-dependent vesicular glutamate. If ischemic release of glutamate and its prevention were nonspecific, there would have been an alteration in the glutamate/aspartate ratio toward the lower end reflecting the increase in cytoplasmic as well as they vesicular glutamate. This was not observed, thus supporting a specific action of CI-977 on the vesicular glutamate. Furthermore, if glutamate release had been nonspecific because of widespread neuronal damage, the structural amino acids should also have been increased. Again, this was not observed, confirming the specific effect of CI-977. We conclude therefore that CI-977 acting via the opioid receptor reduces extracellular glutamate by blocking its presynaptic vesicular release in this ischemic penumbra.

Microdialysis is a developing technique for the management of patients with cerebral ischemia. Our study has confirmed its potential, and we have used microdialysis to establish the mode of action of the opioid agonist CI-977.

References

1. Benveniste, H, Drejer J, Schousboe A, Diemer NH (1984) Elevation of the extracellular concentrations of glutamate and aspartate in rat hippocampus during transient cerebral ischemia monitored by intracerebral microdialysis. J Neurochem 43:1369–1374
2. Butcher SP, Bullock R, Graham DI, McCulloch J (1990) Correlation between amino acid release and neuropathologic outcome in rat brain following middle cerebral artery occlusion. Stroke 21:1727–1733
3. McCulloch J, Bullock R, Teasdale GM (1991) Excitatory amino acid antagonists: opportunities for the treatment of ischaemic brain damage in man. In: Meldrum BS (ed) Excitatory amino acid antagonists. Blackwell, London, pp 287–326
4. Graham DI, Adams JH, Doyle D (1968) Ischemic brain damage in fatal non-missile head injuries. J Neuropsychiatry 39:213–234
5. Graham DI, Ford I, Adams JH, Doyle D, Teasdale GM, Lawrence A, McClennan DR (1989) Ischemic brain damage is still common in fatal nonmissile head injury. J Neurol Neurosurg Psychiatry 52:346–350
6. Persson L, Hillered L (1992) Chemical monitoring of neurosurgical intensive care patients using intracerebral microdialysis. J Neurosurg 76:72–80

7. Hillered L, Persson L, Pontén U, Ungerstedt U (1990) Neurometabolic monitoring of the ischaemic human brain using microdialysis. Acta Neurochir 102:91–97
8. Grotta J (1994) Safety and tolerability of the glutamate antagonist CGS 19755 in acute stroke patients. Stroke 25:255
9. Muir KW, Grosset DG, Gamzu E, Lees KR (to be published) Pharmacological effects of the non-competitive NMDA antagonist CNS 1102 in normal volunteers. Br J Clin Pharmacol
10. Steinberg GK, Bell T (1991) Clinical dose-escalation safety study of the NMDA antagonist dextromethorphan in neurosurgical patients. Stroke 22:141
11. Olney JW, Labruyere J, Price MT (1989) Pathological changes induced in cerebrocortical neurons by phencyclidine and related drugs. Science 244:1360–1362
12. Woods JH, Koek W, France CP, Moersch Baecher JM (1991) Behavioural effects of NMDA antgonists. In: Meldrum BS (ed) Excitatory amino acids antagonists. Blackwell, London, pp 237–264
13. Mackay KB, Kusumoto K, Graham DI, McCulloch J (1993) Focal cerebral ischemia in the cat: pretreatment with a kappa-1 opioid receptor agonist, CI-977. Brain Res 618:213–219
14. Lindroth P, Mopper K (1979) High performance liquid chromatographic determination of subpicomole amounts of amino acid by precolumn fluroesence derivatization with δ-pthaldialdehyde. Anal Chem 51:1667–1674
15. Matsumoto K,, Graf R, Rosner G, Taguchi J, Heiss W-D (1993) Elevation of neuroactive substances in the cortex of cats during prolonged focal ischemia. J Cereb Blood Flow Metab 13:586–594
16. Shimada N, Graf R, Rosner G, Wakayama A, George CP, Heiss W-D (1989) Ischemic flow threshold for extracellular glutamate increase in cat cortex. J Cereb Blood Flow Metab 9:603–606
17. Nicholls D, Attwell D (1990) The release and uptake of excitatory amino acids. Trends Pharmacol Sci 11:462–468

Part 2

Clinical Application of Microdialysis
Technique

Microdialysis for Neurochemical Monitoring in Human Brain Injuries

LARS HILLERED[1,2] AND LENNART PERSSON[1]

Introduction

Based on our experience from studies on ischemic [1] and traumatic [2] brain injuries in the rat, in 1989 we formulated the hypothesis that microdialysis may be a powerful tool for metabolic monitoring and neurochemical studies of acute brain injuries in man. Modern neurointensive care (NIC) is based mainly on neurological, neuroradiological, and neurophysiological diagnostic methods. Methods for direct neurochemical measurements are greatly needed.

During the past decade, important secondary mechanisms of irreversible brain injury following ischemia and trauma have been identified on the basis of extensive experimental research. Excessive lactic acidosis from failing energy metabolism, increased production of oxygen radical species, and the neurotoxic effects of excitatory amino acids [3] are a few examples of such mechanisms. Relatively few studies on the importance of these secondary injury mechanisms have been carried out in patients, mainly because of the limited availability of suitable methods. Microdialysis is a relatively new technique by which important chemical substances can be retrieved from the extracellular fluid (ECF) of the brain (for references, see [4]), for example, energy-related metabolites such as lactate, pyruvate, glucose and hypoxanthine, and neuroactive amino acids. This chapter describes the current status of an ongoing development of microdialysis as a diagnostic tool in NIC. We focus particularly on the search for clinically useful markers of impending and manifest secondary ischemia.

Patients and Methods

Neurosurgical patients with acute brain injuries (head injury or subarachnoid hemorrhage, SAH) requiring NIC were studied.

[1] Department of Neurosurgery
[2] Department of Clinical Chemistry Uppsala University Hospital, S-751 85 Uppsala, Sweden

Sterile microdialysis probes (CMA/10, CMA/Microdialysis, Stockholm, Sweden) with a 4-mm membrane length were inserted into cortical tissue during neurosurgical procedures [5] or in conjunction with a ventriculostomy for routine monitoring of the intracranial pressure [4,6,7]. The probes were perfused with sterile Ringer's solution or artificial CSF (Na^+, 140 mmol/l; Ca^{2+}, 1.2 mmol/L; Mg^{2+}, 0.9 mmol/L; K^+, 2.7 mmol/L; Cl^-, 147 mmol/L) at a rate of 2 μl/min. Lactate and glucose in the dialysate samples were measured at bedside by an enzymatic method (YSI 2700 Select, Yellow Springs Instrument, Yellow Springs, OH, USA). The remaining dialysates were deep frozen and later analyzed by HPLC for lactate, pyruvate, purines (hypoxanthine, inosine, adenosine), and amino acids (see [1]).

These studies were approved by the ethics committee at the Uppsala University Hospital.

Results and Discussion

In a first series of five patients, microdialysis measurements in the exposed cerebral cortex were performed during neurosurgical procedures. Following probe implantation, all metabolites appeared to reach their basal level within 15–30 min [5]. This "implantation artefact" thus seemed to be shorter lasting compared to rat brain [2]. We also found that ischemia caused by blood vessel occlusion during resective surgery was associated with a marked increase in dialysate concentrations of lactate, purines, and neuroactive amino acids [5], as expected from previous animal work [1].

In a series of four patients, long-term measurement (2.3–8.3 days) was performed in the NIC unit. A total of 4447 chemical analyses were carried out [4]. The study demonstrated the technical feasibility of using microdialysis for long-term measurements in NIC patients. Fluctuations in the dialysate levels of energy-related metabolites (lactate, pyruvate, purines) roughly corresponded to clinical events, presumably involving hypoxia/ischemia. Events with intracranial hypertension were associated with markedly increased levels of energy-related metabolites, and a dramatic elevation of the excitatory amino acids (EAAs) glutamate and aspartate. The latter phenomenon is currently thought to be an important mediator of ischemic and traumatic brain damage (i.e., excitotoxicity) [3]. Based on methodological considerations that the probe recovery may vary during the disease process (e.g., because of edema), we proposed that the lactate-to-pyruvate ratio may be a more reliable indicator of hypoxia and ischemia than lactate or hypoxanthine alone. Furthermore, whereas a mild to moderate increase of lactate may merely reflect increased glycolysis, the lactate-to-pyruvate ratio reflects the redox situation of the cells.

In a series of six patients, simultaneous microdialysis and PET (positron emission tomography) was performed during 12 PET sessions [6]. PET was used to characterize the energy metabolic state [cerebral blood flow (CBF), cerebral metabolic rate of oxygen consumption ($CMRO_2$), oxygen extraction ratio (OER)] of the tissue hosting the probe, in order to validate the microdialysis results. The findings support the concept that the dialysate levels of energy-related metabolites, particularly the lactate-to-pyruvate ratio, reliably reflect the energy state of the tissue surrounding the probe. Glutamate and aspartate appear to be useful indicators of severe ischemia. Whereas microdialysis seems to be clearly valuable in global insults, a preceeding identification of "tissue at risk" must be done with such techniques as PET or magnetic resonance (MR) in focal insults.

In a recent series of ten patients with SAH, microdialysis measurements were performed 24 h/day for 6–11 days during NIC [7]. The results from 16 000 chemical analyses were compared with clinical data encompassing neurological state, intracranial pressure, cerebral perfusion pressure, computed tomography (CT) scans, transcranial Doppler measurement, and PET. During emerging ischemia subsequently leading to cerebral infarction of the probe area in one of the patients, the dialysate lactate-to-pyruvate ratio gradually increased, followed by an increase of EAAs. When lactate accumulation was extensive, glucose fell to zero, suggesting the transition from partial to complete ischemia. Brain glucose supply is critically dependent on blood flow. Because blood flow is preserved during hypoxia, the dialysate glucose concentration or the lactate-to-glucose ratio may also help in differentiating between ischemia (reduced blood flow) and arterial hypoxemia as the cause of increased lactate production.

When comparing the dialysate lactate-to-pyruvate ratio with the glutamate concentration, a threshold phenomenon was observed. Thus, at ratios less than 20–25, that is, close to the tentative normal value of 15–20 [4], virtually all glutamate values were low (see following). At moderately elevated lactate-to-pyruvate ratios of 40 and more, increased glutamate levels appeared. Such a threshold relationship was not found between lactate and glutamate. The observation suggests a threshold-type relationship between the degree of energy failure and the ECF level of glutamate. This is in line with the previously reported threshold-type relationship between CBF and ECF glutamate [8] in which increased ECF glutamate concentrations appeared when CBF fell below 35% of control in cat cerebral cortex. The present results support the usefulness of the dialysate lactate-to-pyruvate ratio as an indicator of disturbed brain energy metabolism.

Table 1 shows the mean dialysate glutamate levels over time in the ten SAH patients. A correlation was found between the average dialysate glutamate level and outcome (Glasgow Outcome Scale, 3-month follow-up), the highest levels being seen in patients with poor outcome. In comparison with the tentative normal glutamate level ($<2 \mu mol/l$) estimated in previous studies [4,5], even good recovery patients appeared to have slightly increased extracellular glutamate concentrations. In this context, it is important to note that cerebral infarction was not observed in nine of the ten SAH patients in the probe area according to CT and PET investigations. We

TABLE 1. Mean dialysate glutamate levels in SAH patients ($\mu mol/L$)[a]

GOS	Days after ictus			
	0–4	4–7	>7	0–11
Good recovery (n = 4)	3.6	5.8	3.8	4.5
Moderate disability (n = 3)	6.4*	6.4	7.3*	6.6*
Severe disability (n = 3)	22.4*	26.0*	29.6*	25.6*

[a] The dialysate glutamate concentration in 1600 samples from ten patients with subarachnoid hemorrhage (SAH) and outcome at 3-month follow-up, using Glasgow Outcome Scale (GOS). Asterisk, statistically significant difference between the groups of patients (Student's t test, $P <$ .001).

therefore hypothesize that the "total glutamate burden" may be of importance for the development a more diffuse cortical injury in the frontal lobes of patients after severe SAH.

In conclusion, our microdialysis results from NIC patient studies support the hypothesis that microdialysis may become a valuable tool in neurochemical brain monitoring. The technique appears to have a clear potential for metabolic monitoring, using the dialysate lactate-to-pyruvate ratio and glucose and hypoxanthine levels, for example, and for studying the mechanism of brain injuries using the extracellular accumulation of EAAs.

The success of future clinical development of the microdialysis technique will depend on both the standardization of results from different investigators and the availability of probes, pumps, and fraction collectors designed for clinical use, as well as bedside and on-line analytical methods.

Our most recent results on SAH show a correlation between the ECF glutamate level during the first 11 days after ictus and outcome, suggesting that glutamate toxicity may be an important mechanism underlying cortical brain damage of the frontal lobes resulting in mental impairment, a common sequela after SAH. This novel finding merits further investigation and forms a rationale for future neuroprotective pharmacotherapy after SAH, using glutamate antagonists.

Acknowledgment. This research was supported financially by the Swedish Medical Research Council, the 1987 Foundation for Stroke Research, the Foundation of Erik, Karin & Gösta Selander, and the Astrid Karlsson Foundation.

References

1. Hillered L, Hallström Å, Segersvärd S, Persson L, Ungerstedt U (1989) Dynamics of extracellular metabolites in the striatum after middle cerebral artery occlusion in the rat monitored by intracerebral microdialysis. J Cereb Blood Flow Metab 9:607–616

2. Nilsson P, Hillered L, Ungerstedt U, Pontén U (1990) Changes in cortical extracellular levels of energy-related metabolites and amino acids following concussive brain injury in rats. J Cereb Blood Flow Metab 10:631–637
3. Lipton SA, Rosenberg PA (1994) Excitatory amino acids as a final common pathway for neurologic disorders. N Engl J Med 330:613–622
4. Presson L, Hillered L (1992) Chemical monitoring of neurosurgical intensive care patients using intracerebral microdialysis. J Neurosurg 76:72–80
5. Hillered L, Persson L, Pontén U, Ungerstedt U (1990) Neurometabolic monitoring of the ischemic human brain using microdialysis. Acta Neurochir 102:91–97
6. Enblad P, Valtysson J, Cesarini K, Wärme P-E, Lilja A, Valind S, Andersson J, Hillered L, Persson L (1993) Cerebral metabolism simultaneously monitored by positron emission tomography and intracerebral microdialysis in patients with SAH. Upsala J Med Sci 98(Suppl 52):38
7. Hillered L, Valtysson J, Enblad P, Cesarini K, Wärme P-E, Lewén A, Persson L (1993) Long-term chemical monitoring in neurosurgical intensive care patients by intracerebral microdialysis. Upsala J Med Sci 98(Suppl 52):35
8. Shimada N, Graf R, Rosner G, Wakayama A, George CP, Heiss W-D (1989) Ischemic flow threshold for extracellular glutamate increase in cat cortex. J Cereb Blood Flow Metab 9:603–606

Patterns of Excitatory Amino Acid Release and Ionic Flux After Severe Human Head Trauma

R. Bullock, A. Zauner, O. Tsuji, J.J. Woodward, A.T. Marmarou, and H.F. Young

Introduction

In many of the conditions that result in acute cerebral damage, the role of excitatory amino acids has become the focus of current investigation [1,2]. The demonstration of excitatory amino acid release has been shown in several animal models of brain trauma, and has been associated with both structural damage and metabolic abnormalities [3–5]. These changes may be reversed by administration of excitatory amino acid antagonists, and this group of compounds has shown a greater magnitude of neuroprotective effect than any other series of drugs in the laboratory [3,6]. As part of an ongoing study, we have recently measured release of excitatory amino acids (EAAs) and ions in 17 acutely head-injured patients in our institution, with the aim of determining the circumstances that are responsible for glutamate release and their possible role as an exacerbating factor in causing *secondary* brain damage after severe human head injury.

In this chapter, we describe the patterns and time course of EAA release. The role of associated factors such as structural amino acid release, cerebral oxygen extraction, and concomitant changes in sodium and potassium in the extracellular space are also addressed.

Patients and Methods

The characteristics of the patients in this report are shown in Table 1. In six patients, excitatory amino acids were measured within the hemisphere underlining an acute subdural hematoma, and in one, under an epidural hematoma. In four, microdialysis monitoring was established in edematous cortical tissue, adjacent to a focal cerebral contusion that had been surgically resected. In the remaining five patients, the microdialysis probe was inserted

Division of Neurosurgery, Medical College of Virginia, Box 980631, Richmond, VA, 23298 USA

TABLE 1. Pattern of injury, and EAA release

Pathophysiological category	n	Outcome					Mean glutamate (μmol ± SEM)	Mean aspartate (μmol ± SEM)
		GCS range	Death	VEG	SD	GR/MD		
1. Diffuse injury	4	5–9	2		2	2	2.0 ± 0.8	0.5 ± 0.2
2. Subdural hematoma	2	4–10	2	1	2	1	1.3 ± 0.1	0.4 ± 0.1
3. Epidural hematoma	1	9				1	1.2	0.5
4. Focal contusion	4	6–10				4	27 ± 22	1.2 ± 0.9
5. Patients with major secondary/ ischemic/ hypoxic events (2 diffuse injuries, 4 subdural hematomas)	6	3–6	2	1	2	1	33 ± 14	13 ± 6

GCS, Glasgow Coma Scale; VEG, Vegetative; SD, Severely Disabled; GR/MD, Good Outcome/Minimal Disability. For patients in categories 1 through 4, no secondary ischemic/hypoxic events could be identified.

via a twist drill ventriculostomy opening. In these patients with diffuse injuries who did not undergo craniotomy, the probe was angled at 45° away from the ventriculostomy, and a guide cannula was used to achieve placement of the membrane in cortex.

Microdialysis

A 10-mm flexible sterile probe with external diameter of 0.75 mm was used. The active portion of the probe was inserted into the cortex, which was perfused at 2 μl/min with sterile 0.9% saline. Then 60-μl dialysate aliquots were collected every 30 min into sealed glass tubes using a CMA 170 refrigerated collector system (4°C). Clinical events that took place during microdialysis were logged into a VAX mainframe computer, along with intracranial pressure (ICP), mean arterial blood pressure (MABP), and Cerebral Anteriovenous Oxygen extraction (AJDO$_2$) data.

Probe Calibration and Standardization of Measurement Techniques

After use, each probe was calibrated in vitro by immersion in a bath solution of known glutamate, aspartate, sodium, and potassium concentration. The probes were perfused with 0.9% saline, and recoveries were calculated for the amino acids and ions. For each probe, six estimations were made.
    Recovery rates were as follows:

Excitatory amino acids	43% ± 5%
Sodium	63% ± 4%
Potassium	72% ± 5%

The flame photometry ionic measurement system was also calibrated against known standards, warranted pure by the manufacturer, over a wide range of ion concentrations.

Measurement of Neurochemicals

The excitatory amino acids glutamate and aspartate and the structural amino acids serine and threonine were measured, using high performance liquid chromatography. In alternating aliquots, sodium and potassium were measured using flame photometry.

ICP and CPP Monitoring

In all patients, a ventriculostomy was used to measure ICP and cerebral perfusion pressure (CPP). Continuous data from an arterial line were used to measure MABP, and an oxymetrix continuous oxygen saturation monitoring system was inserted into the jugular bulb for measurement of jugular vein oxygen saturation ($JSATO_2$ and $AVDO_2$). These physiological parameters were continuously acquired by a VAX mainframe computer system, and the data were smoothed to yield graphs for each parameter for 12-h epochs.

Data Analysis

For each of the 17 patients, the graphs for ICP, CPP, MABP, and $JSATO_2$ were obtained, and the mainframe then superimposed the data for excitatory amino acids and structural amino acids upon these curves producing as many as 24 graphs per patient. These graphs were then visually inspected to determine possible relationships. The small number of patients precluded statistical analysis in view of the heterogeneity of the data.

Results

Patterns of EAA Release and Intracranial Pathology

In general, glutamate and aspartate release fluctuated together (see Figure 1). In patients with focal cerebral contusions, EAA release was 6–20 times above the normal level ($\pm 2 mM$), determined from the literature [2]. In these patients, EAA levels in extracellular fluid remained elevated and constant, although slowly declining during the entire monitored period (Fig. 1). In patients with diffuse cerebral injuries, without prior ischemic events or reduced CPP ($n = 4$), the pattern of EAA release was remarkably

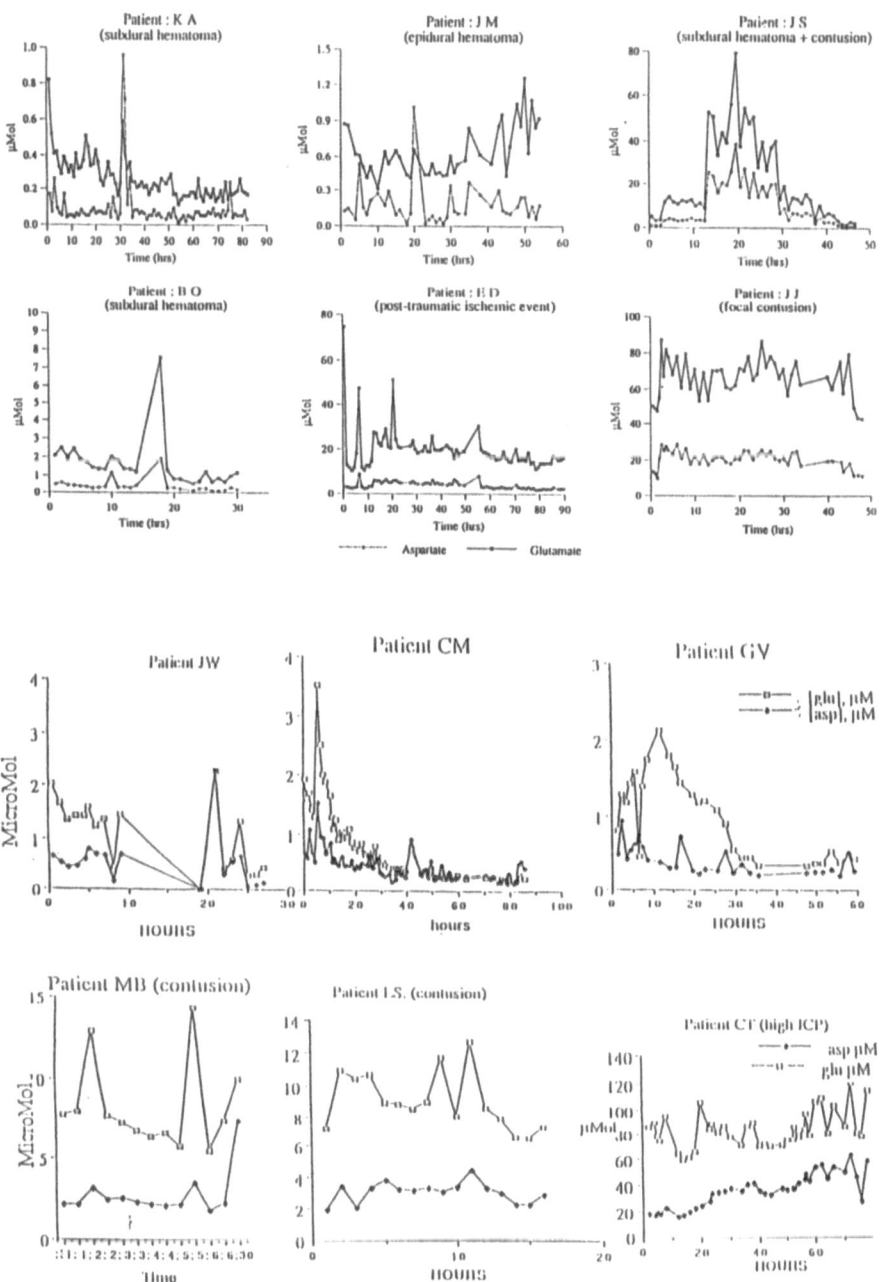

FIG. 1. Patterns of EAA release in 12 patients with severe head injury. Note the different magnitudes of EAA release on the Y axes

constant (Fig. 1 Third row). In these patients, EAA levels were initially 3–4 times above the normal level, but declined over about 6h to within the normal range. The highest levels of EAA release were seen in patients with severe diffuse injuries and prior ischemic events ($n = 4$). These ischemic events were documented as follows: a prolonged hypotensive period >1h, at the scene of the accident, from visceral injuries; low cerebral blood flow (CBF; 6ml/100g min^{-1}, and 20ml/100g min^{-1}) in two patients, and transtentorial herniation, and bilateral fixed pupils, plus hypotension and hypoxia, for 30min. In these patients, EAA release ranged from 20 to 50 times above normal.

In all but 1 of the 17 patients, the EAA trend was one of progressive decline (Fig. 1). In 1 patient, however, EAA rose from 10 times above the normal level to 60 times normal without any measured change in ICP or CPP. The factors leading to this rise in this patient remain unknown.

Time Course

When EAAs were elevated to more than 5 times normal, as seen in the patients with contusions and secondary ischemic injury, they remained high for the entire monitoring period (up to 4 days) in most cases.

Relationship Between Excitatory and Structural Amino Acids

In general, the changes in structural amino acids were parallel to those of the EAAs, but the release of structural amino acids was 5–20 times greater in magnitude.

Relationship Between ICP, CPP, and EAA Release

During 1648 hours of microdialysis for the 17 patients, only 2 patients demonstrated sustained elevations of ICP for longer than 30min. Both these patients died, and in these 2 patients EAA release trended steadily upward to extremely high levels, more than 50 times normal (see, for example, patient CT, Fig. 1). In 6 patients, 18 brief episodes (<5min) of ICP above 40mmHg were noted. However, none of these episodes was associated with EAA release at more than 100% over baseline.

Relationship Between Jugular Desaturations, AJDO$_2$, and EAA Release

In nine patients, graphs of continuous JSATO$_2$ and calculated AJDO$_2$ and CEO$_2$ (cerebral oxygen extraction) were available for comparison with EAA release. In only one of these nine patients was a sustained increased AJDO$_2$ and high CEO$_2$ seen. This patient demonstrated a 15- to 20-fold elevated level of sustained EAA release (patient ED; Fig. 1). In most of the patients with high EAA release and a prior secondary insult, CEO_2 and $AJDO_2$ was low, suggesting a cerebral hyperemic process.

Ionic Changes

The changes in ions in extracellular fluid (ECF) for six patients are shown in Fig. 2.

Potassium

In three patients, K^+ increased to the levels seen in fluid percussion injury in rats (>fivefold increase) [4]. In each of these three, EAAs were more than 50-fold higher than normal. In all three patients, however, the K^+ increases were transient ($\pm 2\,h$) while the EAA increases were sustained (2–4 days). In the remaining patients, K^+ remained below 2.5 meq in the ECF.

Sodium

Striking changes in hour-to-hour Na^+ concentrations were seen (Fig. 2). In general, a tendency to reciprocal changes in Na^+ were seen with respect to K^+. Patients with the most marked hour-to-hour Na^+ fluctuations tended to have high EAAs, but this was not consistent. (For example, contrast JM in Fig. 2, with JJ, and ED).

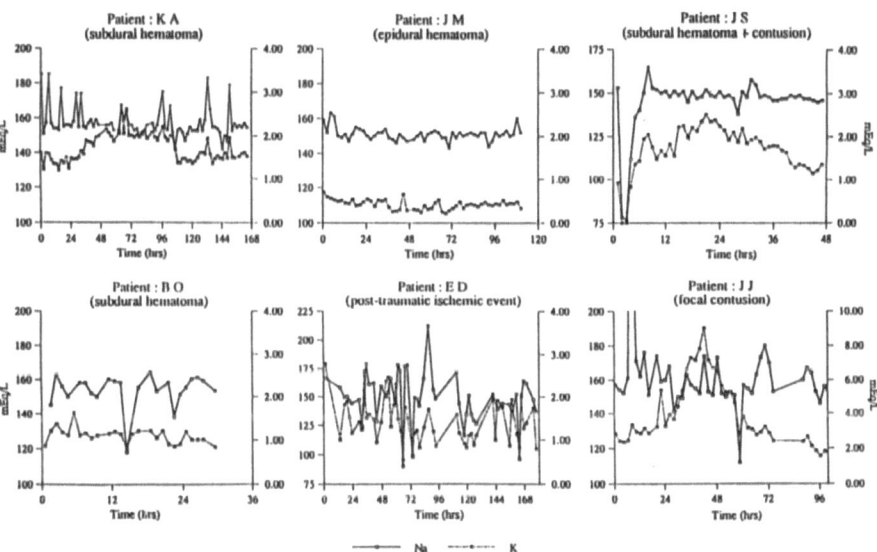

FIG. 2. Patterns of sodium and potassium changes in six patients after severe head trauma (compare with Fig. 1).

Discussion

These descriptive studies are the first in which the patterns and time course of sustained increased EAA release has been documented in severe human head injury. Overall, 10 of these 17 patients (59%) manifested sustained high glutamate levels in the ECF (a 6- to 50-fold increase over normal).

These changes persisted for the duration of monitoring, in most patients. The implications of this data are several:

1. In the majority of patients without secondary ischemic complications, EAA release appears to be a transient phenomenon, as in animal models, persisting in humans for about 6–8 h after injury.
2. In those with focal contusions, causing "low density" on CT, EAA release into the ECF is 6- to 50-fold increased, and persists for the duration of monitoring.
3. In those with secondary ischemic events, EAA release is very high (20- to 50-fold normal) and persistent during a period of days.

Thus it appears that the latter groups would benefit from prolonged therapy with EAA antagonist drugs, while patients without contusions, or secondary insults, may only require these agents to "cover" the first hours after injury. Clearly, further data are needed to validate these concepts. However, our recent animal studies are consistent with the view that secondary ischemic insults are necessary to cause marked increases in EAA release and to cause this release to be sustained [7].

We have recently reported our preliminary findings, which seek to validate the apparent relationship between EAA release and ICP reported by Persson et al. [8,9]. Our data imply that ICP only becomes a significant factor with respect to EAA release when it is sustained at more than 40 mmHg, with concomitant CPP reduction (<40 mmHg) for sustained periods. Brief CPP and ICP fluctuations (<5 min) do not seem to affect EAA release. We hypothesize that severe traumatic shear damage to the brain or major ischemic events early after traumatic brain mjury (TBI) cause massive EAA release and ionic flux, and that in some circumstances the brain is unable, either focally or globally, to restore ion homeostasis and energy substrate delivery. When this occurs focally, ischemic neuronal neurosis and astrocyte swelling (from K^+ buffering) occur. When the process is widespread, then brain swelling and high ICP occur (as seen in patient CT, Fig. 1). This may then jeopardize the CPP and lead to brain death. Our data lead us speculate that EAAs are thus an important factor in exacerbating harmful events after human TBI.

The ionic changes measured in this study support these concepts. The increases in ECF K^+, which only occur in the patients with the highest levels of EAAs, imply close linkage between ion flux and EAAs. We speculate that ECF K^+ never reaches the very brief 40- to 50-meq levels measured by ion-sensitive microelectrodes in TBI models, because astrocyte buffering prevents large, prolonged accumulations of K^+ in the ECF [10].

Our sodium fluctuations are more difficult to interpret. The use of a dialysate fluid (saline) with 154 meq of Na^+ makes these changes less clear. Further studies are needed to validate these events.

These findings reinforce the view that EAA release after trauma is far more than an epiphenomenon, and suggest exciting new approaches for therapy and further studies.

References

1. During MJ, Spencer DD (1993) Extracellular hippocampal glutamate and spontaneous seizure in the conscious human brain. Lancet 341:1607–1610
2. Ronne-Engstrom L, Hillered I. (1992) Intracerebral microdialysis of extracellular amino acids in the human epileptic focus. J Cereb Blood Flow Metab 12:873–876
3. Bullock R, Fujisawa H (1992) The role of glutamate antagonists for the treatment of CNS injury. J Neurotrauma 9:5443–5461
4. Katayama Y, Becker DP, Tamura T, Hovda DA (1990) Massive increases in extracellular potassium and the indiscriminate release of glutamate following concussive brain injury. J Neurosurg 73:889–990
5. Inglis F, Kuroda Y, Bullock R (1992) Glucose hyper-metabolism after acute subdural hematoma is ameliorated by a competitive NMDA antagonist. J Neurotrauma 9:75–83
6. Bullock R (1993) Opportunities for neuroprotective drugs in clinical management of head injury. J Emerg Med 11:23–30
7. Tsuji O, Marmarou A, Bullock R (1994) Microdialysis detection of eletrolytes and amino acid changes following head impact acceleration, coupled with secondary insult. In: 9th International Symposium on Intracranial Pressure (in press)
8. Persson L, Hillered L (1992) Chemical monitoring of neurosurgical intensive care patients using intracerebral microdialysis. J Neurosurg 76:72–80
9. Bullock R, Stout A, Woodward JJ, Tsuji O, Marmarou A, Young HF (1994) EAA release in severe human head trauma: the role of intracranial pressure and cerebral perfusion changes. In: 9th International Symposium on Intracranial Pressure (in press)
10. Nilsson P, Hillered L, Olsson Y, Sheiardown MJ, Hanson AJ (1993) Regional changes in interstitial potassium and clacium levels following cortical compression contusion trauma in rats. J Cereb Flow Metabol 13:183–192

Measurement of Excitatory Amino Acid Release in Glioma and Contused Brain Tissue During Intracranial Surgery

Tatsuro Kawamata, Yoichi Katayama, Kosaku Kinoshita, and Takashi Tsubokawa

Introduction

Excitatory amino acids (EAAs) may act as causal factors in ischemic or traumatic brain damage, according to the concept of excitotoxicity [1–9]. To understand the pathological role of EAAs in the cell injury process of the central nervous system, we have employed the cerebral microdialysis technique to measure the extracellular concentration of EAAs in our laboratory experiments [4,6,10–12]. Recently we have had opportunities to measure EAA levels in brain tumor and contused brain tissue in humans using microdialysis during intracranial surgery. These observations might produce unique opportunities to understand the pathophysiology of human EAA excitotoxicity.

Patients and Methods

Case 1 was a 57-year-old man injured in a traffic accident. The initial computed tomography (CT) scan revealed multiple cerebral contusion and acute subdural hematoma on the right side (Fig. 1). Because the patient's consciousness level progressively deteriorated, surgery was performed. After evacuation of the subdural hematoma, cerebral contusion was recognized in the frontal and temporal cortex. The contusion was more severe in the temporal lobe than in the frontal lobe. The microdialysis probes (membrane length, 3 mm) were placed in the contusion areas in the temporal and the frontal lobe. The tip of the probe was inserted to a 5-mm depth and modified Ringer's solution was perfused at the rate of 5 µl/min for 30 min. Dialysate was sampled every 5 min (sample volume, 25 µl). After completion of the dialysis, the contused brain tissue was surgically removed. The dialysate concentration of glutamate was determined by HPLC with precolumn fluorescence derivatization with o-phthalaldehyde.

Department of Neurological Surgery, Nihon University School of Medicine, 30-1, Oyaguchi, Itabashi-ku, Tokyo 173, Japan

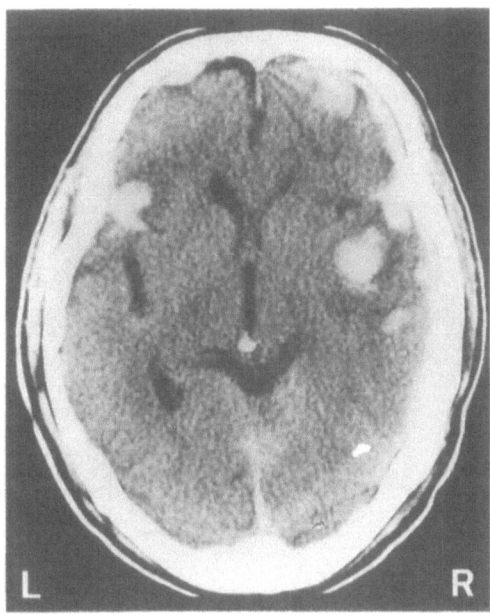

FIG.1. Computed tomography (CT) scan of case 1 demonstrates multiple cerebral contusion and thin acute subdural hematoma

Case 2 was a 38-year-old man who complained of chronic headache. A T_1-weighted magnetic resonance (MR) image revealed a low-intensity mass in the right frontal lobe. A T_2-weighted MR image showed a high-intensity mass of a larger size than that in the T_1-weighted MR image, indicating the existence of peritumoral brain edema (Fig. 2). The patient underwent surgery to remove the tumor. Before the tumor resection, microdialysis probes were placed in the tumor and peritumor area (area of surgical margin) (Fig. 2). Microdialysis was performed before, during, and after tumor resection in the same manner described in case 1. The histological diagnosis was astrocytoma grade 2.

Results

Case 1

The dialysate concentration of glutamate ($[GLU]_d$) showed high levels during the first 10 min after probe insertion, approximately $23 \mu M$ in the frontal lobe and $31 \mu M$ in the temporal lobe. The $[GLU]_d$ gradually decreased and showed stable levels after 15 min after the insertion, approximately $12 \mu M$ and $18 \mu M$, respectively (Fig. 3). Previous studies have reported that $[GLU]_d$ in the normal brain is less than $5 \mu M$; therefore, these $[GLU]_d$ in the contusion are approximately two- to tenfold the normal level.

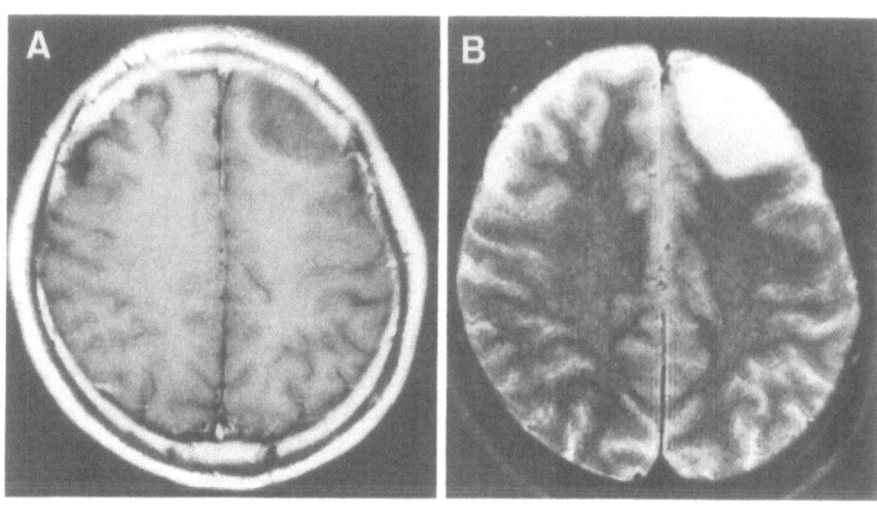

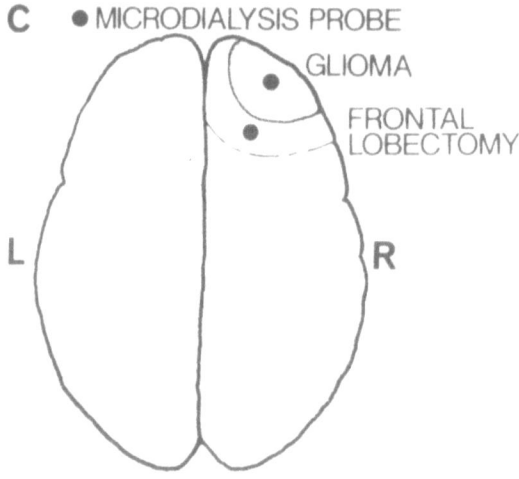

FIG.2. A–C. Case 2. **A** T_1-weighted magnetic resonance imaging (MRI) reveals low-intensity mass lesion in the right frontal lobe. **B** T_2-weighted MRI shows high-intensity mass with perifocal edema. **C** Schema shows location of microdialysis probes in case 2. One probe was placed in the tumor tissue and the other in the peritumor area. *Hatched line*, surgical margin for tumor resection

Case 2

Before tumor resection, the $[GLU]_d$ showed low levels in the tumor tissue and relatively high levels in the peritumor area. During tumor resection, $[GLU]_d$ was markedly increased in the peritumor area, reaching approximately fourfold the pre-resection level. In contrast, changes in $[GLU]_d$ in the tumor tissue during resection were less pronounced (Fig. 4).

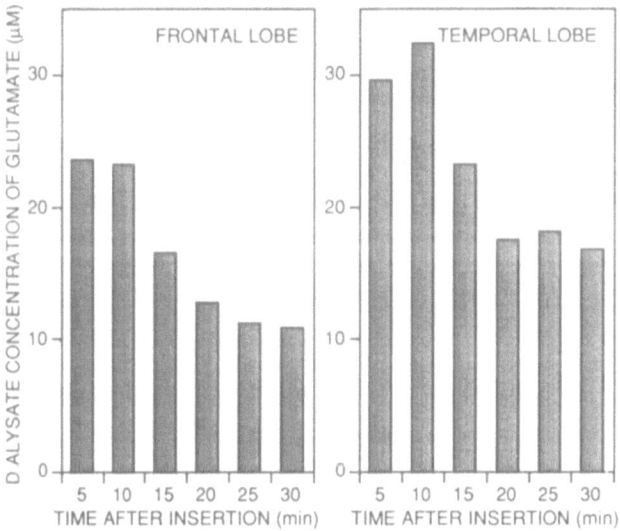

FIG.3. Changes in the dialysate concentration of glutamate ($[GLU]_d$) in the contused brain tissue of the frontal lobe (*left*) and temporal lobe (*right*) in case 1. $[GLU]_d$ was markedly increased in the contusion in both lobes

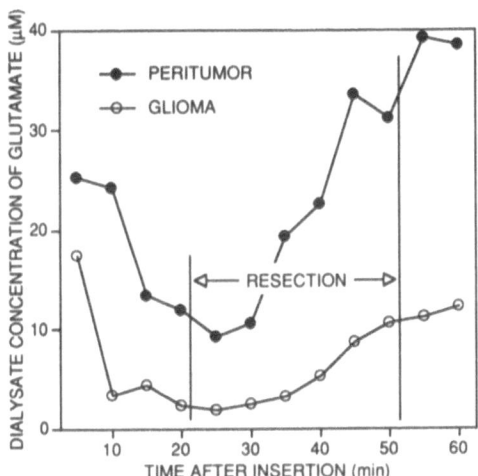

FIG.4. Changes in dialysate concentration of glutamate ($[GLU]_d$) in the tumor tissue and in the peritumor area in case 2 before and during tumor resection. $[GLU]_d$ in the peritumor area was rapidly increased after the beginning of resection (*closed circles*). $[GLU]_d$ in the tumor tissue showed late and slow increase during the resection (*open circles*)

No complications such as infection were observed after the microdialysis procedure in either cases.

Discussion

The results of the current study clearly demonstrated a significant increase in extracellular EAA levels in contused human brain tissue. Because neuronal cells contain high concentrations (millimolar levels) of EAAs in the cytosol, the increase in EAAs levels is most likely caused by the disruption of cell membrane and liberation of cytosolic EAAs to extracellular space. It has been well documented that elevation in extracellular EAAs concentration induces secondary cell damage, according to the concept of excitotoxicity [8]. The EAAs released from contused brain may infiltrate into surrounding brain area and cause secondary cell damage [12].

In case 2, the extracellular glutamate level was markedly increased in the peritumor area immediately after surgical resection (frontal lobectomy). The resection obstructed blood supply to the tumor and peritumor area, resulting in tissue ischemia. It has been well documented that cerebral ischemia induces a rapid increase in EAA levels in the extracellular space [9,11,13,14]. This early rapid increase appears to be a result of Ca^{2+}-dependent exocytotic release of EAAs from the nerve terminals depolarized by ischemic insult [6]. The rapid elevation of glutamate level observed in the peritumor area is, therefore, most likely the result of glutamate release from depolarized nerve terminals to the extracellular space.

During the surgical resection, the extracellular glutamate levels in the tumor tissue did not show rapid elevation as in the peritumor area. Because tumor tissue does not have a neuronal network, exocytotic release of glutamate from nerve terminals, which is typically observed in neurotransmission, could not be induced during the ischemic insult. The $[GLU]_d$ in the tumor tissue, in contrast, exhibited slow and late elevation. Energy depletion caused by ischemia may cause a loss of the electrogenic component maintaining the glutamate gradient across the plasma membrane, and continuous Ca^{2+}-independent flux of glutamate from the cytoplasmic pool may be induced thereby. Loss of function of the glutamate uptake system and breakdown of membrane function resulting from many other causes may also be responsible for a later slow increase in glutamate level in the tumor tissue.

In summary, changes in the extracellular concentration of glutamate during surgical operation were investigated in two clinical cases. The glutamate levels were markedly elevated in contusional brain tissue, approximately two- to tenfold the normal level. The glutamate level following surgical resection of the brain changed differently between the tumor tissue and the peritumor area, suggesting that there are several mechanisms of glutamate release. These results might allow understanding of the pathophysiology of EAA excitotoxicity in humans.

References

1. Benveniste H, Drejer J, Schousboe A, Diemer NH (1984) Elevation of the extracellular concentrations of glutamate and aspartate in rat hippocampus during transient cerebral ischemia monitored by intracerebral microdialysis. J Neurochem 43:1369–1374
2. Choi DW (1987) Ionic dependent of glutamate neurotoxicity. J Neurosci 7:369–379
3. Cotman CW, Iversen LL (1987) Excitatory amino acids in the brain—focus on NMDA receptors. Trends Neurosci 10:263–265
4. Katayama Y, Cheung MK, Alves A, Becker DP (1989) Ion fluxes and cell swelling in experimental traumatic brain injury: the role of excitatory amino acids. In: Hoff JT, Betz AL (eds) Intracranial pressure VII. Springer, Berlin Heidelberg New York
5. Katayama Y, Kawamata T, Maeda T, Ishikawa K, Tsubokawa T (1994) Inhibition of the early free fatty acid liberation during cerebral ischemia by excitatory amino acid antagonist administered by microdialysis. Brain Res 635:331–334
6. Katayama Y, Kawamata T, Tamura T, Becker DP, Tsubokawa T (1991) Calcium-dependent glutamate release concomitant with massive potassium flux during cerebral ischemia in vivo. Brain Res 558:136–140
7. Kawamata T, Katayama Y, Hovda DA, Yoshino A, Becker DP (1992) Administration of excitatory amino acid antagonists via microdialysis attenuates the increase in glucose utilization seen following concussive brain injury. J Cereb Blood Flow Metab 12:12–24
8. Mayer ML, Westbrool GL (1987) Cellular mechanisms underlying excitotoxicity. Trends Neurosci 10:59–61
9. Rothman SM, Olney JW (1986) Glutamate and the pathophysiology of hypoxic-ischemic brain damage. Ann Neurol 19:105–111
10. Katayama Y, Becker DP, Tamura T, Hovda DA (1990) Massive increase in extracellular potassium and the indiscriminate release of glutamate following concussive brain injury. J Neurosurg 73:889–900
11. Katayama Y, Tamura T, Becker DP, Tsubokawa T (1991) Inhibition of rapid potassium flux during cerebral ischemia in vivo with excitatory amino acid antagonist. Brain Res 568:294–298
12. Tanaka H, Katayama Y, Kawamata, T, Tsubokawa T (1994) Excitatory amino acid release from contused brain tissue into surrounding brain areas. Acta Neurochir 60:524–527
13. Hangberg H, Lehmann A, Sandberg M, Nystrom B, Jacobson I, Hamberger A (1985) Ischemia-induced shift of inhibitory and excitatory amino acids from intra- to extracellular compartments. J Cereb Blood Flow Metab 5:413–419
14. Westerberg E, Monaghan DT, Cotman CW, Wieloch T (1987) Excitatory amino acid receptors and ischemic brain damage in the rat. Neurosci Lett 73:119–124

Measurement of Lactic Acid and Amino Acids in the Cerebral Cortex of Head-Injured Patients Using Microdialysis

J. Clay Goodman[1,2], Daniel P. Robertson[1],
Shankar P. Gopinath[1], Raj K. Narayan[1],
Robert G. Grossman[1], Richard K. Simpson Jr.[1],
and Claudia S. Robertson[1]

Introduction

Lactic acidosis and release of excitotoxic amino acids may contribute to secondary brain damage following head injury [1–6]. Microdialysis is one of the most promising new methods for analyzing these neurochemical alterations in the intensive care setting [7–17]. We analyzed the chemical composition of the extracellular space of the brain, which was continuously sampled using microdialysis in 15 brain-injured patients, and correlated these neurochemical data with information regarding intracranial pressure, jugular venous oxygen saturation, clinical events, and patient outcome.

Methods

Microdialysis probes were placed via burrhole in the cerebral cortex. Probes were placed at the time of intracranial pressure monitor placement or at craniotomy for decompression of hematoma or contusion. The cerebral cortex was directly visualized, and the probes were placed in grossly normal-appearing cortex whenever possible. The microdialysis probes were constructed using 30 000 molecular weight cutoff dialysis tubing fashioned into a 5-mm loop. The 5-mm active loop was inserted into the cerebral cortex and was lightly anchored to the dura, allowing some slack in the infusion and collection lines. This allowed the probe to move with the brain rather than extending rigidly into the cortical parenchyma and potentially damaging the cortex. The probe was confined to the cerebral cortex with no significant sampling of subcortical structures. The delicate inflow and outflow lines of the probe ran through a length of clear plastic tubing, which served as a

Departments of [1]Neurosurgery and [2]Pathology, Baylor College of Medicine, One Baylor Plaza, Houston, TX 77030, U.S.A.

protective umbilical cord leading from the probe to the microfraction collector and pump at the bedside (CMA/Microdialysis AB, Stockholm, Sweden). Medical grade 0.9% intravenous infusion saline solution was used as the dialysate. This dialysate is readily available, sterile, pyrogen free, potassium free, and devoid of lactic acid and amino acids. Dialysate was collected in 30-min epochs using a refrigerated bedside fraction collector. The dialysate flow rate was 2 µl/min, and analyte recovery was 9%–11% during in vitro probe calibration against lactate and amino acids.

Organic and amino acid analyses were performed using high-pressure liquid chromatography (HPLC) [15,18–23]. Lactate and pyruvate measurements were performed by HPLC using a 25-µl injection of unprocessed microdialysate onto a BioRad HPX87 anion exchange organic acid column perfused isocratically with dilute sulfuric acid (BioRad Laboratories, Hercules, CA, USA). Detection was performed by ultraviolet (UV) absorbance at 210 nm, using peak area measurement with a three-point standard curve. The method requires no sample preparation when applied to microdialysis specimens, and has a run time of 17 min. The mobile phase is inexpensive and is continuously recycled. This method has been used extensively in the analysis of microdialysate samples.

Amino acid analysis was performed using precolumn phenylisothiocyanate (PITC) derivatization with subsequent gradient programmed reverse-phase chromatography with UV absorbance detection (PICO-TAG, Waters Associates, Milford, MA, USA). Quantitation was done by peak area using a three-point standard curve and internal standard (norleucine). The derivatization is labor intensive, and the reagents and standards are moderately expensive. The mobile phases are expensive, require helium sparging, and are consumed in substantial quantities as the analytical run time is 87 min. We have used this technique extensively for amino acid quantification in microdialysis samples.

A total of 742 h of microdialysis monitoring was performed. Continuous intracranial pressure (ICP), mean arterial pressure (MAP), cerebral perfusion pressure (CPP), and jugular venous oxygen saturation (SjVO$_2$) measurements were obtained concurrently with microdialysis monitoring. The microdialysis sample collection times were linked to the physiological data stream, permiting graphic display of the information using a commercially available scientific graphing software package (SigmaPlot, Jandel Scientific, San Rafael, CA, USA). This form of display facilitates visual correlation of multiple physiological and neurochemical events.

Results

The 15 patients were predominantly young men, reflecting the demographics of head trauma in the United States. Their ages ranged from 15 to 66 years (mean, 38 years), and their injuries included cerebral contusion (7), epidural hematoma (1), subdural hematoma (7), intracerebral hematoma (1), and penetrating gunshot wound (1). Some individuals had multiple types of injury. The admission Glasgow Coma Scores (GCS) ranged from 3 to 15 (mean, 8.4). Four patients with an initial GCS greater than 13 subsequently deteriorated, and all patients in this category had cerebral contusions. The 3-month Glasgow Outcome Scores (GOS) included 2 good recoveries, 3 moderate disabilities, 3 severe disabilities, 1 persistent vegetative state, and 4 deaths. Patients having good recovery or moderate disability were regarded as favorable outcomes, whereas patients having severe disability, persistent vegetative state, or death were tabulated as unfavorable outcomes. Lactate analyses have been completed in 14 of 15 patients, and amino acid analyses have been completed in 7 of 15. No complications resulted from microdialysis monitoring.

Three-month GOS correlated with peak lactate level seen in the microdialysates. Peak lactate levels did not exceed $1.0\,mM$ in the dialysates in the two patients having a good recovery and in two of four having moderate disability at 3 months. Peak lactate values greater than $1.0\,mM$ were seen in all patients having poor outcomes and in two of four patients experiencing moderate disability at 3 months. None of the patients with poor outcomes had peak lactate levels of $1.0\,mM$ or less. The mean value of peak lactate was $0.55\,mM$ in the good recovery patients, $1.25\,mM$ in the moderate disability patients, and $2.45\,mM$ in the severe disability, persistent vegetative, or dead patients. When the patients with good recovery or moderate disability were combined to form a favorable outcome group, the mean peak lactate was $1.0\,mM$. The difference between the peak lactate levels of the favorable and unfavorable outcome groups is statistically significant at the $P = .04$ level. In four cases, the peak lactate levels were so elevated (3.8–$29\,mM$) that we questioned the validity of the result. These patients were not included in the outcome analysis, but interestingly they all fell into the unfavorable outcome category.

The increased peak lactate levels may have resulted from impaired dialysate flow with subsequent increased analyte recovery. We guarded against this possibility by inspecting the microfraction collection vials for uniform sample volume at the time of analysis, but if there were flow stoppages required because of patient manipulation, our analyte recoveries may have been artifactually elevated.

In two instances, elevations of lactate were seen during episodes of jugular venous oxygen desaturation or increased ICP. Additionally, one instance of failure of barbiturate coma to control increased intracranial pressure was accompanied by a progressive elevation of microdialysate lactate. Similarly, in two instances of clinical deterioration caused by coalescence and enlargement of cerebral contusions, increases in lactate were observed.

The excitatory amino acids glutamate and aspartate, the inhibitory amino acid and N-methyl-D-aspartate (NMDA) receptor obligate coagonist glycine, and the putative glial osmoregulatory amino acid taurine were also elevated during pathophysiological events. We have not yet established provisional threshold levels of amino acids correlating with outcome. However, the patients with poor outcomes have larger fluctuations of extracellular amino acid concentrations, expressed as the difference between trough and peak amino acid levels, compared to the good outcome group. In several instances, the excitatory amino acids increased in concert with lactate and corresponded to a physiologically identifiable jugular venous oxygen desaturation or ICP elevation. Importantly, the nonneurotransmitter amino acids such as leucine, isoleucine, and valine, as well as the inhibitory amino acid gamma-amino butyric acid (GABA) failed to increase. Because the elevations were confined to excitatory amino acids, glycine and taurine indicate that the concentration changes were pathophysiological rather than simply reflective of changes in tissue tortuosity.

Maintaining the operation of the microdialysis system was technically demanding, and clinical circumstances controlled the timing of probe placement and removal so that neurochemical monitoring never spanned any patient's entire intensive care course. Opportunities to correlate pathophysiological events with neurochemical alterations were missed when the patients were transported to neuroimaging facilities or operating suites. In correlating long-term clinical outcome with microdialysis monitoring, it is important to realize that crucial neurochemical alterations may occur as the patient is deteriorating before probe placement, during periods of neurosurgical operation or transport, or after the microdialysis is discontinued.

Discussion

Elevations of lactate correlate with pathophysiological events and poor clinical outcome. This neurochemical marker of anaerobic tissue metabolism corroborates the role of ischemic injury in head trauma, as has been suggested by pathological, cerebral blood flow, $SjVO_2$, and positron emission tomography (PET) scan studies. The magnitude of dialysate lactate elevation correlates with outcome, suggesting that the relative severity of ischemic injury affects tissue viability and functional recovery.

Our study also shows that elevations of the excitatory amino acids glutamate and aspartate occur during pathophysiological events, and that there may be a relationship between the magnitude of extracellular amino acid concentration fluctuations and outcome. These findings support the role of excitotoxicity in secondary brain injury. Additionally, the inhibitory amino acid glycine is elevated. This amino acid also may play a role in excitotoxicity because it is an obligatory coagonist of glutamate acting on the NMDA receptor [1,2,5,6,24–26]. The elevation of taurine was unexpected, but is of interest in that this amino acid is believed to play a role in astrocyte osmoregulation, and its elevation may reflect deranged glial volume regulation following head injury [27].

This study demonstrates that neurochemical monitoring using microdialysis is feasible in neurosurgical patients, and can potentially provide understanding of the biochemical events after brain injury. Correlation was obtained between worsening neurological state and elevations of lactic acid and amino acids. If threshold concentrations of these analytes corresponding to tissue damage or poor clinical outcome can be established, it may be desirable to develop on-line analysis systems capable of alerting intensive care physicians to neurochemical deterioration in their head-injured patients.

Acknowledgments. The authors gratefully acknowledge the excellent support of the nursing staff and neurosurgical house officers of the Neurosurgical Intensive Care Unit, Ben Taub General Hospital, Houston, Texas, and the technical staff of the Neurochemical Research Laboratory, Department of Neurosurgery, Baylor College of Medicine. This work was supported by NIH PO1-NS27616.

References

1. Siesjo BK (1992) Pathophysiology and treatment of focal cerebral ischemia: Part I. Pathophysiology. J Neurosurg 77:169–184
2. Siesjo B (1992) Pathophysiology and treatment of focal cerebral ischemia: Part II. Mechanisms of damage and treatment. J Neurosurg 77:337–354
3. Pitts LH, McIntosh TK (1990) Dynamic changes after brain trauma. In: Braakmn R (ed) Head injury (revised series), 13th edn. Elsevier, New York, pp 65–100 (Handbook of clinical neurology, vol 57)
4. Hovda DA, Becker DP, Katayama Y (1992) Secondary injury and acidosis. J Neurotrauma 9(Suppl 1):47–60
5. Globus MYT, Dietrich WD (1992) The role of neurotransmitters in brain injury, 1st edn. Plenum, New York, p 378
6. Benveniste H (1991) The excitotoxin hypothesis in relation to cerebral ischemia. Cerebrovasc Brain Metab Rev 3(3):213–245
7. Hamberger A, Jacobson I, Nystrom B, Sandberg M (1991) Microdialysis sampling of the neuronal environment in basic and clinical research. J Intern Med 230(4): 376–380
8. Hillered L, Persson L, Ponten U, Ungerstedt U (1990) Neurometabolic monitoring of the ischaemic human brain using microdialysis. Acta Neurochir (Wien) 102(3–4):91–97
9. Hillered L, Persson L (1991) Microdialysis for metabolic monitoring in cerebral ischemia and trauma: experimental and clinical studies. In: Robinson TE, Justice JB Jr (eds) Microdialysis in the neurosciences, 1st edn. Elsevier, New York, p 450 (Techniques in the behavioral and neural sciences, vol 7)
10. Hillered L, Kotwica Z, Ungerstedt U (1991) Interstitial and cerebrospinal fluid levels of energy-related metabolites after middle cerebral artery occlusion in rats. Exp Med 191:219–225
11. Lonnroth P (1991) Microdialysis—a new and promising method in clinical medicine. J Intern Med 230:363–364
12. Meyerson BA, Linderoth B, Karlsson H, Ungerstedt U (1990) Microdialysis in the human brain: extracellular measurements in the thalamus of parkinsonian patients. Life Sci 46(4):301–308

13. Persson L, Hillered L (1992) Chemical monitoring of neurosurgical intensive care patients using intracerebral microdialysis. J Neurosurg 76(1):72–80
14. Robinson TE, Justice JB Jr (1991) Microdialysis in the neurosciences, 1st edn. In: Huston JP (ed) Techniques in the behavioral and neural sciences, vol 7, Elsevier, New York, p 450
15. Ronne EE, Hillered L, Flink R, Spannare B, Ungerstedt U, Carlson H (1992) Intracerebral microdialysis of extracellular amino acids in the human epileptic focus. J Cereb Blood Flow Metab 12(5):873–876
16. Ungerstedt U (1991) Microdialysis—principles and applications for studies in animals and man. J Intern Med 230:365–373
17. Whittle IR (1990) Intracerebral microdialysis: a new method in applied clinical neuroscience research (editorial). Br J Neurosurg 4(6):459–462
18. Eklund T, Wahlberg J, Ungerstedt U, Hillered L (1991) Interstitial lactate, inosine and hypoxanthine in rat kidney during normothermic ischaemia and recirculation. Acta Physiol Scand 143(3):279–286
19. Hallstrom A, Carlsson A, Hillered L, Ungerstedt U (1989) Simultaneous determination of lactate, pyruvate, and ascorbate in microdialysis samples from rat brain, blood, fat, and muscle using high-performance liquid chromatography. J Pharmacol Methods 22(2):113–124
20. Inao S, Marmarou A, Clarke GD, Andersen BJ, Fatouros PP, Young HF (1988) Production and clearance of lactate from brain tissue, cerebrospinal fluid, and serum following experimental brain injury. J Neurosurg 69:736–744
21. Nilsson P, Hillered L, Ponten U, Ungerstedt U (1990) Changes in cortical extracellular levels of energy-related metabolites and amino acids following concussive brain injury in rats. J Cereb Blood Flow Metab 19:631–637
22. Robertson CS, Goodman JC, Grossman RG, Priessman A (1990) Reduction in spinal cord post-ischemic lactic acidosis and functional improvement with dichloroacetate. J Neurotrauma 7:1–12
23. Simpson RK, Robertson CS, Goodman JC (1990) Spinal cord ischemia-induced elevation of amino acids: extracellular measurement with microdialysis. Neurochem Res 15(6):635–639
24. Rothman SM, Olney JW (1986) Glutamate and the pathophysiology of hypoxic-ischemic brain damage. Ann Neurol 19:105–111
25. Palmer AM, Marion DW, Botscheller ML, Swedlow PE, Styren SD, DeKosky ST (1993) Traumatic brain injury-induced excitotoxicity assessed in a controlled cortical impact model. J Neurochem 61:2015–2024
26. Tsumoto T (1990) Excitatory amino acid transmitters and their receptors in neural circuits of the cerebral neocortex. Neurosci Res 9:79–102
27. Schousboe A, Pasantes-Morales H (1992) Role of taurine in neural cell volume regulation. Can J Physiol Pharmacol 70(Suppl):356–361

Part 3

Clinical Impact of Jugular Bulb Oximetry

Benefits and Pitfalls of Jugular Bulb Venous Oxygen Saturation Monitoring

N. Mark Dearden

Introduction

Evidence is emerging that substantial ischemic brain damage, which contributes to the morbidity and mortality of critically ill neurosurgical patients, occurs predominantly within the first few hours following brain trauma [1,2,3]. Later ischemic episodes are also reported, however, during intensive care [2,4]. Falling cerebral perfusion pressure (CPP) from systemic hypotension or increased intracranial pressure (ICP) lowers global cerebral blood flow (CBF), while regional ischemia may result from vascular distortion or vasospasm. Boundary zone regional ischemia between anterior and middle cerebral arteries is seen in 22% of brain trauma patients at post mortem.

While the occurrence of early ischemic insults emphasizes the need for improved resuscitation and early evacuation of intracranial hematomas, the reported frequency of ischemic brain insults in critically ill neurosurgical patients highlights a need for early monitoring and correction of cerebral oxygen delivery during both resuscitation and subsequent intensive care. Recent advances in fiberoptic technology have enabled continuous monitoring of jugular bulb venous oxygen saturation (SjO_2), allowing identification and correction of global and occasionally regional cerebral ischemia. This chapter examines the potential advantages and difficulties that may be encountered during SjO_2 monitoring in neurosurgical patients.

Jugular Bulb Venous Oxygen Saturation, Cerebral Blood Flow, and Cerebral Metabolic Rate

The first practical and safe technique of sampling jugular bulb venous blood employed advancing a needle medially into the vein from below and anterior to the mastoid process [5]. Since the description of a Seldinger technique for

Department of Anesthesia, Leeds General Infirmary, Great George Street, Leeds, LS1 3EX, United Kingdom

cannulation of the jugular bulb in 1960 [6], repeated intermittent measurements of CBF, arteriojugular venous oxygen content difference ($AJDO_2$) and arteriojugular venous lactate content difference (AJDL) have been used to monitor neurosurgical patients at risk from cerebral ischemia [7]. $AJDO_2$ (normal range, 4–8 ml oxygen/100 ml blood) depends on the relationship between global cerebral metabolic rate for oxygen ($CMRO_2$) and CBF according to the Fick principle: [$AJDO_2$ (ml oxygen/100 ml blood) = global $CMRO_2$ (ml O_2/100 g per min) * 100/global CBF (ml/100 g per min)]. If SaO_2, PaO_2, hemoglobin concentration level, and the position of the hemoglobin dissociation curve stay unchanged, SjO_2 is proportional to CBF/$CMRO_2$ because $AJDO_2$ = hemoglobin concentration × 1.34 × arteriovenous oxygen saturation difference/100 + ((PaO_2 mmHg − PJO_2 mmHg) * 0.3/100). Normal values for CBF, $CMRO_2$, and SjO_2 are 40–50 ml O_2/100 g per min, 3–3.5 ml O_2/100 g per min and 54%–75%, respectively. The difference between SaO_2 and SjO_2, the cerebral extraction ratio (CEO_2), has been used as a monitor of adequacy of cerebral oxygen delivery and is normally between 25% and 45% [8].

After brain injury, intracranial hemorrhage, or subarachnoid hemorrhage (SAH), $CMRO_2$ falls according to the severity of brain damage; the relationship between the level of consciousness and CBF is variable. Assuming SaO_2 and PaO_2 remain constant, a rise in SjO_2 more than 75% ($AJDO_2$ <4 ml O_2/100 mls blood, CEO_2 ≤22%) suggests a CBF in excess of metabolic requirements. However, SjO_2 alone cannot differentiate relative hyperemia (CBF <50 ml/ 100 g per min) from absolute hyperemia (CBF >50 ml/100 g per min). An SjO_2 below 50% ($AJDO_2$ >7.5 ml O_2/100 mls blood) indicates relative hypoperfusion. An SjO_2 below 40% ($AJDO_2$ ≥9.0 ml O_2/100 mls blood), global cerebral ischemia is likely with increased producion of lactic acid (normal cerebral metabolic rate for lactate is −0.02 μmol/g per min). Because SjO_2 alone is unable to detect regional cerebral ischemia (SjO_2 may be low, normal, or high), the ratio of −AJDL to $AJDO_2$, the LOI, has been used to improve detection of cerebral ischemia. Normal values of LOI lie below 0.03, while ischemia is considered to be present above 0.08 [7,9]. Other factors influence the relationship between CBF and SjO_2, and the clinician must be careful in interpreting data. With developing anemia, if CBF is unaltered, a fall in SjO_2 may occur with an increase in CEO_2 and an unchanged $AJDO_2$. However, if compensatory autoregulation increases CBF in response to decreased oxygen delivery, SjO_2 and CEO_2 are unaltered while $AJDO_2$ falls [10]. Cerebral oxygen delivery is therefore preserved either by increased extraction of oxygen per unit volume of blood or by increased flow of blood.

Anatomy of Jugular Venous Drainage

The jugular bulb is a widening of the rostral internal jugular vein below the jugular formen. Although blood usually drains from both cerebral hemispheres into the right internal jugular vein, predominant drainage to the left also occurs [11,12]. In normal individuals, SjO_2 is the same in both jugular bulbs, but venous drainage may change with intracranial pathology [13,14] (Fig. 1). Many investigators choose to measure SjO_2 from the internal jugular vein on the side of focal pathology [9,15]. Others argue that extra-cranial venous blood enters higher up the internal jugular vein on the right and therefore choose the left jugular bulb as a more accurate reflection of cerebral venous oxygen saturation. Where intracranial pressure monitoring is in situ, an alternative method of selection is to sequentially compress the internal jugular viens and choose the side of greater rise in ICP as representing predominant venous drainage. If an equal rise in ICP is ob-served suggesting communication across the transverse sinus (50% of adults and 75% of children), the right internal jugular vein can be chosen for ease of access. In patients undergoing investigation by cerebral angiography, the side of main venous drainage from an area of interest, such as the site of an aneurysm, may be ascertained.

As the internal jugular vein descends lateral to the internal and common carotid arteries in the carotid sheath to form the brachiocephalic vein by joining the subclavian vein behind the medial third of the clavicle, it receives the inferior petrosal sinus, posterior occipital veins, mastoid emissary veins, pharyngeal plexus, facial veins, lingual vein, superior and middle thyroid veins, and the jugular lymph trunk. Accurate measurement of cerebral venous oxygen saturation necessitates radiological confirmation of the position of the catheter tip high in the jugular bulb, just below the skull base. In this position, about 3% of jugular venous blood arises from extra-cranial sources and the risk of significant contamination of cerebral venous

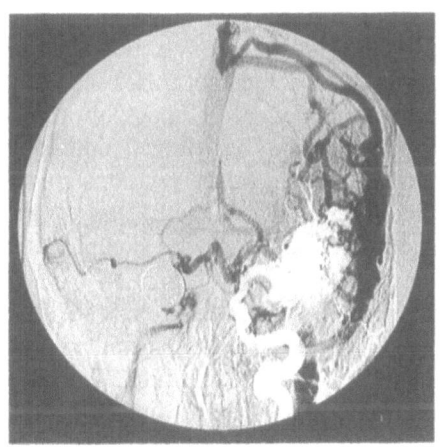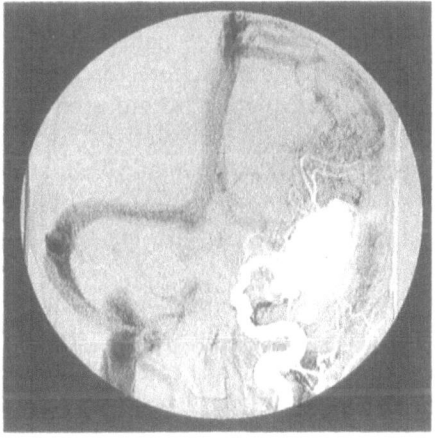

a   b

FIG. 1a,b. Left anteroposterior projection carotid angiogram shows arterial (*white*) and superimposed venous (*black*) phases of injection. **a** An arteriovenous malfor-mation drains predominantly via superficial cerebral veins to the left internal jugular vein. **b** The venous drainage of the left cerebral hemisphere occurs later, mainly down the right internal jugular vein

blood from extracerebral sources during slow venous sampling via the catheter will be minimized. Hemorrhagic diathesis, local infection or trauma, and any impairment to cerebral venous drainage are contraindications to jugular bulb saturation monitoring. Provided these restrictions are observed and the system is continuously flushed with 3 ml/hour of 2 units/ml heparinized saline, impaired cerebral venous drainage based on elevation of ICP is negligible [16] and the risk of significant venous thrombosis is less than 5%, provided the duration of monitoring is less than 7 days. Other rare complications associated with jugular cannulation include, inadvertent arterial puncture, damage to phrenic or recurrent laryngeal nerves, Horner's syndrome, pneumothorax, air embolism and shearing of the Seldinger wire. Fiberoptic catheters require frequent calibration using samples aspirated slowly from the jugular bulb, as described next. If blood cannot be freely aspirated and the obstruction is not rectified, the catheter should be removed to avoid venous thrombosis or embolism.

Fiberoptic Technology for SjO_2 Monitoring

The first description of total internal reflection of light was by John Tyndall at the Royal Institution in 1854. Fiberoptic technology has undergone major advances, with today's finest glass being 10 000 fold more translucent than that of 25 years ago. Fiberoptic-based, continuous jugular venous oximetry improves detection and correction of global cerebral ischemic insults over periodic in vitro analysis because sampling errors from contamination by extracranial blood are more likely at low CBF, and intermittent measurements only monitor momentarily, so transient ischemic insults go undetected [17]. Selected wavelengths of light are transmitted along fiberoptic cables, and the intensity of light reflected from erythrocytes down the fibers is quantified by a photodetector. The intensity of reflected light varies according to the relative concentrations of oxygenated and reduced hemoglobin. Early fiberoptic oximeters used two wavelengths of light but proved unreliable because their mathematical algorithms assumed a linear relationship between the ratio of intensities of light of different wavelengths and oxygen saturation and because changes in hematocrit could not be compensated for automatically.

A three-wavelength device, the Oximetrics 3 system patented by Abbott Critical Care Systems (Chicago, Illinois, U.S.A., permitted accurate, practical, and reasonably reliable monitoring of SjO_2 for the first time. The three wavelengths allowed algebraic solution of oxygen saturation without need to input hematocrit, while the use of a patented digital signal filter eliminated errors invoked from vessel wall artifacts. Reflected light intensity is continuously displayed on the monitor and should always be examined before interpreting the SjO_2 displayed. A bar between two dotted lines is normal, and readings should only be accepted when this state exists (Fig. 2a). High and low reflected light intensities represent vessel wall artifact and catheter obstruction, respectively (Fig. 2b,c). Catheter obstruction associated with therapeutic maneuvers can also be detected by monitoring jugular bulb pressure. Vessel wall artifact can be diminished by leaving the introducer in situ with the catheter tip just protruding from the distal end, while an attached hemostatic valve and catheter contamination sleeve allow sterile

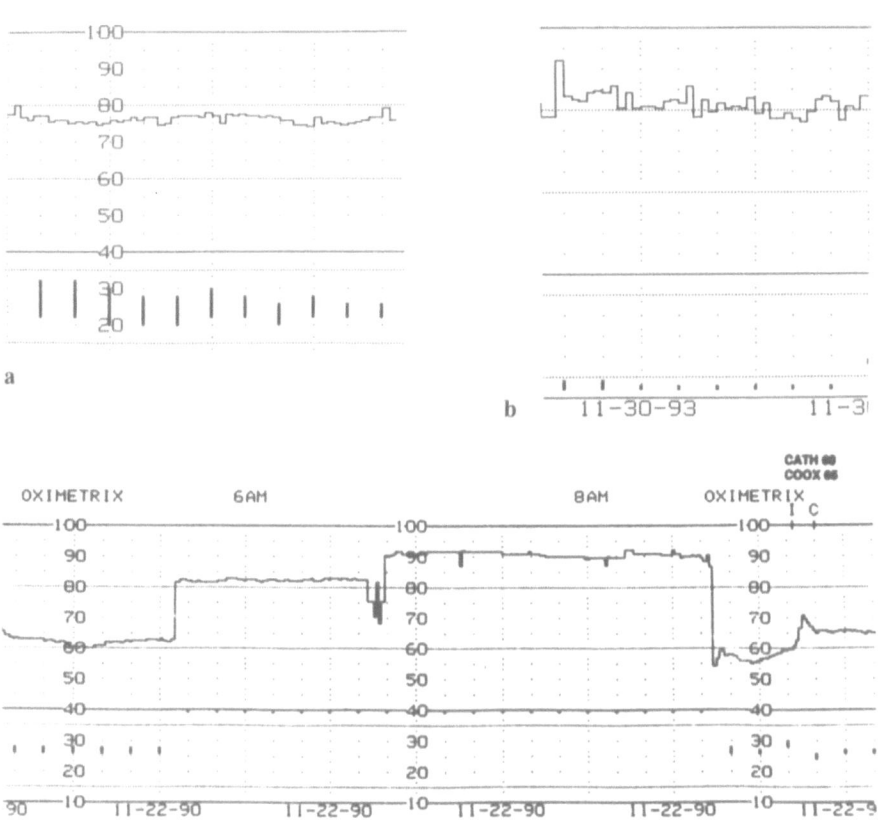

Fig. 2a–c. a A period of acceptable continuous SjO_2 recording using the three-wavelength Oximetrics system. *Upper trace*, SjO_2 between 75% and 80% with characteristic fluctuations in the signal. *Lower display*, vertical bars between two dotted lines indicate adequate light intensity. b *Upper portion* shows what appears to be a reasonable SjO_2 display. However, the lower light intensity bars all lie below the lower dotted line, indicating catheter obstruction. The *upper display* is therefore inaccurate, and patency must be restored or the obstructed catheter should be replaced. c A period of acceptable SjO_2 recording is followed by a sudden increase in the SjO_2 trace associated with turning the patient in bed. The light intensity display changes from adequate to unacceptable, with bars appearing above the upper dotted line indicating high reflected light from vessel wall artifact. Repositioning of the patient some 2 h later restored the signal, and in vivo calibration (I,C) confirmed accurate recording

remanipulation of the catheter [18]. Some authorities have experienced fewer problems with reflected light signals using a pediatric pulmonary artery (Swan Ganz) catheter inserted through a 6 Fr introducer. This arrangement also allows continuous monitoring of jugular bulb temperature. It is possible that algorithms (using jugular bulb temperature) might be used in the future to correct discrepancies between laboratory and monitored SjO_2 caused by the shift in the hemoglobin dissociation curve with temperature.

The Oximetrics 3 System for Measurement of Jugular Venous Oxygen Saturation

The integrity of the whole Oximetrics system can be checked (in vitro) using a pre-insertion calibration before introduction of the catheter into the jugular vein. However, calibration of the catheter must be performed after insertion (in vivo) against a laboratory co-oximeter and repeated every 12 h if accurate recordings are to be achieved [19]. Slow aspiration of blood from the jugular catheter during in vivo calibration, avoiding changes in the displayed SjO_2 or light intensity, should minimize the risk of sample contamination from extracranial sources. A variety of problems have been described during SjO_2

TABLE 1. Technique for establishing SjO_2 monitoring in adults

1. Do pre-insertion calibration of Opticath or pediatric pulmonary artery catheter against standard optical reference.
2. Do venipuncture at or above the level of the thyroid cartilage just lateral to the carotid pulsation with the head in neutral position and patient flat, if intracranial pressure (ICP) allows, aiming toward the external auditory meatus. If the jugular vein is transected before blood can be freely aspirated because of the compressibility of the vein, free flow of blood can be obtained by gently aspirating during slow withdrawl of the needle.
3. Use seldinger technique to insert a Vygon 14 s.w.g, 18-cm catheter (Opticath) or a 10-cm Cordis 5 Fr or 6 Fr percutaneous sheath introducer into the jugular vein to about the skull base; then withdraw about 1 cm.
4. Attach hemostatic valve and contamination sleeve to introducer.
5. Prime and then continuously flush catheter system with heparinized saline.
6. Advance fiberoptic catheter via protective sleeve, hemostatic valve, and introducer until tip abuts the skull base.
7. Withdraw fiberoptic catheter about 0.5 cm, leaving the introducer in situ and maintaining 0.5–1 cm of optical catheter protruding from the introducer tip.
8. Confirm free aspiration of blood via the catheter (if necessary retract the catheter slightly).
9. Verify satisfactory light intensity display (see Fig. 2).
10. Secure with a sterile transparent dressing, noting the length of catheter inserted to allow detection of displacement.
11. Attach pressure transducer to catheter system (optional).
12. Obtain lateral cervical X-ray to confirm correct position.
13. Perform in vivo calibration. Aspirate blood slowly to avoid sample contamination. Adjust catheter reading to match laboratory co-oximeter value.
14. Repeat in vivo calibration 12-hourly.

measurement [20]. Average insertion time for a jugular bulb fiberoptic catheter is about 15 min (range, 5–30 min), depending on the experience of the practitioner. Multiple attempts to cannulate the internal jugular vein are more likely with hypovolemia, head up tilt, and an inexperienced operator. The recommended technique for insertion of an Oximetrics catheter for SjO_2 monitoring is summarized in Table 1.

SjO_2 Measurement for the Detection of Cerebral Ischemia

The potential value of continuously monitoring both CPP and SjO_2 during the intensive care management of neurosurgical patients is the early detection of cerebral hypoperfusion (SjO_2 <50%). A protocol for use when SjO_2 falls below 50% in patients with severe brain trauma, based on the work of Sheinberg and colleagues [17] is (Table 2) and has been used in the management of comatose patients following severe brain trauma, subarachnoid hemorrhage, and intracerebral hemorrhage [21].

TABLE 2. Management protocol for SjO_2 less than 50%

Check Light Intensity Display	
High	Low
Adjust catheter position	Establish catheter patency
	If necessary replace catheter

Verify SaO_2
If <95%, correct

Confirm SjO_2 with Laboratory Co-oximeter
(slow sample rate; avoid changes in displayed light intensity or SjO_2)
If >5% discrepancy, perform in vivo calibration

Measure Arterial and Jugular Lactate Concentration
Calculate LOI to establish presence of ischemia

Measure Blood Hemoglobin Concentration
If <10 g/dl, consider correcting anemia

Measure Arterial $PaCO_2$
If <4 KPa (30 mmHg), correct hypocapnia

Correct Cerebral Hypoperfusion
Increase $PaCO_2$ further
and/or
Raise cerebral perfusion pressure (CPP) (reduce intracranial pressure (ICP)/
correct hypovolemia/raise blood pressure [BP])

Repeat Measurements As Appropriate to Establish Efficacy of Treatment

Jugular Venous Desaturation in Intensive Care

Jugular venous desaturation episodes below 50% have been reported in neurosurgical patients in association with hyperventilation, administration of hypnotic agents, vasospasm, anemia, hypoxemia, and compromised CPP during intensive care [21–23]. In a study of 102 patients with severe brain trauma, 76 episodes of jugular desaturation below 50% for more than 10 min were recorded and verified in 41 patients, mostly during the first 24 h of intensive care. When outcome was evaluated against the number of desaturation episodes in 95 patients at least 3 months post injury, using the Glasgow outcome scale, mortality for none, one, and more than one episode of desaturation was 18%, 46%, and 71%, respectively. The effects of jugular desaturation on dichotomous outcome (good outcome = good recovery or moderate disability; bad outcome = severe disability, vegetative state, or dead) were highly significant ($P < .009$) when analyzed by logistic regression to eliminate the effects of other covariables [2].

During intensive care after severe brain injury, a biphasic relationship exists between SjO_2 and CPP. Below 70 mmHg, SjO_2 is linearly related to CPP ($r = .837$; $P < .0001$); above this threshold, increasing CPP is not associated with a further rise in SjO_2 in most patients [23]. It therefore seems appropriate to maintain CPP above 70 mmHg in adult patients after severe brain trauma in the absence of SjO_2 monitoring to determine the critical CPP below which SjO_2 falls in an individual patient at a particular time.

Jugular Venous Desaturation During Neurosurgery

We have recently studied SjO_2 intraoperatively during clipping of intracerebral aneurysms following subarachnoid hemorrhage (SAH) in 18 patients to date. The side of jugular monitoring was selected from angiographic evidence of the predominant venous drainage of the aneurysm territory. Our preliminary data indicate global cerebral hypoperfusion (SjO_2 <55%) was detectable in 7 of the 18 patients during surgery. Hypoperfusion was corrected on all occasions by increasing mean arterial pressure with intravenous colloid infusion or inotropic agents (dopamine or noradrenaline). On three occasions, a mean arterial pressure in excess of 110 mmHg was needed to restore SjO_2 in patients with preoperative angiographic evidence of severe vasospasm (Fig. 3). Similar observations have been reported in SAH patients during anesthesia and in intensive care [21,24]. The LOI was increased above 0.08 in 4 of the 7 patients during jugular desaturation (below 50%). In a further 2 patients, LOI was increased despite a normal or elevated (>75%) SjO_2, suggesting regional ischemia. Increasing mean arterial pressure reduced LOI in all 6 patients but only below 0.08 in 4.

Neurological status was assessed 24 h postoperatively using the Glasgow outcome scale and the presence or absence of focal neurological defect. Neurological status (good versus bad) was significantly worse in patients

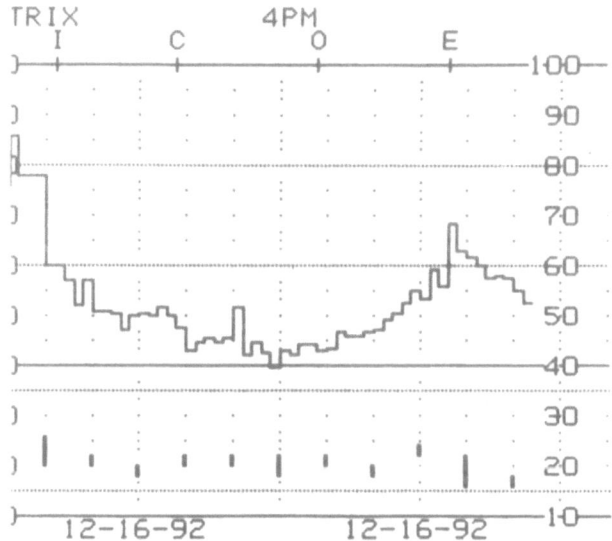

FIG. 3. SjO$_2$ trace from a patient with angiographic evidence of right middle cerebral artery vasospasm undergoing surgery for clipping of a posterior communicating artery aneurysm. After in vivo calibration (I, C), reduction of mean arterial pressure from 120 mmHg to 80 mmHg during deepening of anesthesia with isoflurane 1% resulted in a fall of SjO$_2$ and increase in LOI from 0.07 to 0.10. As PaCO$_2$ was 4.9 kPa and central venous pressure was 12 mmHg, mean blood pressure was increased to 110–120 mmHg (O) using noradrenaline, and this restored SjO$_2$ and reduced LOI to less than 0.08. At (E), PaCO$_2$ was reduced to 4 kPa by hyperventilation, and SjO$_2$ fell. Surgery and postoperative recovery thereafter were uneventful

with an elevated LOI at any time during surgery $(P = .011)$ (good, GCS 15 without neurological deficit; bad, GCS <15 and/or focal neurological defecit) Elevated LOI therefore predicted patients likely to require adjuvant hemodynamic therapy and prolonged invasive monitoring postoperatively (E. Moss, N.M. Dearden, and J.C. Berridge, unpublished work, Jugular Oximetry monitoring during anesthesia for clipping of intracerebral aneurysms, 1994).

Conclusions

Although continuous fiberoptic SjO$_2$ monitoring remains technically difficult and requires vigilance, it does allow an early diagnosis and treatment of global cerebral hypoperfusion and ischaemia in critically ill neurosurgical patients. Concomitant measurements of LOI may allow detection of regional ischemia despite normal or elevated SjO$_2$. Advances in the technology to minimize the problems associated with current fiberoptic catheter systems used in the jugular bulb are urgently required to make SjO$_2$ monitoring easier.

References

1. Gentleman D, Jennett B (1990) Audit of transfer of unconscious patients to a neurosurgical unit. Lancet 335:330–334
2. Robertson CS (1992) Treatment of cerebral ischaemia in severely head injured patients. Br J Intens Care 1(Suppl):12–15
3. Bouma GJ, Muizelaar JP, Stringer WA, Choi SC, Fatouros PP, Young HF (1992) Ultra-early evaluation of regional cerebral blood flow in severely head-injured patients using stable xenon-enhanced computerised tomography. J Neurosurg 77:360–368
4. Jones PA, Andrews PA, Midgley S, Anderson SI, Piper IR, Tocher JL, Housley AM, Corrie JA, Slattery J, Dearden NM, Miller JD (1994) Measuring the burden of secondary insults in head-injured patients during intensive care. J Neurosurg Anesthesiol 6:4–14
5. Robertson CS, Grossman RG, Goodman JC, Narayan RK (1987) The predictive value of cerebral anaerobic metabolism with cerebral infarction after head injury. J Neurosurg 67:361–368
6. Cruz J (1993) Jugular venous oximetry: cerebral oxygenation, monitoring and management. Acta Neurochir (Suppl) 59:86–90
7. Myerson A, Hallorhan RD, Hirsch HL (1927) Technique for obtaining blood from the internal jugular vein and internal carotid artery. Arch Neurol Psychiatry 17:807–808
8. Gejrot T, Lindbom A (1960) Venography of the internal jugular vein and transverse sinuses (retrograde jugularography). Acta Otolaryngol 52:180–186
9. Robertson CS, Narayan RK, Gokaslan ZL, Pahwa R, Grossman RG, Caram P, Allen E (1989) Cerebral arteriovenous oxygen difference as an estimate of cerebral blood flow in comatose patients. J Neurosurg 70:222–230
10. Cruz J, Gennarelli TA (1992) Cerebral extraction of oxygen and related variables in anaemic brain-injured patients. J Neurosurg 76:397a
11. Williams PL, Warwick R, Dyson M (eds) (1989) Gray's anatomy, 37th edn. Churchill Livingstone, New York, pp 793–805
12. Nylin G, Helund S, Regnstrom O (1961) Cerebral circulation studied with labelled red cells in healthy males. Acta Radiol 55:281
13. Lassen NA (1959) Cerebral blood flow and oxygen consumption in man. Physiol Rev 39:183–238
14. Gibbs EL, Lennox WG, Nims LF, Gibbs FA (1942) Comparison of AV differences, oxygen dextrose ratios and respiratory quotients. J Biol Chem 144:325–332
15. Shenkin HA, Spitz EB, Grant FC (1948) Physiologic studies of arteriovenous anomalies of the brain. J Neurosurg 5:165–172
16. Goetting MG, Preston G (1991) Jugular bulb catheterization does not influence intracranial pressure. Intens Care Med 17:195–198
17. Sheinberg M, Kanter MJ, Robertson CS, Contant CF, Narayan RK, Grossman RG (1992) Continuous monitoring of jugular venous oxygen saturation in head injured patients. J Neurosurg 76:212–217
18. DeDeyne C, Poelaert J, Decruyenaere J, Colardyn F (1993) Technical aspects of jugular bulb oximetry. Crit Care Med 21(Suppl 1):205
19. Andrews PJD, Dearden NM, Miller JD (1991) Jugular bulb cannulation: description of a technique and validation of a new continuous monitor. Br J Anaesth 67:553–558

20. Midgley S, Dearden NM (1993) Jugular bulb monitoring; technical considerations. Acta Neurochir (Suppl) 59:91–97
21. Von Helden A, Schneider GH, Unterberg A, Lanksch WR (1993) Monitoring of jugular venous oxygen saturation in comatose patients with subarachnoid haemorrhage and intracerebral haematomas. Acta Neurochir (Suppl) 59: 102–106
22. Andrews PJD, Dearden NM, Miller JD (1991) Comparison of Thiopentone and Propofol at 2 rates of administration in patients with severe head injury. Br J Anaesth 67:212
23. Chan KH, Miller JD, Dearden NM, Andrews PJD, Midgley S (1992) The effect of changes in cerebral perfusion pressure upon middle cerebral artery blood flow velocity and jugular bulb venous oxygen saturation after severe brain injury. J Neurosurg 77:55–61
24. Buckland MR, Batjer HH, Giesecke AH (1988) Anesthesia for cerebral aneurysm surgery. Use of induced hypertension in patients with symptomatic vasospasm. Anesthesiology 69:116–119

Continuous Monitoring of Jugular Venous Oxygen Saturation in Neurosurgical Intensive Care Units

Hiroyuki Yokota[1], Yasuhiro Yamamoto[1], Matoaki Nakabayashi[2], Akira Fuse[2], Kunihiro Mashiko[2], Hiroshi Henmi[2], Toshibumi Otsuka[2], Shiro Kobayashi[3], and Shozo Nakazawa[3]

It is very important for to evaluate cerebral blood flow and cerebral oxygen metabolism of patients who are suffering from severe head injury or severe cerebrovascular disease. It is well known that jugular bulb saturation shows the ratio of cerebral blood flow and cerebral oxygen metabolism. Thus, many trials were carried out to measure jugular bulb saturation to determine cerebral blood flow and cerebral oxygen metabolism. It has been very difficult, however, to measure and record these parameters continuously at bedside. Recent technology now makes it possible to measure and record these parameters at a bedside monitor.

A fiberoptic catheter located at the jugular bulb can detect the oxygen saturation of the jugular vein. The reliability of saturation measured in a fiberoptic catheter was confirmed by Robertson et al. in 1992 [1–3].

Clinical Materials and Methods

Patient Population and Management

Between January 1992 and December 1993, 63 patients measuring less than 8 on the Glasgow Coma Scale (GCS) who had been admitted to the Department of Critical Care Medicine in Nippon Medical School Main Hospital with severe head injury or severe cerebrovascular disease were measured for jugular vein oxygen saturation (SjO_2); 48 of the 63 patients had severe head injury and 15 had severe cerebrovascular disease. For the severe head injury group, 36 patients were classified as focal brain injury and 12 were classified as diffuse brain injury by the criteria established by Gennarelli.

---

[1] Department of Critical Care and Traumatology, Chiba-Hokuso Hospital, Nippon Medical School, 1715, Kamakari, Inba-gun, Chiba 270-16, Japan
[2] Department of Emergency and Critical Care Medicine, and [3] Department of Neurosurgery, Main Hospital, Nihon Medical School, 1-1-5, Sendagi Bunkyo-ku, Tokyo, 113, Japan

SjO$_2$ Measurement Technique

We have measured SjO$_2$ using a fiberoptic catheter for patients who were suffering from a severe head injury of cerebrovascular disease since 1992. For these cases, we continuously recorded intracranial pressure by the subarachniod method. The fiberoptic catheter was inserted percutaneously into the internal jugular vein through a 14-gauge Teflon needle or a 4.5 French introducer. The catheter was inserted on the side on which the intracranial pressure was much greater, as determined by a Queckenstedt's test, or on the right side if the intracranial pressure was not recorded. The top of the catheter was positioned in the jugular bulb, and the position was confirmed by X-ray or digital subtraction angiography.

Results

Head Injury

Of the patients with severe head injury, 36 were classified as focal brain injury and 12 were classified as diffuse brain injury by the criteria established by Gennarelli. The course of SjO$_2$ in severe head injury was classified into four groups: group I included the patients who were always recorded as within 60%–80% of normal SjO$_2$; group II were patients who showed desaturation in SjO$_2$ and were recorded finally within normal ranges; patients who were finally recorded at less than 50% were classified as group III; and those finally recorded at more than 90% of normal SjO$_2$ were classified as group IV. The number and outcome of these patients are shown in Table 1. There were 17 in group I and 15 in group II, and their outcomes were rather good. The patients classified as group III or IV, however, had poor outcomes; none of the patients classified as group III or IV survived.

The reactivity of SjO$_2$ to changes of PaCO$_2$ was examined for eight cases. We defined response to PaCO$_2$ as normal if the level of SjO$_2$ was decreased by hyperventilation. The patients who had normal SjO$_2$ response to changes of a PaCO$_2$ had good outcomes. However, all the patients having abnormal responses to PaCO$_2$ died (Table 2).

TABLE 1. Course of jugular oxygen saturation and outcome

Group	Good	Poor	Dead	Total
I	8	9	0	17
II	6	9	0	15
III	0	0	6	6
IV	0	0	10	10
Total:	14	18	16	48

TABLE 2. CO_2 reactivity and outcome

CO_2 Reactivity	Good	Poor	Dead
Normal	2	4	0
Abnormal	0	1	1
Total:	2	5	1

A Severe Head Injury Case

A 56-year-old man was struck on the head in a traffic accident and was admitted to our hospital at a GCS of 8. He was diagnosed as having an acute subdural hematoma and cerebral contusion, and craniotomy was carried out to remove the acute subdural hematoma. After the operation, intracranial pressure was maintained at less than 20 mmHg, but the level of SjO_2 and local cerebral blood flow recorded by the laser Doppler method gradually decreased. To increase cerebral blood flow and to normalize cerebral metabolism, the mild hyperventilation therapy for his cerebral swelling was stopped. On changing $PaCO_2$ from 35 mmHg to 45 mmHg, SjO_2 returned to a normal level without increasing the level of intracranial pressure (Fig. 1).

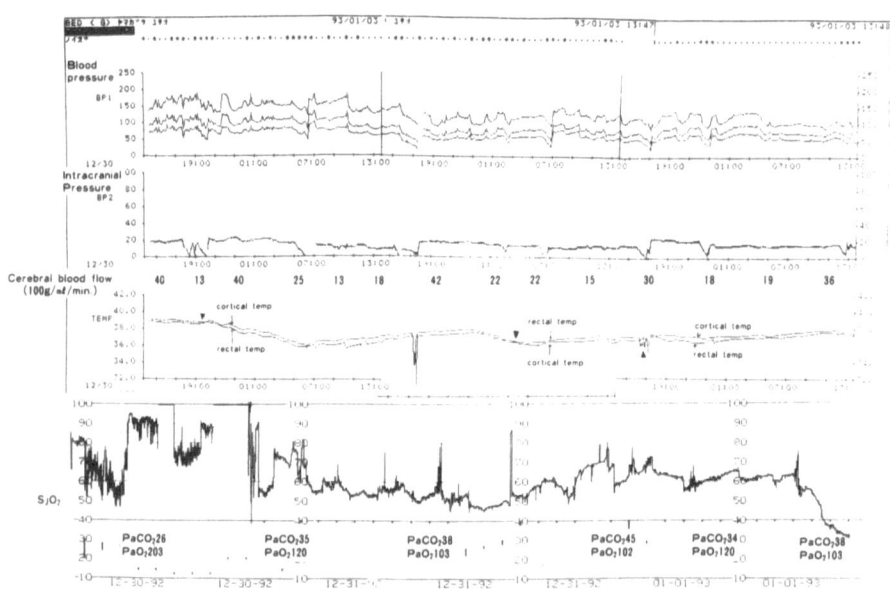

FIG. 1. Laser Doppler recording of a 56-year-old man diagnosed with subdural hematoma and cerebral contusion shows decreased levels of SjO_2 and local cerebral blood flow. To increase cerebral blood flow and to normalize cerebral metabolism, mild hyperventilation therapy for cerebral swelling was stopped

The patient was discharged from our hospital, classed as severe disability on the Glasgow outcome scale, 14 days after his injury.

Cerebrovascular Disease

SjO$_2$ was measured in 16 patients suffering from severe cerebrovascular disease. Of the 16 patients, 9 were diagnosed as suffering subarachnoid hemorrhage caused by a ruptured cerebral aneurysm, 6 patients had hypertensive cerebral hemorrhages, and 1 had cerebral hemorrhage from moya-moya disease. The course of SjO$_2$ was classified as were those of the head injury patients, and the outcomes of these patients were very poor, in group III or IV (Table 3).

A Case of Cerebrovascular Disease

A 64-year-old woman was admitted to our hospital with sudden onset of coma and left hemiplegia. Computed tomography (CT), performed just after her admission, demonstrated a huge hematoma located in the right temporoparietal lobe. Cerebral angiography before surgery showed moya-moya vessels in the bilateral hemisphere. In spite of the cerebral edema shown on CT, intracranial pressure was maintained at less than 20 mmHg by hyperventilation treatment without any sign of desaturation of SjO$_2$ (Fig. 2). It was thought that hyperventilation therapy to prevent cerebral edema for moya-moya disease should not be chosen because of the danger of provoking cerebral vasospasms and cerebral ischemia. In this patient, however, we could treat without any sign of cerebral ischemia, which might be demonstrated by a decrease in SjO$_2$.

In a 64-year-old man suffering from severe subarachnoid hemorrhage caused by the rupture of a cerebral aneurysm, the level of SjO$_2$ remained at 70%–80%, following the sudden onset of desaturation of SjO$_2$. His mean blood pressure was recorded as more than 200 mmHg from 100 mmHg; his pupils were dilatated and showed no response to light. Just after these changes, SjO$_2$ was recorded continuously at more than 90%. From these clinical changes and the serial changes of SjO$_2$ we could determine that the

TABLE 3. Course of jugular oxygen saturation and outcome in cerebrovascular disease

Group	Good	Poor	Dead	Total
I	4	2	0	6
II	1	1	0	2
III	0	0	4	4
IV	0	0	3	3
Total:	5	3	7	15

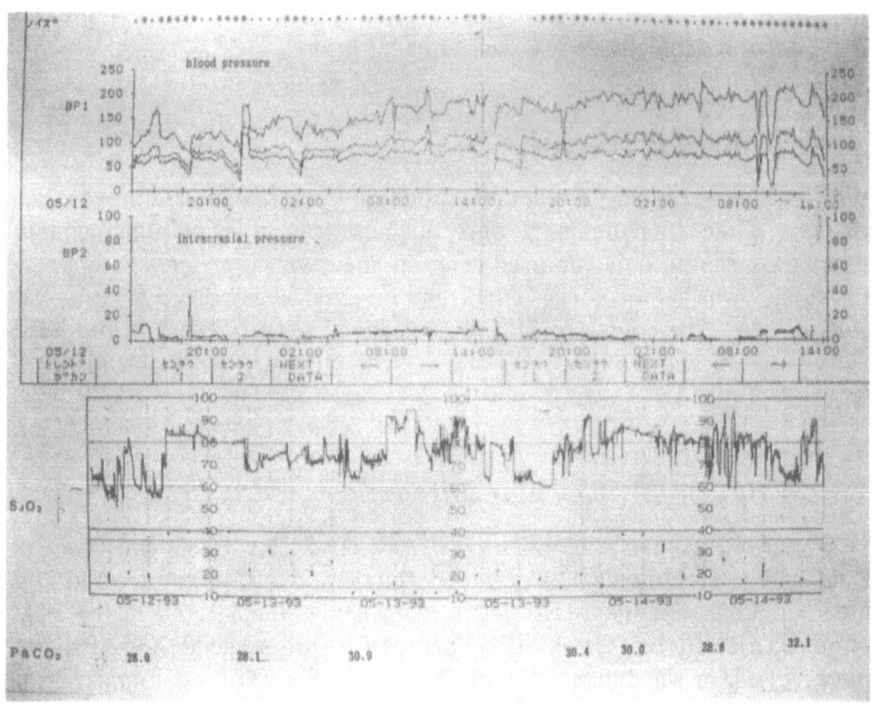

FIG. 2. Laser Doppler recording of 64-year-old woman diagnosed with intracerebral hemorrhage caused by rupture of moya-moya vessels. The patient was treated without any sign of cerebral ischemia, which may be demonstrated by a decrease in SjO_2

cerebral aneurysm was bleeding again and that cerebral blood flow had stopped. As mentioned previously, SjO_2 became greater than 90% in a case of brain death because of the contamination of the external jugular vein.

Discussion

It is well known that jugular bulb saturation demonstrates the ratio of cerebral blood flow and cerebral oxygen metabolism [1]. Thus, many measurements of jugular bulb saturation were carried out to determine cerebral blood flow and cerebral oxygen metabolism [2,3]. SjO_2 is the ratio of cerebral blood flow and cerebral oxygen metabolism. If the level of SjO_2 was recorded within 60%–80%, the balance of cerebral blood flow and cerebral oxygen metabolism were maintained. If SjO_2 was recorded at less than 50%, however, we must consider that the oxygen supply was at a low level compared with the oxygen demand. If SjO_2 was maintained at more than 90%, oxygen supply was too high compared with the oxygen demand

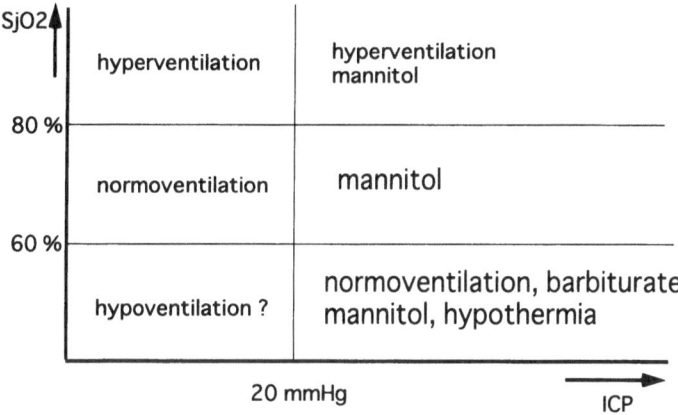

FIG. 3. Protocol for treatment of patients suffering from severe head injuries or cerebrovascular injuries. *ICP*, intracranial pressure

or the external jugular vein might be contaminated. When the oxygen saturation of the external jugular vein is greater than 90%, cases are diagnosed to be brain dead. Indeed, all the patients of group IV were diagnosed as brain death.

For patients suffering from severe head injury and cerebrovascular disease, treatment that takes into consideration intracranial pressure, cerebral blood flow, and cerebral oxygen metabolism is very important and may improve the outcome of these patients. Fig. 3 shows our protocol for the treatment of these patients. For example, if patients have intracranial pressure greater than 20 mmHg and SjO$_2$ less than 60%, we must choose a treatment to improve the cerebral ischemia and increased intracranial pressure, such as normoventilation therapy, mannitol administration, and hypothermia.

Our series suggests that the measurement of SjO$_2$ is useful in the treatment of these patients. We must always remember, however, that SjO$_2$ is influenced by many parameters and has some disadvantages.

1. SjO$_2$ is influenced by the contents of hemoglobin and saturation of arterial blood.
2. SjO$_2$ is not absolute data; it is only the ratio of cerebral blood flow and cerebral oxygen metabolism.
3. In some cases, it is difficult to puncture and insert the opticathether into the internal jugular vein.
4. The level or SjO$_2$ is changed by the position of the patient's head.
5. The SjO$_2$ data may reflect only one hemisphere.

Considering these facts and disadvantages, measurement of SjO$_2$ was very useful in treating and evaluating cases of severe head injury and cerebrovascular disease in neurosurgical intensive care units (ICU).

References

1. Robertson CS, Narayan RK, Gokaslan ZL, Pahwa R, Grossman RG, Allen E (1989) Cerebral arteriovenous oxygen difference as an estimate of cerebral blood flow in comatose patients. J Neurosurg 70:222–230
2. Robertson CS, Contant CF, Gokaslan ZL, Narayan RG, Grossman RG (1992) Cerebral blood flow, arterovenous oxygen difference, and outcome in head injuried patients J Neurol Neurosurg Psychiatry 55:594–603
3. Sheinberg MS, Kanter MJ, Robertson CS (1992) Continuous monitoring of jugular venous oxygen saturation in head-injured patients. J Neurosurg 76:212–217

The Optimal Cerebral Perfusion Pressure for Management of Patients with Severe Brain Injury

K. H. CHAN AND S. C. P. NG

Introduction

The principal goal of management of patients with severe brain injury is to provide an adequate supply of oxygen as well as other important metabolites to the brain. Cerebral ischemia develops when oxygen delivery is impaired. Important causes of brain ischemia include raised intracranial pressure (ICP), decreased cerebral perfusion pressure (CPP), hypotension, and hypoxia.

In the past, reduction of an elevated ICP was the main aim of treatment of cerebral ischemia complicating traumatic brain injury. Recent study, using transcranial doppler monitoring of middle cerebral artery (MCA) blood flow velocity and jugular venous bulb oxygen saturation (SjO_2) measurement for monitoring global oxygen supply and demand ratio, has shown that during ICP reduction therapy, CPP is the most important parameter to monitor [1]. Improvement or maintenance of an adequate CPP was associated with increase in oxygen delivery up to a certain CPP threshold above which further increase in CPP did not improve oxygen delivery. This finding suggests that a critical CPP limit exists for the management of patients with severe brain injury. CPP should be maintained at or above 70 mmHg after severe brain injury [2]. This CPP threshold, however, may vary from time to time in each patient and differ in each individual case. A CPP higher than 70 mmHg may be required in certain situations, for instance, after development of posttraumatic vasospasm [3].

In theory, an increase of CPP is associated with an elevation of oxygen delivery as monitored by SjO_2 measurement if the baseline CPP is below the critical threshold. Above this limit, further increase in CPP would not increase SjO_2. Monitoring the SjO_2 response to stepwise elevation of blood pressure to increase CPP may be used to define this critical CPP limit in each individual patient. The aim of this study was to define the role of

Division of Neurosurgery, Department of Surgery, The University of Hong Kong, Queen Mary Hospital, Pokfulam Road, Hong Kong induced hypertension in the management of patients with severe brain injury.

Patients and Methods

Eight patients with severe closed brain injury, defined as admission postre-suscitation Glasgow Coma Score (GCS) of less than or equal to 8 points with no eye-opening, were studied. There were seven males and one female, with a mean age of 31.6 years (range, 11–68 years). All patients had computerized tomography (CT) scanning on admission, and they were taken to the operating room for treatment of intracranial pathology and placement of an intraventricular catheter for postoperative ICP monitoring.

After surgery, all patients were managed by a standard protocol that included artificial ventilation with muscle paralysis and sedation with continuous infusion of pancuronium and midazolam. The following parameters were monitored continuously:

1. Arterial blood pressure (BP), by an arterial line
2. ICP, by an intraventricular catheter
3. CPP (defined as mean BP minus mean ICP)
4. Arterial oxygen saturation (SaO_2) by pulse oximeter
5. End-tidal carbon dioxide concentration ($EtCO_2$), by capnograph
6. Core body temperature, by a rectal probe
7. MCA flow velocity, by transcranial doppler
8. SjO_2, by the Oximetrix 3 (Abbott Laboratories, North Chicago, USA) system

The SjO_2 was monitored by percutaneous insertion of a Shaw (Abbott Laboratories, North Chicago, USA) 40-cm optical catheter into the jugular venous bulb on the side of predominant venous drainage. The latter was determined by the effects of unilateral compression of each internal jugular vein on the ICP. The side producing the largest rise in ICP represented the side of predominant venous drainage [4]. The tip of the catheter was positioned at the level of the first cervical vertebra. The position of the catheter was always confirmed radiographically. The system was calibrated every 12 h and before each hypertensive study by withdrawing blood slowly from the optical catheter and validation against an in vitro co-oximeter. The catheter was continuously flushed with heparinized saline to prevent blockage. The arteriojugular venous oxygen content difference ($AVDO_2$) was calculated by multiplying the difference between SaO_2 and SjO_2 by the daily hemoglobin concentration, plus 1.39, divided by 100. Global cerebral hyperemia and ischemia were defined as $AVDO_2$ of less than 4 and greater than 9 ml/dl, respectively [5].

Data from the monitors were collected by a bedside microcomputer that sampled data at 1-min intervals. The sampling time could be decreased to 6 s during the study period.

Protocol for Induced Hypertension and Data Collection

After baseline recording of the continuously monitored parameters, the patient's cerebral vascular reactivity to changes in arterial carbon dioxide concentration, as measured by alterations in MCA flow velocity and ICP, was tested by adjusting the dead space [6]. After the CO_2 reactivity test, when the physiological parameters had returned to baseline level, BP was slowly increased by intravenous infusion of phenylephrine (20 mg in 20 ml normal saline). The maximum BP increase was not greater than 30% of the baseline value. Arterial blood gas was determined at the beginning and end of each study. The changes seen in BP, ICP, SjO_2, and MCA flow velocity were recorded by a chart recorder, and data were collected at 6-s intervals by the computer. Measurements of mean BP, ICP, CPP, and SjO_2 were taken at the points of maximum decrease of CPP before phenylephrine and the subsequent maximum increase of CPP after phenylephrine. A change in any monitoring parameter is defined as the greatest postphenylephrine alteration from the last stable prephenylephrine recording observed within a period of 30 min. The phenylephrine test was repeated at least daily for the first 4 days after injury. Statistical analysis was by linear regression, Wilcoxon's rank sum, and t tests.

Results

Twenty-one phenylephrine tests were performed in eight patients. Each patient had at least two tests. There were no significant changes between the values of pH, PaO_2, $PaCO_2$, SaO_2, $EtCO_2$, and temperature before and after phenylephrine. Carbon dioxide reactivity was retained in all but two studies before phenylephrine was administered.

In general, an increase in BP was accompanied by an elevation of CPP and SjO_2 and a reduction in ICP (Table 1). Linear correlation was noted between mean BP ($r = .71$, $P < .0001$) and CPP ($r = .67$, $P < .0001$) and SjO_2. No correlation was observed between ICP and SjO_2 ($r = .17$, $P = $ not significant, NS). An alternative analysis of the CPP/SjO_2 curve showed a

TABLE 1. Changes before and after phenylephrine

	Before	After	Difference	P
Blood pressure (mmHg)	88.74 ± 13.47	123.32 ± 22.82	34.58 ± 12.90	P < .0001
Intracranial pressure (mmHg)	26.26 ± 9.76	19.32 ± 5.95	−6.95 ± 6.65	P = .004
Cerebral perfusion pressure (mmHg)	62.47 ± 16.33	103.89 ± 25.06	41.42 ± 16.43	P < .001
Jugular venous oxygen saturation (%)	64.58 ± 6.81	69.11 ± 7.07	4.53 ± 5.59	P < .01

Mean ± SD.

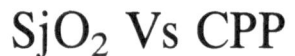

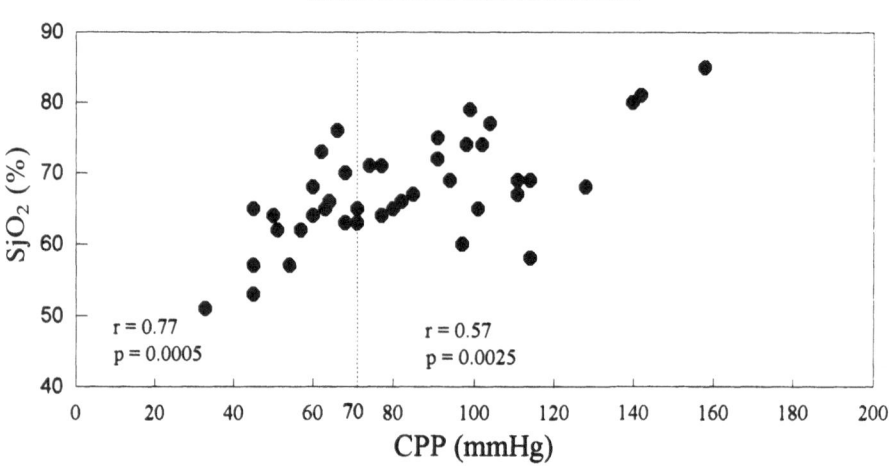

FIG. 1. Cerebral perfusion pressure (*CPP*) versus jugular venous oxygen saturation (*SjO₂*) showing the CPP breakpoint

biphasic relationship with an apparent breakpoint (Fig. 1). Linear regression analysis was applied to different segments of the curve until the most significant correlation coefficient was obtained. Breakpoint was noted at a CPP level of 70 mmHg. As CPP decreased below 70 mmHg, there was a strong correlation between CPP and SjO_2 ($r = .77$, $P = .0005$). Above a CPP level of 70 mmHg, CPP correlated less well with SjO_2 ($r = .57$, $P = .0025$).

Changes of SjO_2 and ICP

Further analysis of the results of induced hypertension showed four patterns of responses in terms of changes in ICP and SjO_2. The first pattern showed an increase in CPP from a low baseline level (mean, 54 mmHg); this was accompanied by a reduction in ICP from a high baseline of more than 20 mmHg (mean, 39 mmHg) and an elevation of SjO_2. As CPP reached the critical level of 70 mmHg, further increase in CPP was not accompanied by a rise of SjO_2, despite further reduction in ICP. In the second type of response, increase of CPP from a baseline value of 60–80 mmHg (mean, 68 mmHg) was associated with an unchanged SjO_2, but a fall of ICP from a high level of greater than 20 mmHg (mean, 35 mmHg). The third pattern showed a fairly constant ICP below 20 mmHg (mean, 18 mmHg) despite an increase in CPP and SjO_2. The latter pattern was observed in studies with loss of carbon dioxide reactivity; increase of BP was accompanied by an elevation of ICP with a resultant unchanged CPP. The SjO_2 change closely followed that of CPP.

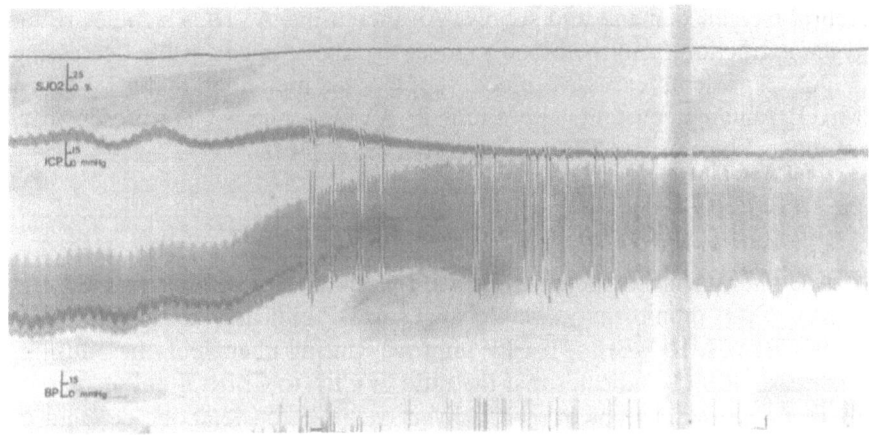

FIG. 2. Polygraphic display of SjO_2, intracranial pressure (*ICP*), and blood pressure (*BP*) changes when ICP rose above 50 mmHg and after induced hypertension

A plateau wave developed on two occasions with ICP rising above 50 mmHg. Induced hypertension resulted in abolition of the ICP wave, and the subsequent ICP was well controlled below 25 mmHg by maintaining the BP with dopamine (Fig. 2).

Discussion

Concepts of Cerebral Autoregulation

The physiological goal of autoregulation is to maintain an adequate cerebral blood flow (CBF) to meet tissue metabolic needs. Oxygen delivery at the tissue level has been shown experimentally to be a strong stimulus to the process of autoregulation [7,8]. Cerebral resistance vessels are sensitive to both changes in CPP and tissue metabolic demands [9]. A clinical definition of autoregulation should incorporate metabolic as well as CPP changes. The lower limit of cerebral autoregulation should be defined as the CPP threshold below which adequate CBF to meet tissue oxygen demands cannot be maintained. In theory, if autoregulation of CBF is preserved, elevation of a reduced CPP will improve CBF until a threshold level of CPP is reached. Further increases in CPP above this threshold will not further augment global CBF. This CPP threshold, therefore, represents the lower limit of autoregulation above which CPP should be maintained during head injury management. The CPP threshold identified in the present study is in accord with the CPP level identified in a previous observational study [2].

The introduction of continuous SjO_2 monitoring allows a real-time assessment of oxygen delivery to the brain. By Fick's principle, $AVDO_2$ represents the ratio between global cerebral metabolic rate of oxygen ($CMRO_2$) and

CBF. A normal $AVDO_2$ value indicates an adequate global balance between cerebral oxygen demand and supply. An increasing $AVDO_2$ signifies rising oxygen extraction from the blood to meet metabolic needs, while decreasing $AVDO_2$ represents excessive blood supply over metabolic demand. When $CMRO_2$ remains constant, alterations in $AVDO_2$ and SjO_2 represent corresponding changes in CBF and oxygen delivery [10].

Relationship between SjO_2 and Changes in BP

Because phenylephrine increases BP with minimal or no effects on CBF and $CMRO_2$, SjO_2 monitoring during changes in BP indicates the overall effect on the $CBF:CMRO_2$ ratio. If CPP improves during phenylephrine infusion, an increase of SjO_2 indicates that the ratio of CBF to $CMRO_2$ has increased, with a global increase of oxygen delivery relative to metabolic demand of the brain. When CPP has surpassed the lower limit of autoregulation, a further increase in CPP would not increase SjO_2. An increase in CPP during induced hypertension without a rise of SjO_2 suggests that the initial CPP is already above the lower threshold of autoregulation and that CBF and oxygen delivery have not changed. When autoregulation is grossly impaired, as in situations of loss of carbon dioxide reactivity, the SjO_2 change will parallel that of CPP, indicating a pressure passive state [11].

ICP Changes During Alterations of BP

If autoregulation is preserved and CBF remains constant, changes in BP can only be offset by alterations in vessel diameter with corresponding changes in cerebral blood volume (CBV) and ICP [12]. An increase of CPP from below the lower limit of autoregulation would lead to compensatory vasoconstriction and fall of ICP. This vasoconstrictive response continues above the lower threshold of autoregulation, resulting in further reduction of ICP. This ICP change to increased BP is more brisk when brain compliance is low, like a high baseline ICP. The change in CBV in these cases will lead to large change in ICP. In situations in which the brain compliance is not critically low, alterations in CBV will not result in large ICP changes. This would explain the lack of ICP reduction in response to phenylephrine when the baseline ICP was low.

Conclusion

The optimal CPP level for management of patients with severe brain injury can be defined, and it should be maintained above 70 mmHg. Induced hypertension may be useful in the treatment of raised ICP after brain injury.

References

1. Chan KH, Dearden NM, Miller JD, Andrews PJD, Midgley S (1993) Multi-modality monitoring as a guide to treatment of intracranial hypertension after severe brain injury. Neurosurgery 32:547–553
2. Chan KH, Miller JD, Dearden NM, Andrews PJD, Midgley S (1992) The effect of changes in cerebral perfusion pressure upon middle cerebral artery blood flow velocity and jugular bulb venous oxygen saturation after severe brain injury. J Neurosurg 77:55–61
3. Chan KH, Dearden NM, Miller JD (1992) The significance of posttraumatic increase in cerebral blood flow velocity: a transcranial doppler ultrasound study. Neurosurgery 30:697–700
4. Dearden NM (1991) Jugular bulb venous oxygen saturation in the management of severe head injury. Curr Opin Anaesth 4:279–730
5. Robertson CS, Narayan RK, Gokaslan ZL, Pahwa R, Grossman RG, Carman P, Allen E (1989) Cerebral arteriovenous oxygen difference as an estimate of cerebral blood flow in comatose patients. J Neurosurg 70:222–230
6. Marmarou A, Bandoh K, Yoshihara M, Tsuji O (1993) Measurement of vascular reactivity in head injured patients. Acta Neurochir (Suppl) 59:18–21
7. Kontos HA, Wei EP, Raper AJ, Rosenblum WI, Navari RM, Patterson JL (1978) Role of tissue hypoxia in local regulation of cerebral microcirculation. Am J Physiol 234:H582–591
8. Kontos HA, Wei EP (1985) Oxygen-dependent mechanisms in cerebral autoregulation. Ann Biomed Eng 13:329–334
9. Paulson OB, Strandgaard S, Edvinsson L (1990) Cerebral autoregulation. Cerebrovasc Brain Metab Rev 2:161–192
10. Gilbert J (1989) Estimation of cerebral blood flow by cerebral venous oxygen difference. J Neurosurg 71:790–791
11. Miller JD, Stanek AE, Langfitt TW (1973) Cerebral blood flow autoregulation during experimental brain compression. J Neurosurg 39:186–196
12. Muizelaar JP, Ward JD, Marmarou A, Newlon PG, Wachi A (1989) Cerebral blood flow and metabolism in severely head-injured children: Part 2. Autoregulation. J Neurosurg 71:72–76

Bilateral Jugular Bulb Oximetry

HIROSHI INAGAWA, YASUSEI OKADA, SOU SUZUKI, KAZUYUKI ONO,
AND KAZUHIKO MAEKAWA

Introduction

Jugular bulb oxygen saturation (SjO_2) monitoring has been proposed as a means of early detection of cerebral ischemia caused by intracranial hypertension. There remain, however, many unsolved problems as to the physiological basis for this monitoring, so that the obtained SjO_2 value sometimes is difficult to interpret. One may ask, for instance, which side of the internal jugular vein is to be cannulated or whether the SjO_2 values obtained from one side really represent whole-brain oxygenation or at least that of the ipsilateral hemisphere. To answer this question, a considerable amount of knowledge about cerebral blood flow distribution and metabolism and their response to various insults must be obtained. Several studies have investigated bilateral jugular bulb oxygenation. The problem of side-to-side discrepancies is still controversial. Our study was planned to observe bilateral SjO_2 in various clinical settings to see whether such discrepancies, if such ever existed, would change our perspective on cerebral oxygenation monitoring.

Patient Population

Between August 1993 and March 1994, 19 comatose patients (17 men and 2 women, average age 48.6 ± 16.0 years) who had been admitted to the University of Tokyo Hospital received bilateral monitoring of SjO_2. These patients included 8 cases of closed head injury, 3 cases of subarachnoid hemorrhage, 5 cases of hypertensive intracerebral hemorrhage, and 3 cases of postresuscitation encephalopathy.

All patients were managed according to our protocol, which aimed at preventing intracranial hypertension and maintaining adequate cerebral per-

Department of Traumatology and Critical Care, Faculty of Medicine, University of Tokyo, 3-1, Hongo 7-chome, Bunkyo-ku, Tokyo 113, Japan

fusion pressure. This protocol included intubation and ventilatory support, intracranial pressure monitoring, administration of osmotic diuretics, and in selected cases of head injury, barbiturate therapy or mild hypothermia. After initial evaluation and clinical procedures had been completed, bilateral jugular venous cannulation was performed by means of Seldinger's maneuver. A fiberoptic catheter (4 Fr or 5.5 Fr) was placed on the side of the most severe injury and a 16-gauge central venous catheter on the other. Placement of the tips of the catheters was verified by X-rays.

As is often noted, the most desirable position of the catheter tip for continuous monitoring is not simply a matter of radiographically (or anatomically) "good" position. To prevent the tip from being contaminated by blood drained from the extracranial origin, catheters should be advanced as far upstream as possible. However, this tends to make the monitoring subject to wall artifact and to result in low signal quality of SjO_2 values. Thus, we chose to draw blood simultaneously from both jugular bulbs and radial artery to measure oxygen saturation using the co-oximeter when the SjO_2 value on the monitor appeared to show significant changes. The rate of drawing blood was intended to be slow enough to avoid extracerebral contamination. Blood gases and blood glucose levels were then determined.

Results

A total of 195 pairs of samples were obtained. The data are summarized in Tables 1–5. Overall mean difference in SjO_2 between the right and the left side was 9.75 ± 11.4 (mean ± SD). Side-to-side difference was calculated by subtracting the smaller number of the two from the larger one. Thus, the difference between mean right SjO_2 and mean left SjO_2 does not necessarily equal mean side-to-side difference. Nine cases of 19 (47%) had a difference of more than 10% in mean SjO_2. The average of the sum of the right minus left SjO_2 was −9.14. Seven patients had a higher mean SjO_2 on the right and 12 patients were higher on the left. Four patients had a space-occupying lesion (SOL) with mass effect on the right and had higher SjO_2 on the left. One patient had an SOL with mass effect on the left and had higher SjO_2

TABLE 1. Side-to-side difference in SjO_2[a]

Range of difference	Mean difference (number of cases)	Maximum difference (number of cases)
>15%	7	12
10%–15%	2	4
5%–10%	5	2
<5%	5	1

[a] Results of 195 paired samples, 10.3 paired samples/patient. Mean difference between jugular bulb oxygen saturation (SjO_2) values, 9.75%.

TABLE 2. Summary of SjO_2 data in head-injured patients[a]

Patient no.	Age/sex	CT findings	GCS on admission	Mean R-SjO$_2$	Mean L-SjO$_2$	Mean difference	Maximum difference	Episode of desaturation
1	20/M	R-SDH contusion	5	65.8	79.9	14.1	39.9	4 (R) <24 h
2	60/M	Skull base fracture, contusion	5	58.2	70.5	12.1	21.5	2 (Bil) <24 h
3	21/M	R-EDH L-SDH	6	60.8	65.2	4.4	13.2	1 (Bil) <48 h
4	59/M	DAI	5	65.1	76.0	15.1	38.9	0
5	34/M	R-SDH L-EDH	9	65.5	62.9	4.1	6.4	0
6	23/M	L-contusion	9	59.5	62.5	3.0	4.6	2 (Bil) <24 h
7	39/M	L-EDH	5	79.6	87.5	8.3	34.5	0
8	67/M	DAI	11	48.5	55.1	6.6	20.7	6 (R,Bil) <180 h

CT, computed tomography; GCS, Glasgow Coma Score; R, right; L, left; Bil, bilateral; SDH, subdural hematoma; EDH, epidural hematoma; DAI, diffuse axonal injury (diagnosis of DAI not based on CT alone).

[a] Desaturation is defined as a drop of SjO_2 below 50%. Removal of hematoma was conducted in patients 3, 5, and 7, surgical decompression in patients 5 and 7, barbiturate therapy in patients 1, 2, and 5, and mild hypothermia in patients 2, 5, and 7.

TABLE 3. Summary of SjO$_2$ data in patients with hypertensive intracerebral hematoma (ICH)

Patient no.	Age/sex	Site	GCS on admission	Surgical decompression	Mean R-SjO$_2$	Mean L-SjO$_2$	Mean difference	Maximum difference	Episode of desaturation
1	47/M	R-putamen	6	(+)	56.9	54.9	5.6	13.2	4 (R2B2)
2	59/M	R-thalamus	8	(−)	56.9	60.8	5.2	45.6	6 (R2L1B3)
3	56/F	R-putamen	4	(−)	68.6	78.4	18.2	64.1	1 (R)
4	47/M	L-putamen	9	(+)	51.1	66.4	15.3	21.3	3 (R)
5	73/M	L-putamen	4	(−)	73.1	59.9	18.1	47.0	2 (L)

Patient no. 1 developed large left low-density area because of spasm following the episode of desaturation. Right SjO$_2$ also dropped, but was above 50%.
Patient no. 3 died before operation was conducted.

TABLE 4. Summary of SjO$_2$ data in patients with subarachnoid hemorrhage (SAH)

Patient no.	Age/sex	Aneurysm	ICH	GCS on admission	Mean R-SjO$_2$	Mean L-SjO$_2$	Mean difference	Maximum difference	Episode of desaturation
1	54/M	R-IC-PC ruptured	(−)	6	68.5	66.3	5.3	10.6	1 (L) 260 h
2	59/F	A-com ruptured	(−)	10	61.6	60.4	3.8	7.3	0
3	44/M	Not investigated	R-frontal	4	59.3	45.3	26.4	54.9	7 (R2L3B1) <36 h

R-IC-PC, right internal carotid-posterior communicating; A-com, Anterior communicating.

TABLE 5. Summary of SjO_2 data in patients with postresuscitation encephalopathy

Patient no.	Age/sex	Cause of arrest	Intracranial SOL	Out-come	Mean R-SjO_2	Mean L-SjO_2	Mean difference	Maximum difference
1	45/M	Hanging	(−)	PV	88.4	85.0	3.4	11.0
2	67/M	Suffocation	(−)	GR	43.5	69.1	25.6	49.8
3	?/M	Unknown	(−)	D	43.3	69.7	26.4	37.8

PV, persistent vegetative state; GR, good recovery; D, death.

on the left. Three patients had an intracerebral hematoma (ICH) without surgical decompression; all of these had lower SjO_2 on the side of the ICH. Three patients with a left SOL had surgical decompression and had higher SjO_2 on the side of the decompression. Three postresuscitation patients had no SOL, but two had higher SjO_2 on the left.

Discussion

Our results demonstrate an average of 9.8% difference in SjO_2 values between the right and the left hemisphere. This value is greater than that of reported previously by Stocchetti et al. [1], who demonstrated that the source of discrepancies was upstream of the sigmoid sinus. He attributed those discrepancies to the incomplete mixing of the venous cerebral blood (at the level of superior and inferior sagittal sinuses and straight sinus). If this is the case, it is supposed that blood drained from either hemisphere flows mostly into the ipsilateral sigmoid sinus. This would support the idea that SjO_2 on one side is more representative of ipsilateral hemispheric oxygenation than of whole-brain oxygenation.

From the anatomical standpoint, sigmoid sinus blood flow is considered to have two major origins, namely the dural sinus and the superficial cerebral vein, such as the vein of Labbe. The latter drains directly into the ipsilateral sigmoid sinus. Therefore, increased contribution of this vein caused by redistribution of intracerebral venous flow in the presence of an SOL may partly account for the discrepancies in SjO_2. Thus, we can hypothesize that when there is increased difference in SjO_2, each SjO_2 will represent ipsilateral hemispheric oxygenation. This speculation, of course, remains to be proved.

Another possibility is that susceptibility to ischemia is different between hemispheres from the beginning. Posthypoglycemic right hemiplegia has been documented [2]. We also observed a case of postresuscitation right hemiparesis following ventricular fibrillation caused by acute myocardial infarction. These facts may suggest that the motor cortex of the left hemisphere may be more vulnerable to ischemic insults than the right. Two cases of postresuscitation encephalopathy showed a left-side-dominant SjO_2 pattern, although laterality was less expected in this type of global ischemia.

Technical errors such as inappropriate positioning of the catheter tip and rapid withdrawal of blood are also possible. But if this were the case with all the discrepancies we showed, the accuracy of the data obtained through the conventional method of placing tips, which most investigators used, would also be anything but satisfactory. We believe that this kind of error contributed little, if any, to our results.

The important problem is that the great difference in SjO_2 may confuse clinical judgment. Figure 1 shows the course of bilateral SjO_2 in a patient with right acute subdural hematoma (SDH). Within 48 h after injury, right SjO_2 was below 50% without any drop in SaO_2, which suggested desaturation [3], while left SjO_2 stayed about 80%, which was disproportionately high relative to $PaCO_2$, intracranial pressure (ICP), and the radiographical finding (brain swelling). This outstanding discrepancy began to diminish, however, with the initiation of barbiturate therapy against intracranial hypertension refractory to osmotic diuretics. If the left SjO_2 values were free from extracerebral contamination, what did this discrepancy mean?

Assuming that each side of SjO_2 is representative of ipsilateral hemispheric oxygenation, these data can be interpreted as ischemia on the side of SDH and hyperemia (or at least the state of abundant flow) on the other side. From the standpoint of respiratory quotient (RQ) as shown in Fig. 2, the initial RQs on both sides nearly equal 1.0, indicating that glucose is the substrate of metabolism in both hemispheres. This is compatible with the nature of blood drained from the brain. If one looks at the oxygen–glucose index (OGI) as an indicator of aerobic metabolism of glucose as shown in Fig. 3, however, OGI on the left side shows a consistently lower value compared with the right, the more ischemic side. Judging solely from the standpoint of aerobic utilization of glucose, these results are quite contrary to what we would expect.

So far we are not able to give a satisfactory explanation for these results. Errors may lie in the assumption or in the choice of parameters, but

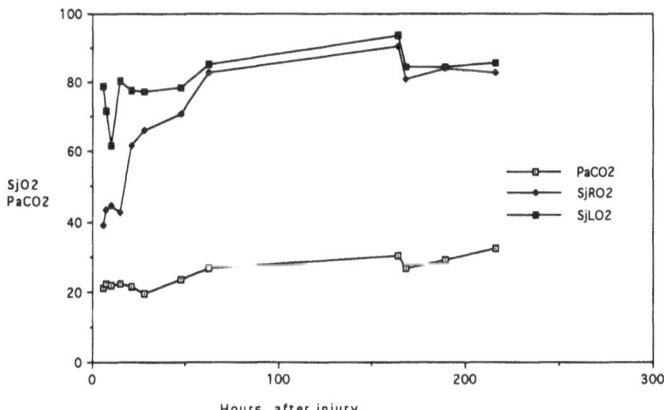

FIG. 1. Time course of bilateral jugular bulb oxygen saturation and arterial carbon dioxide tension. With the initiation of pentobarbital, the left SjO_2 began to rise without significant change in $PaCO_2$

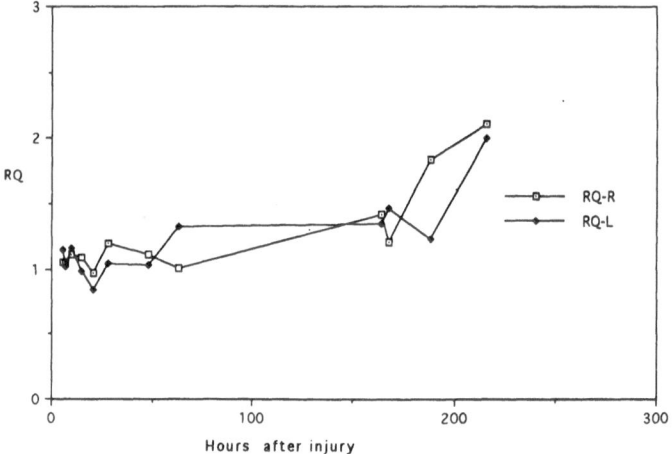

FIG. 2. Time course of bilateral respiratory quotient (*RQ*) calculated from O_2 content and total CO_2 data obtained from radial artery and both jugular bulb blood samples. *L*, left; *R*, right

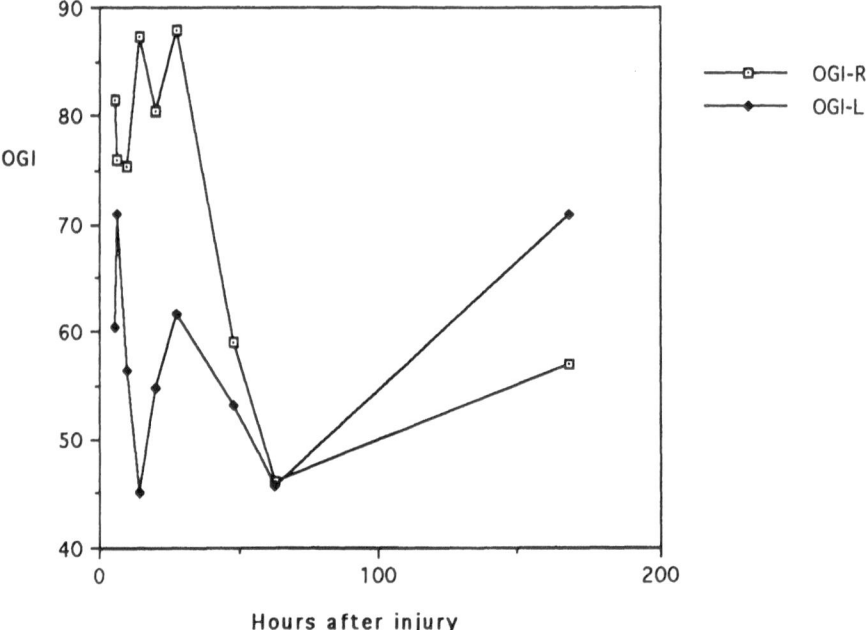

FIG. 3. Time course of bilateral oxygen-glucose index (OGI).

$$OGI = \frac{\text{arteriojugular oxygen difference (mmol/dl)}}{6 \times \text{arteriojugular glucose difference (mmol/dl)}} \times 100$$

In normal subject, OGI equals 100%. Decline in OGI indicates anaerobic glycolysis

obviously it is difficult to know more about what is happening in the brain so long as we stick to a single parameter of SjO_2. For this monitor to be valid, some other parameters must be observed in combination with SjO_2.

In answering the question about the choice of the side to be monitored, there are two different views according to the goal of monitoring. If SjO_2 differs from side to side and jugular venous flow is also different, SjO_2 on the side of greater flow is more representative of "global" oxygenation. Therefore, when the goal is to evaluate global oxygenation, Dearden's approach [4] may be appropriate. If the goal is to detect ischemia, the approach of placing the catheter on the side of most severe injury is thought to be acceptable, because SjO_2 tends to be lower on the side of radiologically detectable lesions than on the other side.

Because the fact that SjO_2 sometimes differs from side to side seems to make the interpretation all the more complicated, it does not follow that this monitoring is of limited validity. Indeed, the presence or absence of the side-to-side difference might reflect some underlying mechanisms that would give us a new insight into the black box of the brain. Future investigations should therefore focus not merely on finding out how much SjO_2 is adequate or how much is too much, but also on determining how SjO_2 in conjunction with other modalities can serve to detect changes in cerebral metabolic status.

References

1. Stocchetti N, Paparella A, Bridelli F, Bacchi M, Piazza P, Zuccoli P (1994) Cerebral venous oxygen saturation studied with bilateral samples in the internal jugular veins. Neurosurgery 34(1):38–44
2. Takamatsu K, Takizawa, T, Miyamoto T, Taguchi A, Hoshino H (1994) A case of hypoglycemic hemiplegia. Shinkeinaika 40:81–84
3. Sheinberg M, Kanter MJ, Robertson CS, Contant CF, Narayan RK, Grossman RG (1992) Continuous monitoring of jugular venous oxygen saturation in head-injured patients. J Neurosurg 76:212–217
4. Dearden NM (1991) Jugular bulb venous oxygen saturation in the management of severe head injury. Curr Opin Anesthesiol 4:279–286

Causes and Treatment of Desaturation in SjO_2 Monitoring

MOTOAKI NAKABAYASHI, HIROYUKI YOKOTA, AKIRA FUSE,
HIDETAKA SATO, SHIGEKI KUSHIMOTO, KAZUYOSHI KATO,
AKIRA KUROKAWA, HIROSHI HENMI, AND TOSHIFUMI OTSUKA

Introduction

To minimize secondary brain damage, which greatly influences prognosis during brain damage, it is necessary to avoid the state of ischemia as much as possible because ischemia is an important factor in secondary brain damage. On the other hand, because ischemia has various causes, gaining an understanding of its pathology and deciding on a course of treatment is certainly not easy. In an attempt to resolve this problem, continuous monitoring of jugular bulb venous oxygen saturation (SjO_2) has recently attracted considerable attention. SjO_2 reflects the status of total brain oxygen metabolism because its value is determined by the ratio between cerebral blood flow and brain oxygen metabolism.

It is also possible to assess whether ischemia is occurring by monitoring SjO_2 at the time of brain damage. According to the results of past treatment performed at this institution using SjO_2 for severe head injuries and cerebrovascular disorders, there were a significant number of cases in which SjO_2 demonstrated low values. This chapter therefore describes a discussion of whether the desaturation in SjO_2 is occurring in various situations together with representative symptoms selected from our clinical experience.

Desaturation

The definition of desaturation, which was confirmed by Robertson, is as follows: when the display value on an Oximetrix 3 screen at bedside falls below 50%, and at the same time, actual measured oxygen saturation, as determined by drawing blood from a catheter and measuring with a hemo-oxymeter, is confirmed to fall below 50%, we refer to the resulting condition as desaturation when these parameters have been confirmed.

The following paragraphs describe representative cases presenting desaturation that we have observed at our institution.

Department of Emergency and Critical Care Medicine, Nihon Medical School

Case 1

This patient was diagnosed as having acute subdural hematoma and cerebral contusion. Craniotomy was performed immediately. Monitoring of SjO_2 was started immediately before surgery. As shown in Fig. 1, the initially measured SjO_2 value was 40%, indicating desaturation. Although SjO_2 temporarily increased following rapid administration of mannitol, it had again fallen to the 30% level at the start of surgery.

The value of SjO_2 rose to more than 50% when the hematoma was removed just after opening the dura mater, and ischemia was thought to have improved. However, acute brain swelling was observed simultaneously with opening of the dura mater. SjO_2 values again fell below 40% at the time of closure of the scalp. The patient was evaluated as having suffered postsurgical brain death, and eventually died.

Case 2

In this case of pontine hemorrhage, $PaCO_2$ exhibited an extreme decrease because of excessive hyperventilation therapy, and SjO_2 temporarily fell below 50%. As a result of resetting the respirator mode, SjO_2 normalized at

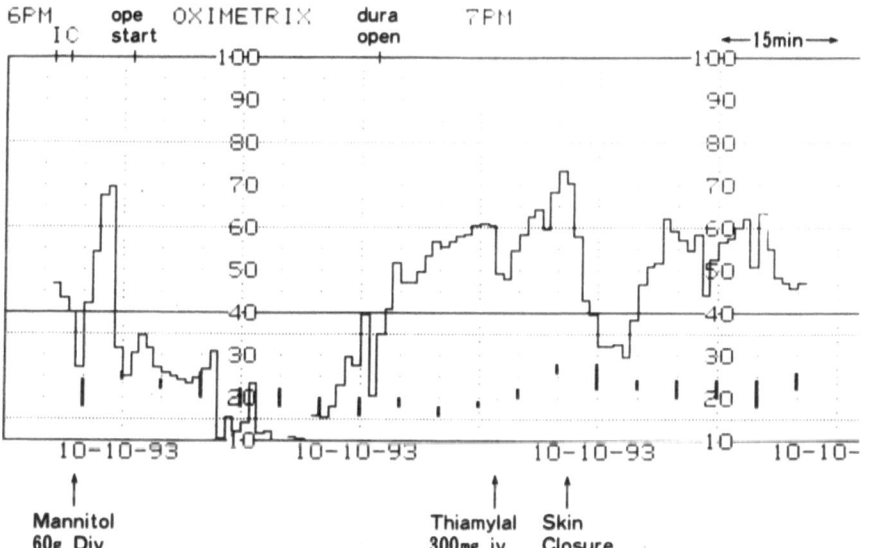

FIG. 1. Intraoperative changes in SjO_2 due to anti-intracranial hypertensive management. SjO_2 rises after i.v. injection of mannitol, dural opening, and i.v. bolus injection of thiamyral. These changes indicate some treatments against intracranial hypertension raise SjO_2 and improve intracranial ischemia

the level of 60%. This was considered to have been a case of desaturation from cerebral ischemia caused by hypocapnemia (Fig. 2).

Case 3

This case was diagnosed as cerebral contusions. The initial level for intracranial pressure (ICP) was 20 mmHg and SjO_2 was 32%. The setting of the respirator was changed to improve the ischemia in consideraton of the SjO_2 values, and hyperventilation therapy was discontinued. As a result, ICP increased remarkably, to 48 mmHg. When hyperventilation therapy was implemented to lower ICP, SjO_2 again decreased. Ultimately, the patient was controlled at ICP of 21 mmHg and SjO_2 of 41%. This case illustrates an example of the difficulties encountered when determining whether SjO_2 values or ICP values should be given priority (Fig. 3).

Case 4

This case was diagnosed as brain contusion complicated with multiple trauma such as fractured pelvis, bilateral and multiple fractured ribs, hemopneumothorax, and fractured femur. The patient exhibited hemorrhagic shock at the time of arrival, and blood pressure continuously remained below 100 mmHg. Hemoglobin concentration was also decreased. Although increased ICP was not observed, an ischemic state of the brain was determined to be present because of decreased blood pressure and decreased hemoglobin concentration. SjO_2 values changed in the same manner accompanying fluctuations in blood pressure at that time as shown

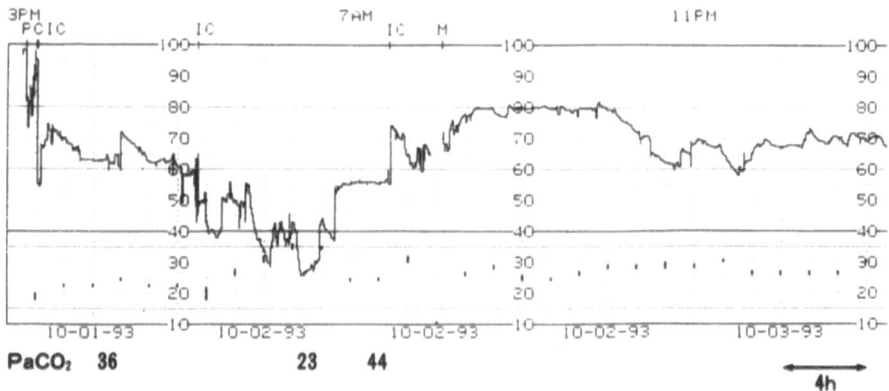

FIG. 2. Relation between SjO_2 and $PaCO_2$. In normocapnic state, SjO_2 is within normal range, but in hypocapnic state, SjO_2 indicates ischemic condition. Resetting of ventilator changes SjO_2 value from under 50% to over 50%

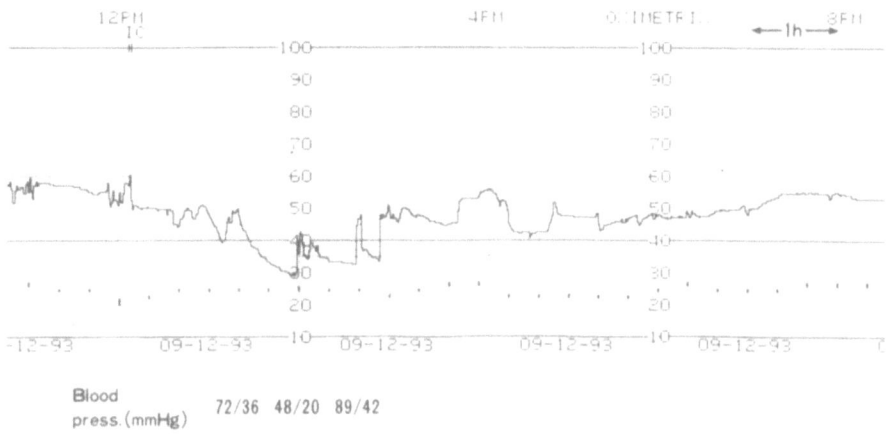

Blood
press.(mmHg)   72/36 48/20 89/42

FIG. 3. Relation between SjO$_2$ and blood pressure. In hypotensive state, SjO$_2$ is low and lower blood pressure causes SjO$_2$ value to deteriorate

in Fig. 4. This case supported the belief that hemoglobin concentration may be strongly involved in the cause of desaturation.

Discussion

Based on the theory behind this parameter, SjO$_2$ values are determined by various factors. However, desaturation encountered in the clinical setting can be theoretically perceived in the manner shown in Fig. 5. These causes are thought to be predictable to a certain extent from the underlying disorder and its pathology.

For example, in the case of head trauma accompanying multiple trauma, desaturation occurs caused by shock or anemia caused by hemorrhage. In patients having space occupational lesions, increased ICP causes a decrease in cerebral blood flow, thereby causing desaturation. On the other hand, artificial extreme hyperventilation can also result in desaturation as a result of lowering cerebral blood flow volume.

In the four cases described in this report, each of the causes of desaturation was inferred to be as described below;

Case 1: Intracranial Hypertension
Case 2: Decreased CBF due to Hypocapnea
Case 3: Combined Case 1 & 2
Case 4: Decreased oxygen transport due to hemorrhagic shock

In case 1, although ICP was not actually measured, it was interpreted that the increase in intracranial pressure during the course of surgery resulted in the ischemia. SjO$_2$ values improved from the ischemic state in response to mannitol, and ischemia was improved by opening of the dura. Thus, it can

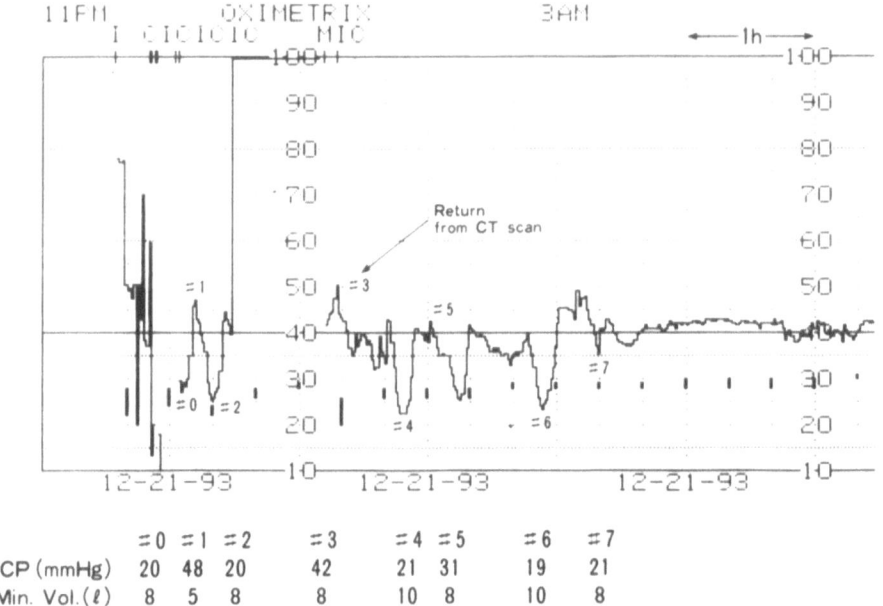

FIG. 4. Relation between minute volume of ventilator, SjO$_2$, and PaCO$_2$. Low minute volume causes intracranial hypertension, but does not indicate ischemic state in SjO$_2$ value. High minute volume causes release of intracranial hypertension, but indicates ischemic state in SjO$_2$ value

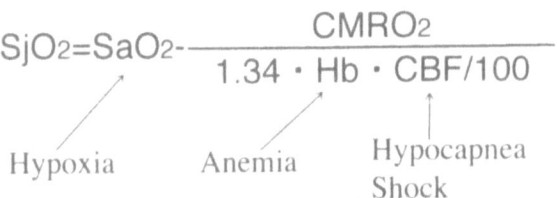

FIG. 5. Causes of desaturation. In the clinical setting, decreased SjO$_2$ is caused by hypoxia, anemia, hypotension, and intracranial hypertension. In these instances some factors are correctable in the intensive care unit, so that cerebral ischemia is avoidable in some cases

be seen that the intracranial environment changed on a real-time basis as a result of surgical manipulation.

In case 2, excessive hyperventilation brought about a decrease in cerebral blood flow. This was thought to then cause the desaturation.

In case 3, cerebral ischemia progressed when hyperventilation therapy was selected to lower ICP in brain swelling. In the treatment of cases that present with brain swelling, the subject of whether SjO$_2$ values or ICP should be given priority requires additional investigation of more cases.

Case 4 was that of a patient with multiple trauma who had suffered from hemorrhagic shock. In cases of trauma to the head accompanying multiple trauma, adequate evaluation and treatment may not be possible because priority must be placed on cardiopulmonary resuscitation. In such cases, it is important to gain as much information about the intracranial environment as possible. It is therefore thought that monitoring of SjO$_2$ values could be used in these cases in the future. Although the majority of such patients whom we have encountered have died of rapidly progressing shock, because there were also cases in which SjO$_2$ values decreased, the possibility was suggested that ischemia could be improved by relieving shock.

Many of the cases demonstrating desaturation that we encountered were caused by factors similar to those presented in this chapter, namely increased ICP, hyperventilation, and shock. However, it is thought that some of those cases could have been treated or problems prevented by specifying the cause of the desaturation. In other words, decreases in oxygen transport function such as anemia and lowered blood pressure, as well as decreases in cerebral blood flow caused by hyperventilation, can be avoided during the course of treatment.

The definition of desaturation at our institution is indicated in Fig. 6. We have encountered a significant number of cases in which previously stable values suddenly began to fluctuate. This was frequently encountered during changes in body position or endotracheal aspiration. When there are no significant changes in vital signs or neurological findings, it is considered to

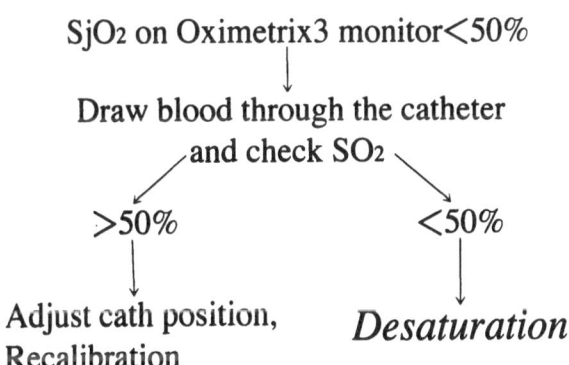

FIG. 6. Observation of desaturation. When SjO$_2$ decreases below 50% on the monitor, real blood oxygen saturation must be checked. Blood sampling through the catheter is carried out and blood saturation is checked by cooxymeter. If the cooxymeter shows the same values as the monitor, it is actual desaturation, but if the cooxymeter shows different values than the monitor, adjustment of the catheter tip or recalibration must be performed

be possible to evaluate whether fluctuations in values are true fluctuations or those resulting from shifts in the location of the catheter from the changes in SjO_2 values before and after the fluctuations. It is also necessary to move the neck while viewing light intensity or flush the catheter so that values coincide with immediately previous values. Naturally, blood samples should always be drawn for confirmation when the patient's condition has changed or in cases in which ischemia is suspected. It is additionally important to confirm those values with a hemooxymeter.

There are several problems as described below with respect to the desaturation described in this chapter. These problems include whether it is valid to define desaturation with a cutoff value of 50%, whether desaturation represents true ischemia locally or throughout the entire brain, whether the extent of that ischemia really has an effect on vital prognosis or functional prognosis, and whether improvement of ischemia while monitoring SjO_2 improves the patient's prognosis. We believe that it is necessary to further examine these questions following additional studies on a larger number of cases.

Problems about desaturation

1. Is it appropriate to define desaturation as less than 50%?
2. Dose desaturaton in SjO_2 monitoring mean real cerebral ischemia?
3. Dose desaturation make prognosis worse?

Conclusion

This chapter describes clinical cases of desaturation encountered at this institution that exhibited decreased SjO_2 values. The causes of that desaturation were estimated from each of the pathological states.

1. The major causes of desaturation consisted of increased intracranial pressure, hyperventilation, and hemorrhagic shock.
2. Desaturation caused by some of these causes is thought to be treatable or preventable.

Evaluation of Continuous Monitoring of Jugular Venous Oxygen Saturation, Regional Cerebral Oxygen Saturation, and Electroencephalography Power Spectrum for Intraoperative Cerebral Ischemia

Yoshihiro Ikuta[1], Tatsuhiko Kano[1], Eiji Abe[2], Mari Seshita[2], and Kanemitsu Higashi[1]

Introduction

Brain damage caused by ischemia during reconstructive surgery of the main cerebral arteries is a most serious complication. Because neurological signs and symptoms of ischemic lesions are masked under anesthesia, an alternative measure is required for monitoring cerebral function.

Electroencephalography (EEG) has been used as an intraoperative monitor to detect the early stages of ischemia in the cerebral hemisphere. Jugular bulb venous oxygen saturation (SjO_2), although invasive, is a reliable monitor of global cerebral oxygenation, reflecting the overall balance between cerebral oxygen supply and demad. Continuous monitoring of SjO_2 with fiberoptic catheters has been applied to patients with head injuries or to those undergoing cardiac or aortic arch surgery with cardiopulmonary bypass [1]. Recently, a noninvasive method of continuously monitoring regional cerebral oxygen saturation (rSO_2) by spectroscopy of reflected near infrared light has been reported [2].

In this study, we evaluated these three methods of continuous cerebral monitoring for the detection of intraoperative cerebral ischemia.

---

[1] Surgical Center, Kumamoto University Hospital, 1-1-1 Honjo, Kumamoto 860, Japan
[2] Department of Anesthesiology, Kumamoto University Hospital, 1-1-1 Honjo, Kumamoto 860, Japan

Subjects and Methods

After approval from the Institutional Ethics Committee on Human Research, 28 patients (16 men and 12 women) with a mean age of 57.6 ± 3.2 years (range 18–79 years) were studied. The subjects underwent bypass grafting for aortitis syndrome or giant cerebral aneurysm (4 patients), endoarterectomy for internal carotid or vertebral artery stenosis (3 patients), aortocoronary bypass graft or valve replacement (4 patients), and resection and grafting for thoracic aortic aneurysm (TAA) including the aortic arch (17 patients). Informed consent for intraoperative cerebral monitoring was obtained from all subjects. Seven patients in the former two groups received isoflurane/N_2O anesthesia supplemented with an ordinal dose of fentanyl (5–10 µg/kg), and the remaining 21 patients in the latter two groups received fentanyl (30–80 µg/kg) anesthesia supplemented with isoflurane. Replacement of TAA including the arch with an artificial vessel was planned under mild hypothermic femorofemoral venoarterial partial bypass (F-F bypass) or moderate hypothermic F-F total bypass. In addition to moderate hypothermia, selective cerebral perfusion (SCP) was conducted to ameliorate ischemic brain damage in critical cases (14/17 patients).

EEG and its power spectrum were observed with frontooccipital or frontoparietal bipolar leads on both sides by using a two-channel monitor (OEE-7120, Nihon Kohden, Tokyo, Japan) ($n = 21$). SjO_2 was continuously measured with an oximeter (Oximetrix, Abbott, North Chicago, USA) through a 4 Fr fiberoptic catheter (Opticath, Oximetrix) introduced to the internal juglar bulb by a retrograde approach under fluoroscopy ($n = 13$) and rSO_2 by nearinfrared spectroscopy (INVOS 3100, Somanetics, Troy, Mo, USA) through a probe placed on the forehead ($n = 10$). SjO_2 was calibrated in vivo and rSO_2 in vitro.

Results were expressed as means ± SE. Values before F-F bypass, under partial F-F bypass, and under total F-F bypass were compared using Wilcoxon's signed ranks test, and significance was defined as $P < .05$. Linear regression analysis was also performed and the correlation coefficient calculated.

Results

EEG slowing on the operating side, that is, laterality, was seen in 1 of the 21 patients with EEG power spectrum monitoring. It appeared not during cross-clamping of the main cerebral artery but after declamping. Near the end of the left internal carotid endarterectomy, a temporary shunt tube bridging the distal and proximal sites along the artery was pulled out; immediately after this, EEG slowing on the operating side became distinct. Postoperatively, this patient had sensory and motor disturbances on the right side, and cerebral thrombus of clots detached on extubation from the tip of the shunt tube was suspected to be the most likely cause. In 8 of the 21 patients who underwent moderate hypothermia at about 20°C during F-F bypass, the EEG was almost flat and thus was unavailable as a monitor during such hypothermic periods.

SjO_2 under moderate hypothermic total F-F bypass plus SCP reponded well to changes in SCP flow rate and also in the oxygen fraction of the artificial lung. SjO_2 was useful for adjusting SCP flow rate and oxygen fraction even during periods of moderate hypothermia. SjO_2 generally showed a sharp increase and decrease with the initiation of cooling and rewarming, respectively, during F-F bypass. A representative case is shown in Fig. 1. A linear correlation ($r = -.68$) was observed between SjO_2 and arterial blood temperature during F-F bypass (Fig. 2) and it was not uncommon for the arterial blood temperature to rise to nearly 40°C during the rewarming phase, although the period of such hyperthermia was short.

SjO_2 below 50% was observed during surgery in 6 of the 13 patients with continuous SjO_2 monitoring. These 6 patients all received resection and grafting for TAA including the aortic arch under initiation of F-F bypass, and SjO_2 decreased further, to below 40%, in 3 of these 6 patients. No neurological disturbance was observed postoperatively in 4 patients whose durations of SjO_2 below 50% (>40%) were less than 20 min even under normothermic conditions, and in 1 patient in whom SjO_2 below 50% (>40%) for 60 min and SjO_2 below 40% (>30%) for 150 min were forced under moderate hypothermia. The remaining patient was exposed to 390 min of

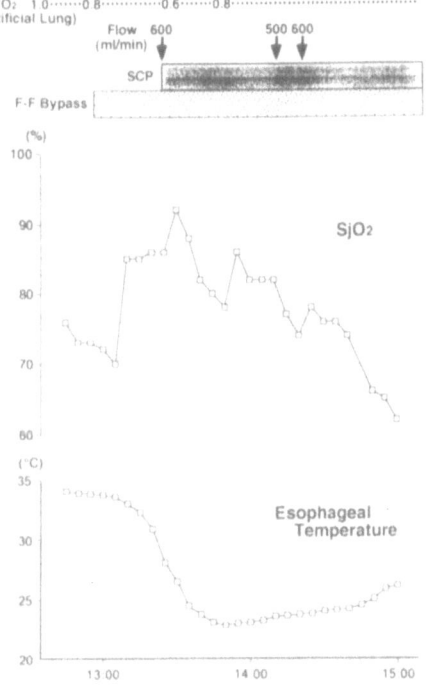

FIG. 1. Influences of oxygen fraction (FO_2) of the artificial lung, selective cerebral perfusion (SCP) flow and esophageal temperature on SjO_2 in a patient (59-yr-old man) undergoing thoracic aortic aneurysm surgery under femorofemoral venoarterial partial (F-F) bypass and SCP. When the oxygen fraction was lowered from 0.8 to 0.6 or SCP flow was reduced from 600 to 500 ml/min, SjO_2 decreased promptly. An increase in SjO_2 with cooling and a decrease in SjO_2 with rewarming were also seen.

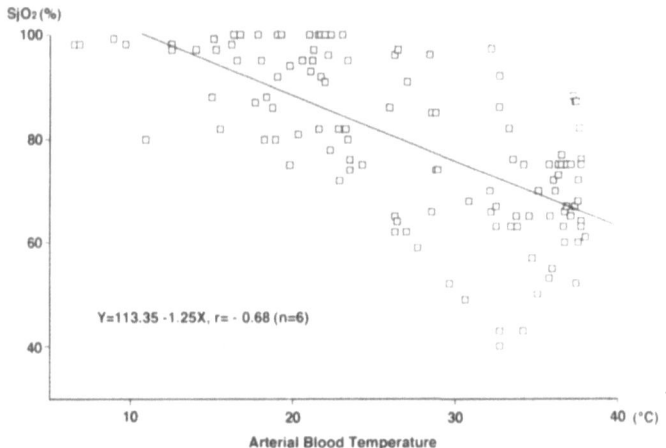

FIG. 2. Correlation of SjO$_2$ with arterial blood temperature under F-F bypass ($n = 6$)

SjO$_2$ below 50% (>40%) and 150 min of SjO$_2$ below 40%, and died within 48 h postoperatively without recovering consciousness.

SjO$_2$ and rSO$_2$ were measured simultaneously in four patients. Plotting of the corresponding SjO$_2$ and rSO$_2$ values revealed that SjO$_2$ (25%–100%) was distributed over a wider range than rSO$_2$ (25%–89%) (Fig. 3). There was no significant correlation between SjO$_2$ and rSO$_2$ during the course of surgery of these three patients. However, a good correlation ($r = -.92$) between SjO$_2$ and rSO$_2$ was seen in one of the four patients (Fig. 4). Both SjO$_2$ and rSO$_2$ decreased with the initiation of F-F partial bypass under normothermia, although those decreases were not statistically significant. Subsequent cooling through the F-F bypass induced a significant increase in both SjO$_2$ and rSO$_2$ (Fig. 5). Transient reductions in SjO$_2$ followed by rSO$_2$ were observed shortly after returning the ordinate blood pathway from SCP in another of the four patients, and SjO$_2$ and rSO$_2$ were subsequently above 60%. Three days after the operation, disturbances in aspiration and eye movement became apparent in this patient, and magnetic resonance imaging (MRI) revealed a brainstem infarction extending from the medulla through the midbrain.

FIG. 3. Distribution of simultaneously recorded SjO$_2$ and rSO$_2$ ($n = 3$)

FIG. 4. A good correlation between SjO$_2$ and rSO$_2$ was observed in a patient (38-yr-old woman) under F-F bypass and SCP

FIG. 5. Influences of body temperature and hemodilution on SjO$_2$ (*left*) and rSO$_2$ (*right*) ($n = 4$). Hb, hemoglobin; *, $P < .05$, vs before F-F bypass; **, $P < .01$, vs before F-F bypass; #, $P < .05$, vs partial F-F bypass; ##, $P < .01$, vs partial F-F bypass

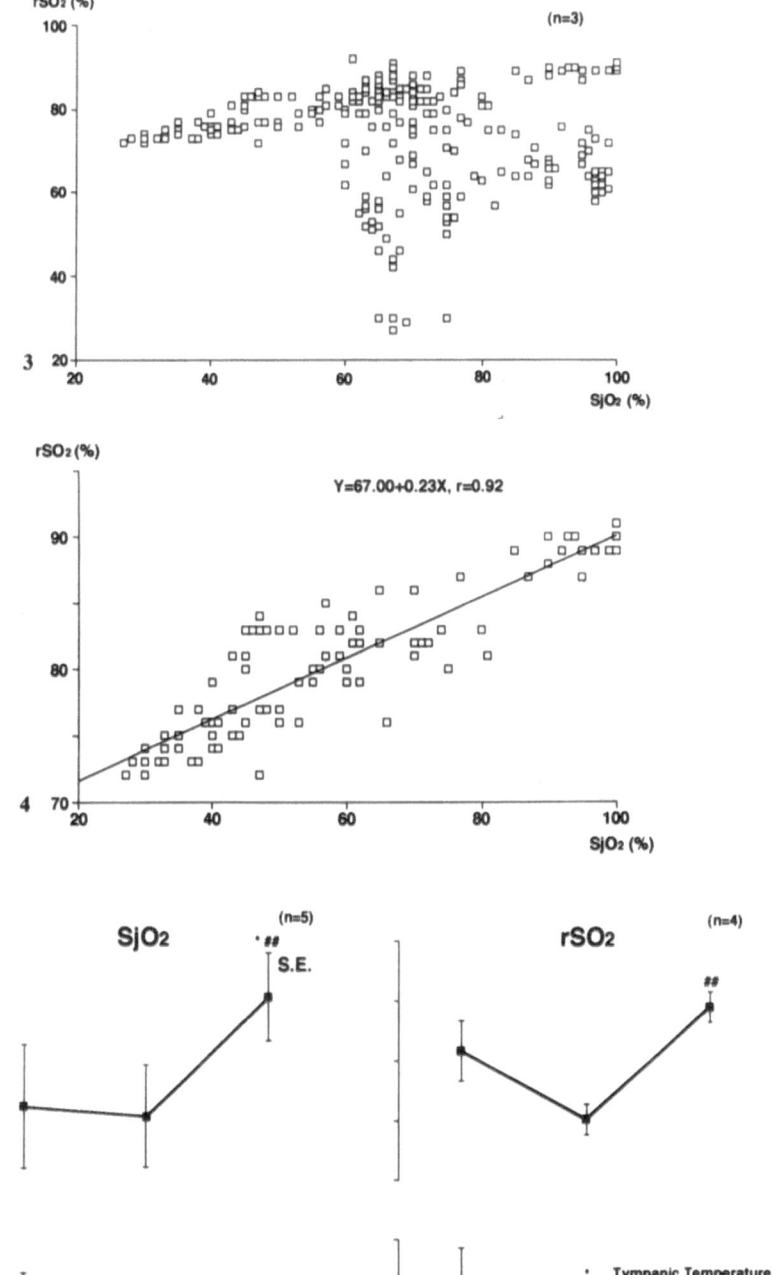

Discussion

Laterality in EEG or EEG power spectrum is clinically useful for detecting ischemia in the cerebral hemisphere. Heparinization has been used in cases requiring placement of a temporary shunt tube because of the probability of clot or thrombus formation. Body temperature is a crucial factor for EEG monitoring under hypothermic extracorporeal cardiopulmonary bypass; a body temperature of at least 20°C is needed for EEG monitoring because the electrical activities of the brain are almost completely suppressed below this temperature.

Continuous SjO_2 monitoring provided useful real-time information regarding overall cerebral oxygen balance even under moderate extracorporeal circulation. SjO_2 seems, therefore, to be one of the most reliable methods for clinically monitoring global cerebral ischemia, although it is invasive. Nakajima et al. [1] compared SjO_2 determined using a catheter oximeter with a concurrent laboratory co-oximeter value and reported that continuous SjO_2 monitoring is accurate and reliable even under moderate hypothermia and hemodilution during extracorporeal circulation.

The current results with SjO_2 monitoring indicate that care should be taken to avoid rapid rewarming through the F-F bypass. The observed reductions in SjO_2 during the rewarming phase seem to reflect excessive oxygen demand compared with oxygen supply under hyperthermic conditions. Rapid rewarming with blood at an excessively high temperature may induce cerebral oxygen deficiency and exacerbate postperfusional cerebral damage. In the current study, a patient with a 20-min exposure of SjO_2 below 50% under normothermic anesthesia was free from postoperative neurological disturbance, as was another patient with 60 min of SjO_2 below 50% (>40%) and 150 min of SjO_2 below 40% (>30%) under moderate hypothermia. Degree and duration of SjO_2 reduction and body temperature at this time seem to be the main factors regulating postischemic cerebral disfunction. The size of our population was too small to infer any safety criteria for a limit in SjO_2 reduction.

SjO_2 was ditributed over a wider range compared with simutaneously measured rSO_2, suggesting SjO_2 was a more sensitive parameter with which to monitor ischemic insult. There was no significant correlation between the whole SjO_2 and rSO_2 obtained from three patients in the course of surgery. However, both SjO_2 and rSO_2 decreased after initiation of F-F bypass, increased with cooling, and decreased with rewarming. Reductions in SjO_2 and rSO_2 observed shortly after the initiation of F-F partial bypass under normothermic conditions may be explained by hemodilution, that is, a decrease in oxygen capacity. Parallel fluctuations between SjO_2 and rSO_2 including a transient drop, presumably because of thrombus formation, were seen only in one patient. This case indicated that it might be possible to replace the invasive monitoring of SjO_2 with the noninvasive determination of rSO_2, although further refinements and validation are needed before introduction of rSO_2 into routine clinical use.

In conclusion, laterality in EEG power spectrum was useful and practical to detect ischemia in the cerebral hemisphere if body temperature remained normothermic or mildly hypothermic. Continuous SjO_2 monitoring was indicative of the overall cerebral oxygen balance, even under moderate hypothermia and hemodilution during extracorporeal circulation, and there was a linear correlation between SjO_2 and arterial blood temperature. SjO_2 often fell below the precooling level during the rewarming phase through F-F bypass. Five of six patients with SjO_2 below 50% developed no neurological disturbance postoperatively, but the remaining patient died without recovering consciousness. Noninvasive rSO_2 monitoring showed parallel changes to those observed by the invasive determinations of SjO_2 in one of four patients in whom both parameters were simultaneously recorded throughout surgery, although relative changes in rSO_2 were less than those in SjO_2.

References

1. Nakajima T, Ohsumi H, Kuro M (1993) Accuracy of continuous jugular bulb venous oximetry during carodiopulmonary bypass. Anesth Analg 77:1111–1115
2. McCormick PW, Stewart M, Goetting MG, Balakrishnan G (1991) Regional cerebrovascular oxygen saturation measured by optical spectroscopy in humans. Stroke 22:596–602

Jugular Bulb Oxygen Saturation and Oxygen Consumption in Patients Receiving Barbiturate Therapy

Toshiaki Ikeda, Kazumi Ikeda, Narihiro Yoshimatsu, Hideto Kaneko, Masatoshi Sugi, Tohru Iizuka, Yoshiyuki Kameyama, and Nagao Ishii

Introduction

Jugular bulb oxygen saturation ($SjVO_2$) is thought to indicate the ratio of cerebral blood flow to cerebral metabolic rate of oxygen consumption ($CMRO_2$). Continuous monitoring of $SjVO_2$ has been used in the management of severe head injury patients in intensive care units. The purpose of this study was to evaluate the influence of $SjVO_2$ and oxygen consumption (VO_2) under barbiturate therapy in patients with various types of intracranial hemorrhage.

Materials and Methods

Comatose patients (Glasgow Coma Scale [GCS] score less than 8) who had various types of cerebral hemorrhage and were receiving thiopental sodium as barbiturate therapy in our intensive care unit were studied between December 1993 and March 1994. The four men and two women (average age, 54 years) had respective diagnoses of acute subdural hematoma caused by a motor vehicle accident, subarachnoid hemorrhage caused by a ruptured aneurysm, hypertensive intracranial hematoma, subcortical hematoma, and, in two cases, cerebellar hematoma (Table 1). A 5.5 Fr fiberoptic oxygen saturation catheter (Abbott Laboratories, North Chicago, USA) was inserted through a 6.0 Fr peel-away introducer into each patient's right internal jugular vein to measure $SjVO_2$. The tip of the catheter was positioned in the jugular bulb, as confirmed by radiography. The catheter was calibrated by in vitro calibration before insertion. VO_2 was determined by a metabolic computer (Deltatrack, Helsinki, Finland) under mechanical ventilation at less than 50% oxygen concentration. The times of $SjVO_2$ and VO_2 determinations were as follows: (1) during 5 mg/kg/h of thiopental sodium administration; (2) during 3 mg/kg/h of thiopental sodium administration; and (3) 12 h

Department of Anesthesiology, Hachioji Medical Center, Tokyo Medical College, 1163, Tate-machi, Hachioji, Tokyo 193, Japan

TABLE 1. Cases of barbiturate therapy

Case	Sex	Age	Weight (kg)	Diagnosis	Consciousness level	Outcome[a]
1	M	48	60	Acute subdural hematoma	E2V2M3	GR
2	F	54	65	Subarachnoid hemorrhage	E1V2M3	GR
3	M	54	68	Intracerebral hematoma	E1V1M3	VS
4	M	29	50	Subcortical hematoma	E1V2M3	GR
5	M	59	70	Cerebellar hematoma	E1V1M4	VS
6	F	79	39	Cerebellar hematoma	E1V1M3	VS

[a] GR, good recovery; VS, vegetative state.

after discontinuation of each barbiturate, respectively. SjVO$_2$ and VO$_2$ were determined each minute for 120 min at steady state.

Case 1

A 48-year-old man, who had a head injury from a motor vehicle accident, was transferred to our hospital with a GCS score of 7 (E2: Eyes open to pain, V2: Best verbal response is inappropriate words, M3: Best motor response is decorticate rigidity). Cranial computed tomography (CT) showed acute subdural hematoma on the left side and traumatic subarachnoid hemorrhage on the right side. Emergency surgery was performed to evacuate the hematoma. Immediately after the operation, cranial CT revealed the midline deviated to the right side and a ventricular hemorrhage. To reduce both cerebral swelling and cerebral metabolism, 5 mg/kg/h of barbiturate therapy was administered. The dosage was reduced to 3 mg/kg/h 2 days after the operation. SjVO$_2$ during administration of 5 mg/kg/h of thiopental sodium varied from 55% to 80%, and VO$_2$ was 233 ± 17 ml/min (Fig. 1). During administration of 3 mg/kg/h of thiopental sodium, SjVO$_2$ was about 60% and VO$_2$ was 261 ± 23 ml/min. After barbiturate therapy, SjVO$_2$ varied from 40% to 60% and at the same time the value of VO$_2$ was 280 ± 26 ml/minute.

Case 3

A 54-year-old man who had intracerebral hemorrhage caused by hypertension, confirmed by cranial CT, was admitted to our intensive care unit with severe coma (E1, V1, M3). His pupil size was 4.5 mm on the right side and 4.0 mm on the left side, with no response to light at intensive care unit (ICU) admission. Mechanical ventilation was performed to maintain appropriate PaCO$_2$ and PaO$_2$ with 50% oxygen concentration. To reduce intracranial pressure and induce sedation, 5 mg/kg/h of thiopental sodium and 1.0 mg/kg/h of vecuronium bromide were administered Fig. 2. Also, a calcium antagonist (nicardipine) was administered intermittently via a peripheral vein to prevent hypertension. An emergency CT stereotactic operation was performed, and 29 ml of hematoma fluid was evacuated.

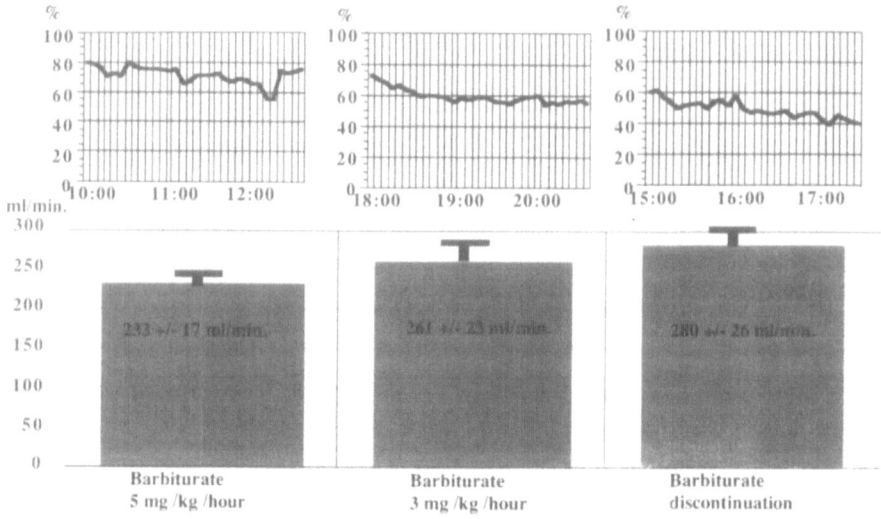

FIG. 1. Changes in jugular bulb oxygen saturation (SjVO₂) and oxygen consumption (VO₂) during barbiturate therapy in a patient with acute subdural hematoma (case 1)

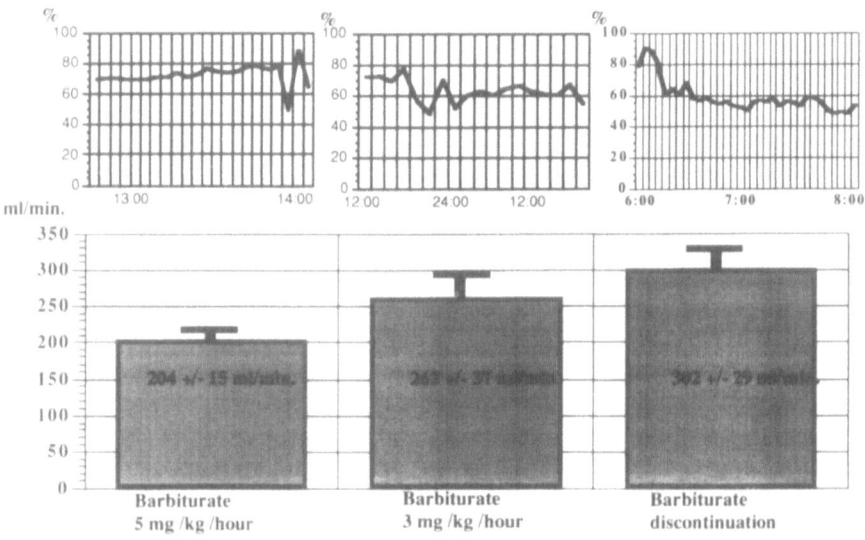

FIG. 2. Changes in SjVO₂ and VO₂ in a patient with intracranial hematoma during barbiturate therapy (case 3)

After this operation, 5 mg/kg/h of thiopental sodium was administered under mechanical ventilation. During barbiturate administration, SjVO₂ maintained above 60%. With subsequent 3 mg/kg/h of barbiturate therapy, SjVO₂ varied from 50% to 60%. After discontinuation of thiopental sodium,

SjVO$_2$ was 40%–60%. The value of VO$_2$ was 225 ± 18 ml/min with 5 mg/ kg/h of barbiturate therapy. After barbiturate therapy, VO$_2$ was 251 ± 29 ml/min. This was a remarkable increase in VO$_2$ compared to the values during barbiturate therapy for coma.

Case 4

A 29-year-old man who had abruptly convulsed and lost consciousness in his house was transferred to our hospital by ambulance. His initial GCS was 6 (E1, V2, M3). Cranial CT showed a subcortical hematoma on the left side and diffuse brain swelling (Fig. 3). The patient was intubated, and respiration was maintained by mechanical ventilation (slight hyperventi- lation: pH 7.513; PaCO$_2$, 33 mmHg; PaO$_2$, 121 mmHg). Barbitrate therapy was commenced with 5 mg/kg/h of thiopental sodium after ICU admission, and mannitol and methylprednisolone were also administered to reduce intracranial pressure. A CT stereotactic operation was performed to eva- cuate the hematoma. During 5 mg/kg/h of barbiturate therapy, SjVO$_2$ varied from 55% to 62%, and with subsquent 3 mg/kg/h of barbiturate therapy, SjVO$_2$ was 51%–60%; after discontinuation of barbiturate therapy, SjVO$_2$ declined to 45%. VO$_2$ was not determined in this case.

Case 6

A 79-year-old woman who had lost consciousness (initial GCS, 5) because of a cerebellar hematoma that was confirmed by CT scan, was admitted to ICU (Fig. 4). A tracheal tube was inserted at the emergency unit, and mechanical

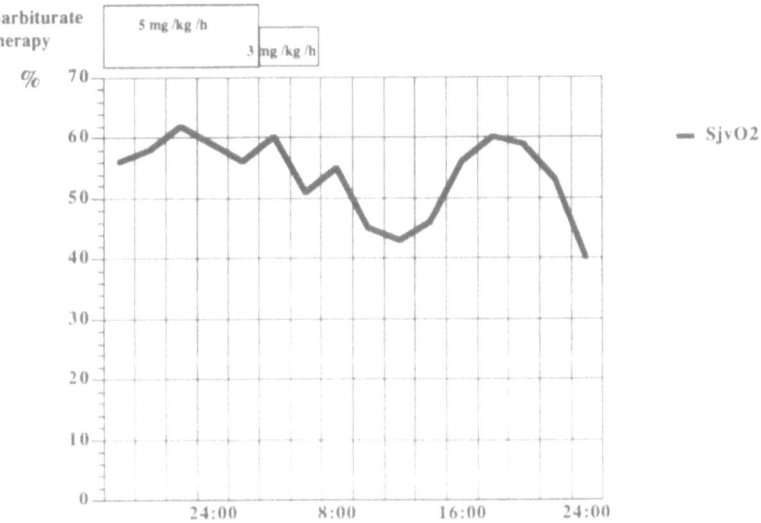

FIG. 3. Changes in SjVO$_2$ in a patient with subcortical hematoma (case 4)

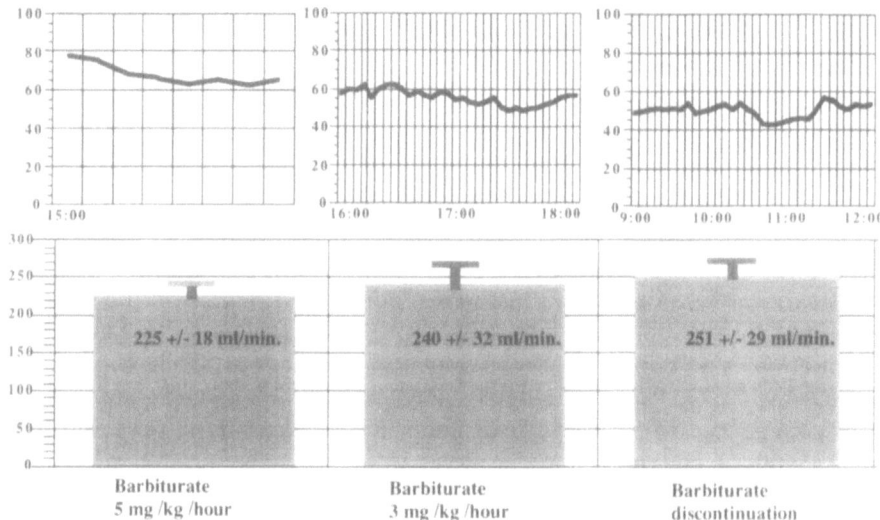

FIG. 4. Changes in $SjVO_2$ and VO_2 during barbiturate therapy in a patient with cerebellar hemorrhage (case 6)

ventilation was started with $3\,cmH_2O$ of positive end-expiratory pressure (PEEP); $5\,mg/kg/h$ of barbiturate therapy was commenced to prevent increased intracranial pressure. During $5\,mg/kg/h$ of thiopental sodium administration, $SjVO_2$ remained above 60%; with $3\,mg/kg/h$ of barbiturate therapy, $SjVO_2$ varied from 50% to 60%. After barbiturate therapy, $SjVO_2$ declined to 40%–60%. On the other hand, VO_2 was $225 \pm 18\,ml/min$ under $5\,mg/kg/h$ of thiopental sodium administration and increased 12% to $251 \pm 29\,ml/min$ after discontinuation of barbiturate therapy.

Discussion

It would be useful to measure cerebral blood flow (CBF) as an indicator of cerebral pathological conditions because ischemia is the final common pathway for the production of damage. Ischemia involves an inappropriately low CBF for the metabolic requirements of the brain. Measurement of CBF alone would be a useful indicator of the onset of damage, providing the metabolism was always at the same level. However, positron emission tomography studies have shown that metabolism may vary considerably in response to various stimulations and different pathological situations [1]. Therefore, the ideal situation would include simultaneous measurement of both CBF and cerebral metabolism. The blood obtained from the jugular venous bulb is considered to be mixed venous blood from the whole brain. Shenkin et al. [2] reported that the mean influx rate from extracerebral parts to the jugular bulb was 2.7%, so the tip of the catheter should be inserted to the jugular bulb in as high a position as possible.

In this study, SjVO$_2$ values were relatively stable because of a relative suppression of CMRO$_2$ compared with CBF during barbiturate therapy for coma. VO$_2$ increased and SjVO$_2$ decreased with declining dosage of thiopental sodium. Also, barbiturate therapy affected VO$_2$, which indicated an increase in oxygen consumption of 12% to 50% following barbiturate therapy discontinuation. The insertion technique into the jugular venous bulb is not very difficult if care is taken not to puncture the carotid artery. However, the value of SjVO$_2$ alone does not reflect the local cerebral pathophysiological conditions. Changes in SjVO$_2$ should be considered along with general cerebral metabolism, especially oxygen consumption.

References

1. Garlick R, Bihari D (1987) The use of intermittent and continuous recordings of jugular venous bulb oxygen saturation in the unconscious patient. Scand J Clin Lab Invest 47(Suppl) 188:47–52
2. Shenkin HA, Harmel MH, Kety SS (1948) Dynamic anatomy of the cerebral circulation. Arch Neurol Psychiatry 60:240–252

Does the Transient Decrease in Mixed Venous Oxygen Saturation and Jugular Venous Hemoglobin Saturation During the Rewarming Phase in a Cardiopulmonary Bypass Merely Reflect a Recovery of the Metabolic Rate? A Case Report

H. Okamoto[1], K. Irita[1], T. Taniyama[2], T. Kawasaki[1], Y. Kai[1], and S. Takahashi[1]

Introduction

Maintaining the balance between oxygen supply and demand during a cardiopulmonary bypass (CPB) is a key issue in the anesthetic management of cardiovascular surgery. Although many reports have described this balance at a constant, low body temperature, little is known about the balance during the cooling and the rewarming phase of CPB. Nakajima et al. [1] reported that jugular venous hemoglobin saturation (SjO_2) decreased during the rewarming phase of CPB, and that rapid rewarming produced a pronounced decrease in SjO_2. We analyzed retrospectively the intraoperative changes in SjO_2, mixed venous oxygen saturation ($S\bar{v}O_2$), and oxygen consumption ($\dot{V}O_2$) in three patients who underwent reconstruction of the thoracic aorta, two of whom developed postoperative neurological deficits.

Patients and Methods

Patient profiles are shown in Table 1. The preoperative arterial blood pressure was controlled adequately by anti-hypertensive drugs. High doses of fentanyl ($68-101\,\mu g \cdot kg^{-1} \cdot min^{-1}$) were given for anesthesia. CPB was

[1] Department of Anesthesiology and Critical Care Medicine and [2] Intensive Care Unit, Faculty of Medicine, Kyushu University, 3-1-1 Maidashi, Higashi-ku, Fukuoka 812, Japan

TABLE 1. Clinical information

Patient	Case 1	Case 2	Case 3
Age	72	72	67
Sex	Male	Female	Male
Height (cm)	155	151	168
Weight (kg)	54	46	54
Diagnosis	Descending aortic aneurysm	Descending aortic aneurysm	Aortic arch aneurysm
Preoperative complications	Hypertension Cerebral infarction Carotid aneurysm Renal dysfunction	Hypertension Hyperlipidemia	Hypertension Cerebral infarction Abdominal aneurysm Renal failure
Preoperative medications	Metoprorol Bunazosin Nicardipine Benidipine Nicorandil	Metoprorol Metolazone Captopril	Metoprorol Manidipine Hydralazine
Preoperative mean arterial pressure (mmHg)	75–110	75–105	80–95
ASA physical status	3	2	3
Duration of CPB (min)	180	227	196
Duration of SCP (min)	22	31	108
Postoperative neurological complications	EEG abnormality (spike wave) Right lower hemiplegia	None	Disorientation

ASA, American Society of Anesthesiologists; CPB, cardiopulmonary bypass; SCP, selective cerebral perfusion; EEG, Electroencephalogram.

maintained using an arterial line filter, a nonpulsatile pump, and a membrane oxygenator primed with crystalloid solution. The pump flow rate was kept about $66\,ml\cdot kg^{-1}\cdot min^{-1}$. Selective cerebral perfusion (SCP) was employed at a flow rate of $5-8\,ml\cdot kg^{-1}\cdot min^{-1}$. Acid–base status was maintained according to alpha-stat regulation. Although all patients were weaned successfully from CPB, two patients (case 1 and case 3) developed postoperative neurological deficits.

Cardiac output (CO) was measured by the thermodilution technique before and after CPB and was calculated from the pump flow rate during CPB. $\bar{S}vO_2$ and SjO_2 were monitored continuously with oximetry catheters (OPTICATH, Abbot, North Chicago, IL, USA) connected to an oximeter (OXIMETRIX 3, Abott). During CPB, $\bar{S}vO_2$ was measured using a oxygen saturation monitor (SM-0100, Bentley Laboratory, San Diego, CA, USA) placed on the venous side of the CPB. $\dot{V}O_2$ was calculated using Fick's equation. Dissolved oxygen was neglected because mixed venous oxygen tensions were not available. Blood lactate concentrations were determined using Diagluca (Toyobo, Osaka, Japan).

Results

In all three cases, $S\bar{v}O_2$ started to increase immediately after the initiation of cooling, followed by a decrease after the initiation or rewarming (Fig. 1). SjO_2 changed in a similar manner, especially in case 1. $\dot{V}O_2$ decreased rapidly after cooling began, and then increased abruptly after the initiation of rewarming. Cooling by CPB also induced an increase in blood lactate concentration, which persisted until the end of CPB. These changes again were most obvious in case 1. Although the changes in oxygen delivery ($\dot{D}O_2$) during the cooling phase seemed to be almost the same in all three

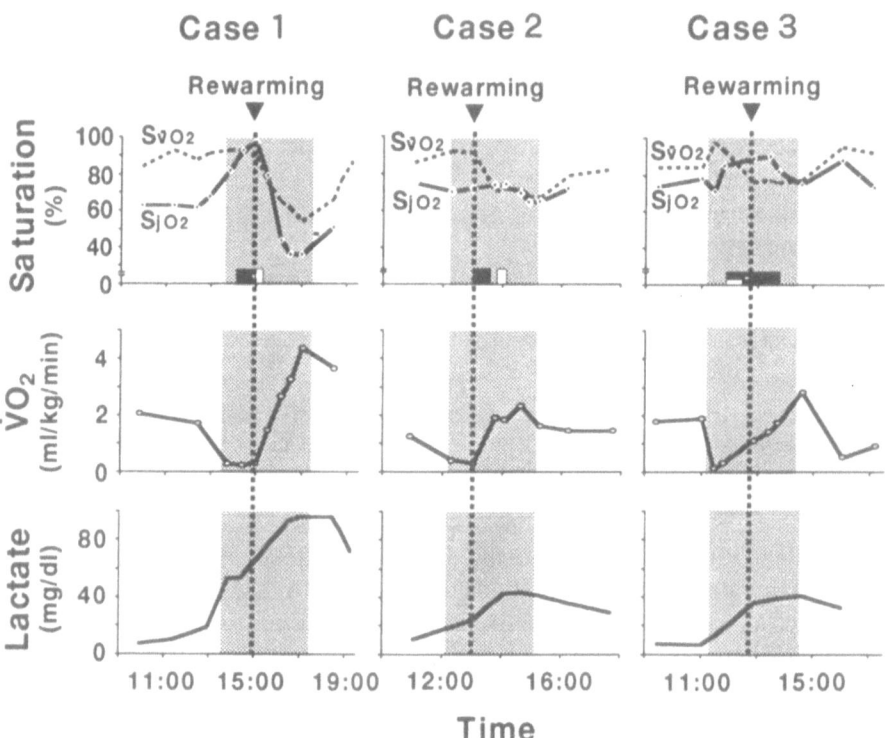

FIG. 1. Changes in mixed venous oxygen consumption oxygen saturation ($S\bar{v}O_2$), jugular venous hemoglobin saturation (SjO_2), oxygent consumption ($\dot{V}O_2$) values, and blood lactate concentrations for all three cases. $S\bar{v}O_2$ started to increase immediately after the initiation of cooling and to decrease after the initiation of rewarming. The change in SjO_2 was similar to that in $S\bar{v}O_2$ with the exception of the time period during selective cerebral perfusion (SCP). $\dot{V}O_2$ decreased soon after the initiation of cooling, and then increased abruptly after the initiation of rewarming. Cooling by cardiopulmonary bypass (CPB) also induced an increase in blood lactate concentrations, which persisted until the end of CPB. These changes were most obvious in case 1. *Shaded areas*, CPB; *black areas*, SCP; *white areas*, circulatory arrest of lower body

cases, overconsumption of oxygen was obvious in case 1 (Fig. 2). VO_2 during the rewarming phase was much higher than that during the cooling phase at the same rectal temperatures of 25°C and 30°C, respectively (Fig. 3). Cooling by CPB also induced an increase in blood lactate concentration,

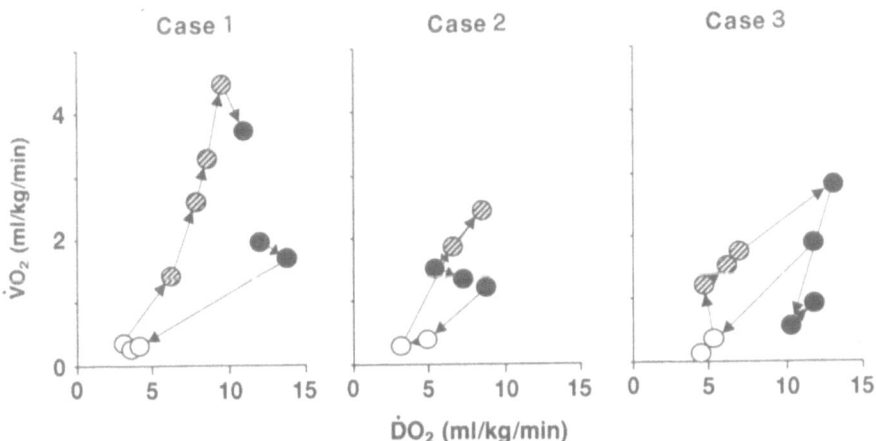

FIG. 2. Relationship between oxygen delivery ($\dot{D}O_2$) and $\dot{V}O_2$. Overconsumption of oxygen was observed during the rewarming phase of CPB. $\dot{D}O_2$ changed between 3 and 14 ml/kg·min. *Black circles*, pre- and post-CPB; *white circles*, cooling; *shaded circles*, rewarming

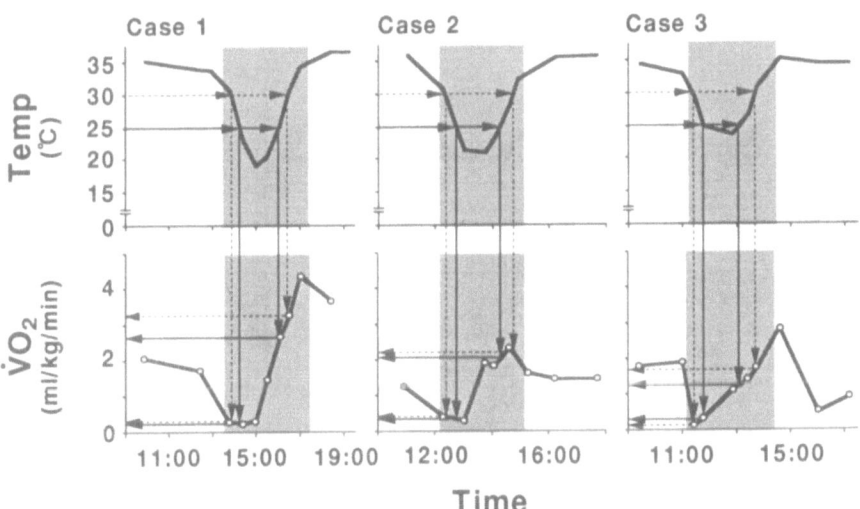

FIG. 3. Differences in $\dot{V}O_2$ values between the cooling and the rewarming phase at rectal temperatures of 25°C and 30°C, respectively. $\dot{V}O_2$ values during the rewarming phase were much higher than those during the cooling phase

which persisted until the end of CPB (see Fig. 1). Furthermore, the maximum VO_2 values during the rewarming phase corresponded with the speed of rewarming, while the minimum SjO_2 and $S\bar{v}O_2$ values varied inversely with the rewarming speed (Fig. 4).

Discussion

We observed overconsumption of oxygen during the rewarming phase of CPB. An increase in $\dot{V}O_2$ during the rewarming phase has been generally believed to result from an increase in metabolism in accordance with a rise in body temperature, an increase in oxygen delivery by red cell transfusion, a rightward shift of the oxygen dissociation curve, and some changes in the distribution of blood flow. The reperfusion-induced increase in the production of active oxygen may contribute to the overconsumption. The following observations indicate that oxygen debt develops during the cooling phase of CPB, and is compensated during the rewarming phase: (a) an immediate increase in blood lactate concentrations after the initiation of cooling, (b) the clear difference in $\dot{V}O_2$ values between the cooling and the rewarming phase at the same temperature, and (c) overconsumption of oxygen during the rewarming phase. We speculate that the oxygen debt might be caused by several factors, including a leftward shift of the oxygen dissociation curve, maldistribution of organ blood flow, and an insufficient $\dot{D}O_2$ during the cooling phase. Although Shibutani et al. [2] reported a critical $\dot{D}O_2$ of $8.2\,\text{ml}\cdot\text{min}^{-1}\cdot\text{kg}^{-1}$ in cardiac patients anesthetized with a moderate dose of fentanyl, critical $\dot{D}O_2$ values at lower body temperatures are unknown. The incidence of postoperative neurological deficit has been reported to be low

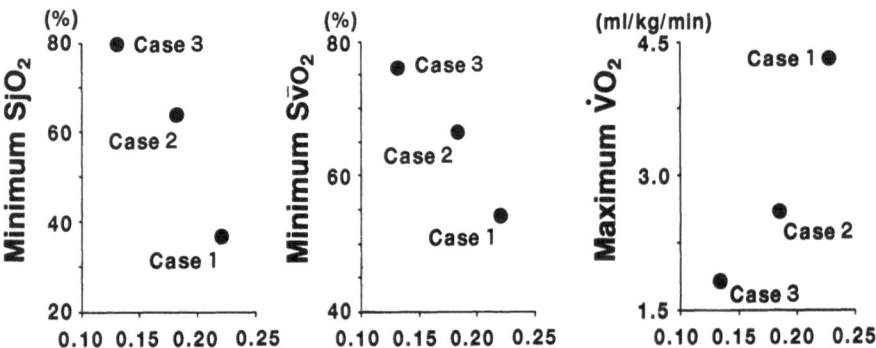

Rewarming speed of rectal temperature (°C/min)

FIG. 4. Scattergrams of minimum SjO_2 and $S\bar{v}O_2$ and maximum $\dot{V}O_2$ during the rewarming phase plotted against the speed of rewarming from a rectal temperature of 25°C to 30°C. The minimum SjO_2 and $S\bar{v}O_2$ varied inversely. and the maximum $\dot{V}O_2$ varied directly with rewarming speed in alpha-stat regulation rather than in pH-stat regulation [3]. It might be possible, however, that alpha-stat regulation limits organ blood flow during the cooling phase, resulting in oxygen debt.

Our findings coincide with those of Nakajima et al., who reported that more rapid warming induced a sharper decrease in SjO_2 [1]. Although the causes of postoperative neurological deficits in our patients could not be ascertained, an increase in $\dot{V}O_2$ in the brain during the rewarming phase might have caused the damage, or have exacerbated the damage caused by surgical procedures. Because the oxygen extraction ratio in the heart is higher than that in the brain, overconsumption of oxygen in the heart, if it occurs, may also have a deleterious effect on weaning from CPB. Further studies are required to clarify oxygen supply/demand balance during the cooling and the rewarming phase of CPB.

In summary, we examined the changes in $\dot{V}O_2$ during reconstruction of the thoracic aorta using hypothermic CPB in three patients. After initiating rewarming, the $\dot{V}O_2$ started to increase abruptly, and exceeded the pre-CPB levels. It is suggested that this overconsumption of oxygen might be caused by oxygen debt accumulated during hypothermia and the speed of rewarming. Because any imbalance in oxygen supply and demand would potentially exacerbate CPB-associated tissue damages, continuous monitoring of $S\bar{v}O_2$ and SjO_2 seems mandatory.

References

1. Nakajima T, Kuro M, Hayashi Y, Kitaguchi K, Uchida O, Takaki O (1992) Clinical evaluation of cerebral oxygen balance during cardiopulmonary bypass: on-line continuous monitoring of jugular venous oxyhemoglobin saturation. Anesth Analg 74:630–635
2. Shibutani K, Komatsu T, Kubal K, Sanchala V, Kumar V, Bizzarri DV (1983) Critical level of oxygen delivery in anesthetized man. Crit Care Med 11:640–643
3. Stephan H, Weyland A, Kazmaier S, Henze T, Menck S, Sonntag H (1992) Acid-base management during hypothermic cardiopulmonary bypass does not affect cerebral metabolism but does affect blood flow and neurological outcome. Br J Anaesth 69:51–57

Jugular Bulb Oximetry in Patients with Cerebral Arteriovenous Malformation

Teruyasu Hirayama, Yoichi Katayama, and Takashi Tsubokawa

Introduction

Arterial blood flow directly through a shunt theoretically does not deliver oxygen to the brain tissue. The draining veins of an arteriovenous malformation (AVM) contain highly oxygenated blood [1], as evidenced by the intraoperative finding commonly denoted as red veins [2]. The jugular bulb oxygen saturation (SjO_2) has been demonsttrated to reflect global cerebral hyperemia or ischemia sensitively [3–6]. In addition, fiberoptic technology is now available for continuous monitoring of SjO_2 [3–5].

We have monitored SjO_2 during a preoperative embolization procedure [7–9] in a consecutive series of large AVMs to estimate the shunt flow ratio. Hyperemic complications may well be reduced by staged preoperative embolization [7–9], avoiding abrupt changes in shunt flow ratio. The aim of the present study was to determine whether SjO_2 sensitively reflects changes in the shunt flow ratio during embolization procedures.

Patients and Methods

Patient Selection

We treated 15 patients with large AVMs in whom the SjO_2 was measured continuously during planned preoperative embolization. While the maximum diameter of a "large" AVM has been defined variably by different authors (range, >4–6 cm) [10–12], the AVMs with a maximum diameter greater than 4 cm were included in the present study.

The AVM volume was calculated as the product of the three angiographic diameters multiplied by 0.52 with correction for the magnification factor according to the methods reported by Fult and Kelly [13] and Pasqualin et al. [14].

Department of Neurological Surgery, Nihon University School of Medicine, Tokyo 173, Japan

Embolization Procedure

We employed N-butyl-cyanoacrylate (NBCA), polyfilament polyethylene threads (PPTs; diameter, $300\,\mu m$; length, $5-10\,mm$), or polyvinyl alcohol particles (PVAs) as embolization materials. Embolization was performed several times, each procedure separated by 1 week, through one to three feeding arteries at each session. The embolization materials were injected via a Tracker microcatheter, usually until the mean blood pressure of the feeding artery was elevated to approximately $80\,mmHg$.

Oxygen Saturation Measurements

A fiberoptic catheter system (4 Fr., Opticath and Oximetrix III Systems, Abbott Laboratories, USA)[1] was used for the continuous measurement of SjO₂. The tip of the catheter was placed in the jugular bulb. The catheter was placed on the dominant side, determined on the basis of the findings of CT scans and previous angiography. The oxygen saturation of the systemic arterial blood (SaO₂) was monitored by pulse oximetry at the finger.

Shunt Flow Ratio

The SjO₂ in cases of AVM represents a composite of the oxygen saturation of the shunt flow (SjSO₂) and of the perfusion flow (SjPO₂). Thus:

$$SjO_2 \cdot (F_{shunt} + F_{perfusion}) = SjSO_2 \cdot F_{shunt} + SjPO_2 \cdot F_{perfusion} \quad (1)$$

Equation 1 can be rewritten as

$$F_{perfusion} = F_{shunt}\,(SjSO_2 - SjO_2)/(SjO_2 - SjPO_2) \quad (2)$$

The shunt flow ratio can thus be expressed as

$$F_{shunt}/(F_{perfusion} + F_{shunt}) = (SjO_2 - SjPO_2)/(SjSO_2 - SjPO_2) \quad (3)$$

Because blood flowing directly through the shunt does not deliver oxygen to the brain tissue, the saturation of this blood flowing through the shunt can be assumed to be the same as the saturation of the systemic arterial blood (SaO₂). Then, Equation 3 can be rewritten as

$$F_{shunt}/(F_{tissue} + F_{shunt}) = (SjO_2 - SjPO_2)/(SaO_2 - SjPO_2) \quad (4)$$

The SjPO₂ can be assumed to be within the range of 50% to 75% when the brain is not globally ischemic (see following). The shunt flow ratio can therefore be evaluated from the SaO₂ and SjO₂ measurements.

Results

The SjO₂ determined for withdrawn jugular bulb blood before embolization ranged from 58% to 97% (mean $\pm$ SD $= 84.1\% \pm 12.7\%$), showing a significant positive correlation with the AVM volume ($r = .66$, $P < .001$).

The SjO$_2$ was significantly greater in patients with AVMs demonstrating clinical or angiographic steal (93.6% ± 4.4%) than in those with no clinical or angiographic steal (75.9% ± 11.8%; P < .002, unpaired t test; Fig. 1).

The SjO$_2$ decreased following embolization in association with an increase in the circulation time, the disappearance of early draining veins from the AVM, and evidence of steal on angiography. Although the embolization was not complete in many cases in this study because of the large AVM volumes, the SjO$_2$ determined for jugular bulb blood withdrawn at the end of the final embolization procedure ranged from 54% to 91% (74.2% ± 10.9%), which was significantly lower than that observed before embolization (P < .0001, paired t test; Fig. 2).

When PPTs were employed, a gradual decrease in SjO$_2$ was noted as the number of injected PPTs increased. SjO$_2$ did not return to the original level within the period of observation ranging up to 2 h, insofar as an appropriate amount of embolization material was injected. The decrease in SjO$_2$ was roughly correlated with an increase in circulation time, disappearance of early draining veins from the AVM, and evidence of steal on angiography.

Discussion

Oxygen Saturation in the Jugular Bulb

This study demonstrated that SjO$_2$ was markedly elevated in cases with a large AVM volume. As preoperative embolization of the AVM progressed, the value SjO$_2$ decreased. The decrease in SjO$_2$ was correlated with an

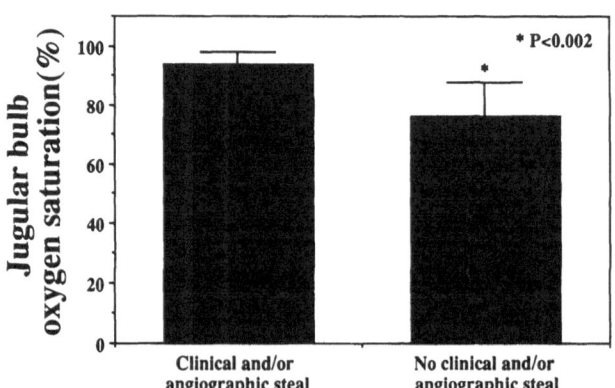

Fig. 1. Comparison between jugular bulb oxygen saturation in patients with arteriovenous malformations (AVMs) demonstrating clinical or angiographic steal and that in those with no clinical or angiographic steal. The SjO$_2$ was significantly greater in patients with AVMs demonstrating clinical or angiographic steal (93.6% ± 4.4%) than in those with no clinical or angiographic steal (75.9% ± 11.8%; P < .002, unpaired t test)

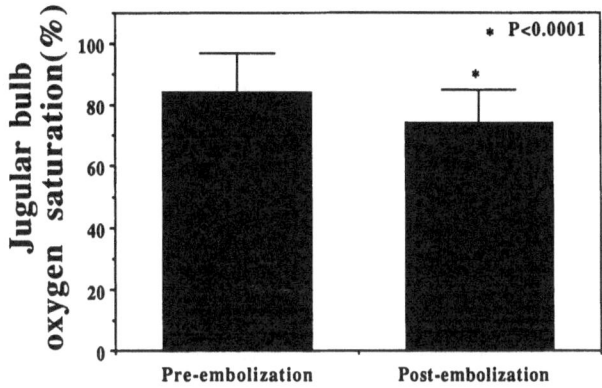

Fig. 2. Comparison between jugular bulb oxygen saturation observed before embolization and that determined after embolization. The SjO_2 determined after embolization (74.2% ± 10.9%) was significantly lower than that observed before embolization (84.1% ± 12.7%; $P < .0001$, paired t test)

increase in circulation time, disappearance of early draining veins from the AVMs, and angiographic steal, supporting the hypothesis that a high SjO_2 in cases with AVMs reflects drainage from the shunt. The initial slow and later rapid decreases in SjO_2 can be accounted for by an exponential decrease in shunt flow as the embolization progressed.

Estimation of the Ratio of Shunt Flow to Total Flow

SjO_2 normally varies between 60% and 75%, and decreases to approximately 50% before the brain becomes globally ischemic [3–6]. In cases with AVMs, perfusion flow may be reduced by steal. More oxygen is taken up the brain tissue from the limited flow, so that $SjPO_2$ may be lowered. It can be assumed, therefore, that $SjPO_2$ in cases of AVM ranges from 50% to 75% unless the brain is globally ischemic. Batjer et al. [15] reported an augmented vasodilatory reactivity in hypoperfused territories adjacent to high-flow AVMs. Their finding suggests that vessels in the hypoperfused territories are still capable of dilating with further increase in metabolic demand, supporting the assumption that $SjPO_2$ in such cases is between 50% and 75%.

Based on these values and Equation 4, the shunt flow ratio can be estimated from the observed SjO_2 together with the SaO_2. For example, an SjO_2 of 90% indicates that the shunt flow ratio is within the range of 0.6 to 0.8. Estimation of the shunt flow ratio in cases with AVMs from the SjO_2 is thus relatively simple. Furthermore, data from repeated measurements are readily available insofar as the catheter resides in the jugular bulb. This technique currently appears to represent the most practical means for estimating the shunt flow ratio. Continuous monitoring of SjO_2 employing a fiberoptic catheter during the embolization procedure provided real-time information regarding the progress of embolization of the AVMs.

Conclusion

In contrast to angiographic assessment with a catheter selectively placed in a single feeding artery, changes in the shunt flow ratio as a whole can be detected by SjO_2. This technique has practical utility for real-time evaluation of the progress of embolization.

References

1. Bauer BL, Beck B, Moessler U (1975) Investigation on volume and pressure overloading of the heart in cerebral angiomas. In: Pia HW, Gleave JRW, Grote E, Zierski J (eds) Cerebral angiomas.Springer, Berlin, pp 101–110
2. Feindel W, Yamamoto YL, Hodge CP (1971) Red cerebral veins and the cerebral steal syndrome. Evidence from fluorescein angiography and microregional blood flow by radioisotopes during excision of an angioma. J Neurosurg 35:167–179
3. Cruz J, Miner ME, Allen SJ, et al (1990) Continuous monitoring of cerebral oxygenation in acute brain injury: injection of mannitol during hyperventilation. J Neurosurg 73:725–730
4. Robertson CS, Grossman RG, Goodman JC (1987) The predictive value of cerebral anaerobic metabolism with cerebral infarction after head injury. J Neurosurg 67:361–368
5. Sheinberg M, Kanter MJ, Robertson CS, et al (1992) Continuous monitoring of jugular venous oxygen saturation in head-injured patients. J Neurosurg 76:212–217
6. Sutton LN, McLaughlin AC, Dante S, et al (1990) Cerebral venous oxygen content as a measure of brain energy metbaolism with increased intracranial pressure and hyperventilation. J Neurosurg 73:927–932
7. Kusske JA, Kelly WA (1974) Embolization and reduction of the "steal" syndrome in cerebral arteriovenous malformations. J Neurosurg 40:313–321
8. Pelz DM, Fox AJ, Vinuela F, et al (1988) Preoperative embolization of brain AVMs with isobutyl-2-cyanoacrylate. AJNR 9:757–764
9. Spetzler RF, Martin NA, Carter LP, et al (1987) Surgical management of large AVMs by staged embolization and operative excision. J Neurosurg 67:17–28
10. Drake CG (1979) Cerebral arteriovenous malformations: considerations for and experience with surgical treatment in 166 cases. Clin Neurosurg 26:145–208
11. Spetzler RF, Martin NA (1986) A proposed grading system for arteriovenous malformations. J Neurosurg 65:476–483
12. Wilson CB, U HS, Domingue J (1979) Microsurgical treatment of intracranial vascular malformation. J Neurosurg 51:446–454
13. Fult D, Kelly DL Jr (1984) Natural history of arteriovenous malformations of the brain: a clinical study. Neurosurgery 15:658–662
14. Pasqualin A, Barone G, Cioffi F, et al (1991) The relevance of anatomic and hemodynamic factors to a classification of cerebral arteriovenous malformations. Neurosurgery 28:370–379
15. Batjer HH, Devous MD Sr, Meyer YJ, et al (1988) Cerebrovascular hemodynamics in arteriovenous malformation complicated by normal perfusion pressure breakthrough. Neurosurgery 22:503–509

Part 4

Jugular Bulb Oximetry in Head Injured Patients

$SjVO_2$ Monitoring in Head-Injured Patients

CLAUDIA S. ROBERTSON

Introduction

Studies of head-injured patients have demonstrated that a reduced cerebral blood flow (CBF) is associated with a poor neurological outcome [1]. Jugular venous oxygen saturation ($SjVO_2$) is theoretically a useful monitor for cerebral hypoxia and ischemia because it reflects the balance between oxygen delivery to the brain and oxygen consumption by the brain. Because both delivery and consumption parameters can be abnormal after a head injury, the relative balance between these two parameters is often more valuable information than the absolute level of either of the parameters alone. Any disturbance that increases cerebral oxygen consumption or decreases oxygen delivery may decrease $SjVO_2$. The purpose of this study was to examine the incidence and causes of jugular venous desaturation detected with continuous monitoring of $SjVO_2$.

Methods

Patient Population

Adult patients with severe head injury (Glasgow Coma Score, GCS ≤ 8) were studied during the first 5–10 days after injury. Patients with contraindications to a jugular catheter, such as those with spinal cord injury or severe coagulopathy, were excluded from the study.

Technique of $SjVO_2$ Monitoring

Fiberoptic Oxygen Saturation Catheters

The earliest oxygen saturation catheter that was used for continuous $SjVO_2$ monitoring was a 4 Fr umbilical artery catheter. The catheter was not

Department of Neurosurgery, Baylor College of Medicine, Scurlock Tower 6560 Fannin, Suite 944, Houston, Texas 77030 USA designed for use in the jugular bulb, and performance was less than optimal [2,3]. Recently, additional catheters have become available for regional oxygen saturation monitoring (Baxter Critical Care, Baxter Healthcare, Valencia, CA, USA). An evaluation of the new regional oxygen saturation catheters in 18 patients demonstrated better performance than that reported with the umbilical artery catheters (Table 1). Of the 197 comparisons of $SjVO_2$ measured by the catheter and from a blood sample drawn through the catheter, 80% of the catheter values were within 4 saturation units of the blood sample value and did not require recalibration of the catheter. In the current study, the first 132 patients were monitored with the umbilical artery catheter, and the most recent 45 patients were monitored with the regional oxygen saturation catheter.

Insertion of the Jugular Bulb Catheter

Several conventions have been used to determine which internal jugular vein is to be catheterized. If the injury is diffuse, then there is general agreement that the catheter should be placed on the side of the dominant venous drainage, which in most cases is the right side. Two methods are commonly used to verify which internal jugular vein accommodates the highest flow. The first method approaches the problem from a functional standpoint by employing sequential manual compression of each internal jugular vein [4]. The vein that, on compression, elicits the greater elevation in intracranial pressure is identified as the dominant side carrying the largest portion of cerebral venous outflow. The second method utilizes the admission head computed tomography (CT) scan to visualize which of the two jugular foramina is the largest, assuming that the larger foramen houses the largest jugular bulb [5].

If the injury is focal, some investigators have placed the catheter on the side of the most severe injury, arguing that this gives the best chance of obtaining the most abnormal values; others continue to place the catheter on the dominant side, arguing that this monitors the greatest portion of the brain and gives the highest blood flow, which may improve performance of the continuous oximetry catheters. The recent bilateral catheterization studies by Stocchetti et al. [5] suggest that there is not a reliable way to determine which internal jugular vein will have the most abnormal values, and therefore that the latter convention may be the most logical. For this study, the catheter was placed on the dominant side.

TABLE 1. Performance parameters for the new regional oxygen saturation catheters

Catheter type	Number of comparisons	Difference between catheter and blood sample SO_2 value	95% Confidence limits
Regional oxygen saturation catheter	197	-0.8 ± 8.0	1.2

Maintenance of the Jugular Bulb Catheter

Once inserted, the catheter is connected to a continuous flush device to keep the lumen patent. To minimize the risk of thrombosis of the vein, no medications or KCl are given through the catheter. The catheter is used only for SjVO$_2$ monitoring and blood sampling.

SjVO$_2$ monitoring has been used for as long as 14 days, although the average length of monitoring is 4–5 days. As with all intravascular catheters, the risk of infection increases with the duration of the monitoring. Some routine should be practiced, such as changing catheters every 5 days in patients who require prolonged monitoring. In addition, catheters should be removed earlier if there is suspicion of catheter sepsis or thrombosis of the internal jugular vein.

Normal SjVO$_2$ Values

Gibbs et al. [6] studied 50 normal young males and observed their SjVO$_2$ to range from 55% to 71% (mean, 61.8%). This is lower than normal mixed venous oxygen saturation, suggesting that the brain normally extracts oxygen more completely from arterial blood than do many organs.

Average SjVO$_2$ Values After Head Injury

In head-injured patients, the range for SjVO$_2$ is considerably wider than in normals. In the Ben Taub General Hospital (BTGH) series of patients with continuous measurement of SjVO$_2$ for the first 5–10 days after a severe head injury, the SjVO$_2$ averaged 68.1% $\pm$ 9.7% (range, 32%–96%) in 1329 measurements. The partial pressure of jugular venous oxygen (PJVO$_2$) averaged 37 $\pm$ 7 torr (range, 22–85 torr). These mean values are slightly higher average values than those reported in normal adults, and the range is much wider.

Diagnosis and Management of Jugular Venous Desaturation

Whenever SjVO$_2$ falls below 50%, the catheter light intensity value is checked to exclude poor catheter position as the cause. If the light intensity is unsatisfactory, the patient's head or the catheter may be repositioned. If the catheter position is determined to be correct, a sample of blood is withdrawn through the jugular venous catheter to verify appropriate calibration of the catheter. If the SjVO$_2$ value measured by the Co-Oximeter differs by more than 4% from the catheter value, then the catheter is recalibrated. If the SjVO$_2$ is confirmed to be less than 50%, then the cause of desaturation is systematically sought. Causes for a reduced arterial oxygen content are examined first. Arterial hypoxia is ruled out by measuring arterial oxygen saturation. If SaO$_2$ is less than 90%, the condition is corrected by increasing fractional inspired oxygen concentration (FiO_2) or adding positive end-expiratory pressure (PEEP). Hemoglobin concentration is measured to ensure that values are at least 9 mg/dl. If arterial oxygen content is not sufficiently reduced to explain the desaturation, then treatable causes of a reduced CBF are sought. Hypocapnia, hypotension, and intracranial hypertension are sought and appropriately treated. Cerebral vasospasm might be considered in cases in which no other systemic cause can be found and where intracranial pressure (ICP) is not sufficiently increased to impair cerebral perfusion pressure (CPP).

Results

One hundred seventy-seven patients had continuous monitoring of $SjVO_2$. The average age of the patients was 32.9 ± 14.7 years; 158 (89.3%) were men. Of the patients, 150 (84.7%) had closed head injuries and 27 (15.3%) had gunshot wounds; 134 (75.7%) of the patients were in coma (GCS ≤8) on admission to the hospital; and 43 (24.3%) had an initial GCS >8 but deteriorated within the first 48 h. The mean GCS was 6.8 ± 3.1 in the emergency room (ER) and 7.0 ± 2.6 on day 1 after injury.

Every attempt was made to start $SjVO_2$ monitoring as soon after admission as possible. The $SjVO_2$ catheter was inserted an average of 19.3 ± 31.8 h after admission to the neurological intensive care unit (NICU); 141 (79.7%) were inserted within 24 h of admission. One hundred and fifty-five (88%) catheters were placed on the right side, and 22 (12%) were on the left. Patients were monitored for an average of 97.1 ± 76.3 h.

One hundred and twelve episodes of jugular desaturation ($SjVO_2$ values less than 50%) were identified and confirmed by blood sampling in 69 (39%) of the 177 patients. Forty-three patients had one episode of desaturation, 15 patients had two episodes, 8 patients had three episodes, 1 patient had four episodes, 1 patient had five episodes, and 1 patient had six episodes. The causes of the episodes of jugular desaturation have been both systemic and cerebral (Table 2).

The occurrence of at least one episode of jugular desaturation was twice as common in patients with a reduced CBF, 70% compared to 29% in patients with a normal CBF and 34% in patients with an elevated CBF. This suggests that a reduced CBF does, in fact, predispose a patient to develop ischemia, and may explain the previously observed relationship between a reduced CBF and a poor outcome.

The relationship between outcome and transient jugular desaturation was examined in these 177 patients (Table 3). Sixty-four (36.1%) of the patients had a favorable outcome (good recovery or moderate disability), 56 patients (31.6%) were severely disabled or vegetative, and 57 (32.2%) died. There was a strong association between the occurrence of jugular desaturation and a poor neurological outcome ($P < .001$). Mortality rate was 21% in patients with no desaturations, compared to 37% in patients with one episode of

TABLE 2. Causes of episodes of jugular desaturation in 177 patients with severe head injury

Number of episodes	Cause of episodes
Systemic causes:	
16	Hypotension
6	Hypoxia
28	Hypocarbia
1	Anemia
Cerebral causes:	
53	Intracranial hypertension
1	Vasospasm
Both systemic and cerebral causes:	
7	Combinations of decreased cerebral perfusion pressure (CPP), hypocarbia, and anemia

TABLE 3. Relationship between the occurrence of episodes of jugular venous desaturation and neurological outcome

3-Month Glasgow Outcome Scale	Number of episodes of desaturation		
	None	One	Multiple
Good recovery/moderate disability	47 (44%)	13 (30%)	4 (15%)
Severe disability/vegetative	38 (35%)	14 (33%)	4 (15%)
Dead	23 (21%)	16 (37%)	18 (69%)
Total	108 (100%)	43 (100%)	26 (100%)

desaturation and 69% in patients with multiple episodes of desaturation. The percentage of patients with a poor neurological outcome (severely disabled, vegetative, or dead) was 56% in patients with no desaturations, 70% in patients with one desaturation, and 85% in patients with multiple desaturations.

The total time that SjVO$_2$ was less than 50% was significantly longer ($P = .002$) in the patients who died than in the patients who survived. The total duration of all episodes of desaturation averaged 1.3 ± 0.3 h in the patients who died, compared to 0.4 ± 0.2 h in patients with a good recovery or moderate disability and 0.4 ± 0.1 h in patients with a severe disability or vegetative.

Several factors including age, severity of injury, and type of injury are known to determine outcome from severe head injury. To examine the effect of these factors on the relationship between neurological outcome and jugular desaturation, logistic regression analysis was used. The final best fit model showed that even when adjusted for these determinants of outcome, the number of desaturations still has a significant association with outcome. One episode of desaturation doubled the risk of a poor outcome, and multiple episodes of desaturation were associated with a 14-fold increase in the risk of a poor outcome.

Discussion

Potential Complications of SjVO₂ Monitoring

Potential complications can be divided into two categories: those associated with insertion of the catheter, including carotid artery puncture, injury to nerves in the neck, and pneumothorax; and those associated with the catheter remaining in the jugular vein including infection, increase in ICP, and thrombosis.

Carotid puncture is the most common complication associated with the internal jugular vein catheterization, but rarely has a serious consequence, and the risk can be minimized by always making certain that the puncture is lateral to the carotid pulsation. In a study of 123 pediatric patients, Goetting and Preston [7] documented only 4 (3%) accidental carotid punctures while attempting to cannulate the internal jugular vein. Stocchetti et al. [8] recorded puncture of the carotid artery in 2 of 45 (4%) attempts. There were no sequelae in either of these series. Most arterial punctures can be managed conservatively without sequelae by applying local pressure for 10 min.

Line sepsis is a complication that is commonly associated with all types of indwelling catheters. Most studies have reported an overall rate of 0–5 episodes of infection per 100 catheters [9]. In the study by Goetting and Preston [7], no cases of line sepsis were observed over a mean catheter duration of 2.5 ± 1.6 days. In the Stocchetti study [8], catheter-induced infection occurred in 1.8% of 45 patients. Proper sterile technique in placement and maintenance of the jugular bulb catheter should minimize this risk.

Intracranial pressure can be increased by maneuvers that obstruct venous return from the brain, and it is reasonable to be concerned that a catheter in the jugular vein might raise ICP. The 4 Fr catheter that is used for SjVO₂ monitoring, however, is quite small relative to the lumen of the internal jugular vein. Stocchetti et al. [8] reported that there was a slight increase "of no clinical significance" during catheter insertion. Goetting and Preston [10] found no evidence that jugular bulb catheterization caused sufficient jugular venous obstruction to exacerbate elevated ICP.

Limitations of SjVO₂ Monitoring

The major limitations of SjVO₂ to detect cerebral hypoxia/ischemia are the anatomical restrictions. SjVO₂ is a monitor of global cerebral oxygenation. Regional ischemia can be present and not be detected by changes in SjVO₂. Also, because jugular venous blood may not be truly mixed cerebral blood, ischemia could occur in a part of the brain being drained by the opposite jugular vein. In addition, as CBF decreases, the amount of extracerebral contamination may become proportionally greater. This can artificially increase SjVO₂.

Nevertheless, with these limitations in mind, transient ischemic episodes can still be detected with this monitoring technique. Early detection of ischemia allows early treatment, hopefully before cerebral function is compromised.

Acknowledgments. This work was supported by NIH grant #PO1-NS26716.

References

1. Gopinath SP, Robertson CS, Contant CF, Hayes C, Feldman Z, Narayan RK, Grossman RG (1994) Jugular venous desaturation and outcome after head injury. J Neurol Neurosurg Psychiatry 57:717–723
2. Andrews PJ, Dearden NM, Miller JD (1991) Jugular bulb cannulation: description of a cannulation technique and validation of a new continuous monitor. Br J Anaesth 67:553–558
3. Sheinberg M, Kanter MJ, Robertson CS, Contant CF, Narayan RK, Grossman RG (1992) Continuous monitoring of jugular venous oxygen saturation in head-injured patients. J Neurosurg 76:212–217
4. Dearden NM (1991) Jugular bulb venous oxygen saturation in the management of severe head injury. Curr Opin Anaesth 4:279–286
5. Stocchetti N, Paparella A, Bridelli F, Bacchi M, Piazza P, Zuccoli P (1994) Cerebral venous oxygen saturation studied using bilateral samples in the jugular veins. Neurosurgery 34:38–44
6. Gibbs EL, Lennox WG, Nims LF, Gibbs FA (1942) Arterial and cerebral venous blood. Arterial-venous differences in man. J Biol Chem 144:325–332
7. Goetting MG, Preston G (1990) Jugular bulb catheterization: experience with 123 patients. Crit Care Med 18:1220–1223
8. Stocchetti N, Barbagallo M, Gordon CR, Mensi F, Paparella A, Piazza P, Serioli T (1991) Arterio-jugular difference of oxygen and intracranial pressure in comatose, head injured patients: I. Technical aspects and complications. Minerva Anestesiol 57:319–326
9. Seneff MG, Rippe JM (1985) Central venous catheters. In: Rippe JM, Irwin RS, Alpert JS, Dalen JE (eds) Intensive care medicine. Little, Brown, Boston, pp 16–33
10. Goetting MG, Preston G (1991) Jugular bulb catheterization does not increase intracranial pressure. Intensive Care Med 17:195–198

Intraoperative Monitoring of Jugular Venous Oxygen Saturation in Patients with Severe Head Injury

S.P. Gopinath, A.M. Ritter, and C.S. Robertson

Introduction

Recent studies have suggested that secondary insults occuring during the early hospitalization period and resulting in hypoxia/ischemia of the brain may significantly contribute to a poor outcome [1,2,3]. The continuous monitoring of jugular venous oxygen saturation ($SjVO_2$) has been shown to be useful in the identification of causes and in early treatment of jugular venous oxygen desaturation episodes [2,4].

Recently, cerebral blood flow (CBF) measurements have demonstrated significantly low values in patients with intracranial hematomas on admission to the hospital. However, because these CBF techniques are not continuous, it has not been possible to study the effects of hematoma evacuation on the reduced CBF [5–7].

The purpose of this study was to use continuous monitoring $SjVO_2$ to observe the consequences of surgery on relative CBF adequacy.

Methods

Six adult patients with a traumatic intracranial hematoma requiring surgery had a retrograde internal jugular bulb fiberoptic catheter inserted after obtaining consent from a relative. The catheter position was confirmed by radiography. Five patients had intracerebral hematoma, and one had a gunshot wound. The catheter reading during surgery was confirmed by obtaining a blood sample from the fiberoptic jugular catheter. $SjVO_2$ values obtained before and after evacuation of the hematoma were compared using a paired t test.

Department of Neurosurgery, Baylor College of Medicine, 6560 Fannin #944, Houston, Texas, 77030 USA

Results

The SjVO$_2$ values before opening of the bone flap and dural flap were less than 50% in four patients. All six patients had some increase in SjVO$_2$ as the intracranial hematoma was evacuated. In some patients, the increase in SjVO$_2$ was noticed as soon as the dural flap was opened, while in other patients the improvement was observed as the hematoma was being evacuated. Values for SjVO$_2$ are summarized in Table 1.

Figures 1 and 2 show examples of intraoperative SjVO$_2$ tracings in two patients with intracranial hematoma. In the first patient, the computed tomography (CT) scan taken on day 4 showed an intracerebral hematoma, and the SjVO$_2$ had dropped to less than 50% before surgery. When the dura was opened, the SjVO$_2$ value rose to more than 50%. In another patient who had an intracerebral hematoma, on the day-4 CT scan the intracranial

TABLE 1. Values for jugular venous oxygen saturation (SjVO$_2$) before and after evacuation of intracranial hematoma in six patients

Patient number	SjVO$_2$ value before craniotomy	Intraoperative SjVO$_2$ value after bone/dural opening
1	41.0	63.0
2	47.7	57.4
3	53.2	59.8
4	46.4	63.8
5	63.7	73.3
6	48.8	57.6
Mean	50.1 ± 7.7	62.5 ± 5.9

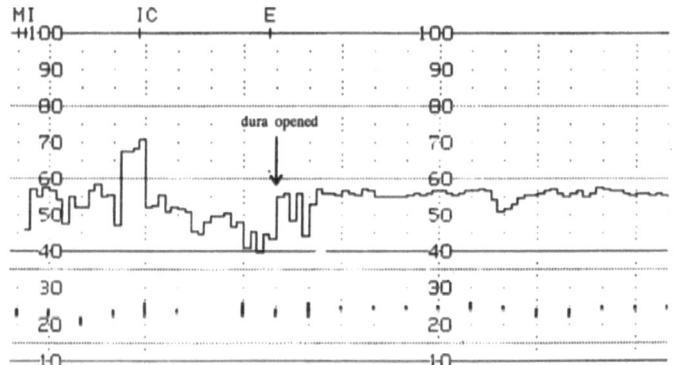

FIG. 1. A 23-year-old who was admitted with a small contusion following an automobile accident. On the fourth day after the injury, his intracranial pressure (ICP) increased and a repeat computed tomography (CT) scan showed coalescence of the contusion into an intracerebral hematoma. He was taken to surgery for evacuation of the hematoma. Intraoperative tracing showed an increase in SjVO$_2$ as the dura was opened

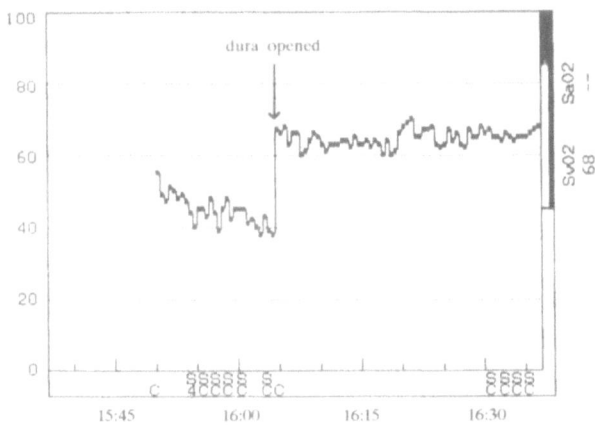

FIG. 2. A 37-year-old was admitted with a small contusion from an assault. Glasgow Coma Scale score was 13 on admission to the hospital. On the fourth day after the injury, he stopped following commands, and a repeat CT scan showed coalescence of the contusion into an intracerebral hematoma. He was taken to surgery for evacuation of the hematoma. Intraoperative tracing showed a marked increase in $SjVO_2$ as the dura was opened

pressure (ICP) was high and the $SjVO_2$ was less than 50%. As soon as the dura was opened, the $SjVO_2$ value improved dramatically.

Discussion

The continuous intraoperative monitoring of jugular venous oxygen saturation showed low $SjVO_2$ in five of six patients with intracranial hematoma, suggesting a relative inadequacy of CBF. The increase in the $SjVO_2$ value with evacuation of the hematoma suggests that the hematoma was causing the reduced cerebral oxygenation.

Acknowledgments. This work was supported by NIH grant #PO1-NS27616.

References

1. Contant CF, Robertson CS, Golpinath SP, Narayan RK, Grossman RG (1993) Determination of clinically important thresholds in continuously monitored patients with head injury. J Neurotrauma 10 (Suppl 1):S57
2. Gopinath SP, Robertson CS, Contant CF, Hayes C, Feldman Z, Narayan RK, Grossman RG (1994) Jugular venous desaturation and outcome after head injury. J Neurol Neurosurg Psychiatry 57:717–723

3. Piek J, Chesnut RM, Marshall LF, van Berkum-Clark M, Klauber MR, Blunt BA, Eisenberg HM, Jane JA, Marmarou A, Foulkes MA (1992) Extracranial complications of severe head injury. J Neurosurg 77:901–907
4. Sheinberg GM, Kanter MJ, Robertson CS, Contant CF, Narayan RK, Grossman RG (1992) Continuous monitoring of jugular venous oxygen saturation in head injured patients. J Neurosurg 76:212–217
5. Bouma GJ, Muizelaar JP, Choi SC, Newlon PG, Young HF (1991) Cerebral circulation and metabolism after severe traumatic brain injury: the elusive role of ischemia. J Neurosurg 75:685–693
6. Bouma GJ, Muizelaar JP, Stringer WA, Choi SC, Fatouros P, Young HF (1992) Ultraearly evaluation of regional cerebral blood flow in severely head injured patients using xenon-enhanced computerized tomography. J Neurosurg 77:360–368
7. Schroder ML, Muizelaar JP, Kuta AJ (1994) Documented reversal of global ischemia immediately after removal of an acute subdural hematoma. J Neurosurg 80:324–327

Multimodal Evaluation of Cerebral Oxygen Metabolism Disturbances in Patients with Severe Head Injury: Special Reference to Cerebrovascular CO_2 Reactivity

TOSHIYUKI SHIOGAI, AKIO NOGUCHI, EISHI SATO, AND ISAMU SAITO

Introduction

In the management of severe head injury patients, hyperventilation (HV) routinely has been used for reduction of intracranial pressure (ICP) or improvement of cerebral acidosis that might otherwise increase the risk of ischemic brain damage [1,2]. Cerebrovascular CO_2 reactivity induced by HV, which has a direct relationship with reduction of cerebral blood flow (CBF) and ICP [3], also has been suggested to have a close relationship with the prognosis of patients with severe head injuries [4,5]. This study was aimed at evaluating disturbances in cerebral oxygen metabolism and cerebral hemodynamics, and related factors, on the basis of CO_2 reactivity induced by HV in comatose patients with severe head injuries. To this end, we have introduced and analyzed a computerized multimodal system for continuously monitoring jugular bulb venous oxygen saturation (SjO_2), arterial oxygen saturation measured by pulse oximeter (SpO_2), transcranial Doppler (TCD), end-tidal CO_2 partial pressure ($PetCO_2$), ICP, cerebral perfusion pressure (CPP), and Fourier-transformed quantitative electroencephalogram (qEEG) [6].

Patients and Methods

The subjects were 16 patients with severe head injury aged from 15 to 72 years (mean, 41). On the basis of neuroimaging techniques, injury was classified as focal in 11 cases and diffuse in 5 cases. Glasgow Coma Scale (GCS) scores were 8 or less. Cerebral CO_2 reactivity tests were evaluated by mean velocity in the middle cerebral artery (Vm) on TCD and SjO_2, and correlations of SjO_2 with TCD parameters, ICP and CPP, and qEEG were

Department of Neurosurgery, Kyorin University School of Medicine, 6-20-2 Shinkawa, Mitaka, Tokyo 181, Japan

analyzed during HV. Data acquisition was carried out every 2 min for 30–40 min, and this was performed 1 to 5 times for each patient (total, 38 times) within 2 weeks after injury. SpO$_2$ was maintained at more than 97% during the tests.

The test results were classified on the basis of minimum SjO$_2$ during HV into an ischemic group (SjO$_2$ <55%; n = 13), a normal group (SjO$_2$, 55%–70%; n = 13), and a hyperemic group (SjO$_2$ ≥70%; n = 12). EEG was recorded in the parietal scalp (P3–A1 or P4–A2 montage) ipsilateral to TCD monitoring. qEEG was calculated by power spectral analysis, displayed on the compressed spectral array (CSA) to eliminate artifacts, and evaluated by serial changes of total power and absolute power bands 0–4 Hz, 4–8 Hz, 8–12 Hz, and 12–30 Hz (δ, θ, α, and β, respectively) (Fig. 1).

Differences in basic factors among the three groups such as age, GCS, type of injury (focal or diffuse), barbiturate therapy, and Glasgow outcome scale (GOS) at 1 month after injury, and correlations with SjO$_2$, were evaluated in terms of (1) Vm and CO$_2$ reactivity (ΔVm/ΔCO$_2$, ΔSjO$_2$/ΔCO$_2$), (2) ICP and CPP, (3) pulsatility index (PI = peak systolic velocity − end diastolic velocity/Vm) and estimated cerebrovascular resistance (CVR = CPP/Vm), and (4) total power (TP) and α power of qEEG.

In statistical analysis, differences in means were tested using the one-way analysis of variance (ANOVA), and differences in proportions were examined with the Kruskal–Wallis test.

Results

a. Basic factors among the three groups (Table 1): no significant differences were observed among the three groups with respect to age, GCS, barbiturate therapy, and GOS. Focal injury was relatively frequent in the ischemic group, but there was no significant difference in injury type among the three groups.

b. CO$_2$ reactivity and ICP and CPP (Table 2): no significant differences among the three groups were observed during CO$_2$ reactivity tests in terms of minimal and maximal PetCO$_2$ and ΔCO$_2$, mean ICP and CPP, and ΔICP and ΔCPP. ΔICP and ΔCPP tended to be high in the normal group, but not in the ischemic and hyperemic groups. Also, no significant differences in response to Vm were observed among the three groups. The SjO$_2$ response, however, was significantly high ($P < .05$) in the order of frequency (ischemic > normal > hyperemic).

c. Correlation of TCD parameters, ICP and CPP, with SjO$_2$ (Table 3): significant correlations with Vm ($P < .05$), CVR ($P < .01$), and PI ($P < .05$) were observed frequently in the ischemic group, less often in the normal group, and rarely in the hyperemic group. Correlation with ICP was also frequently identified in the ischemic group, followed by the normal group, but rarely in the hyperemic group. Correlation with CPP noticeably was rare in all three groups.

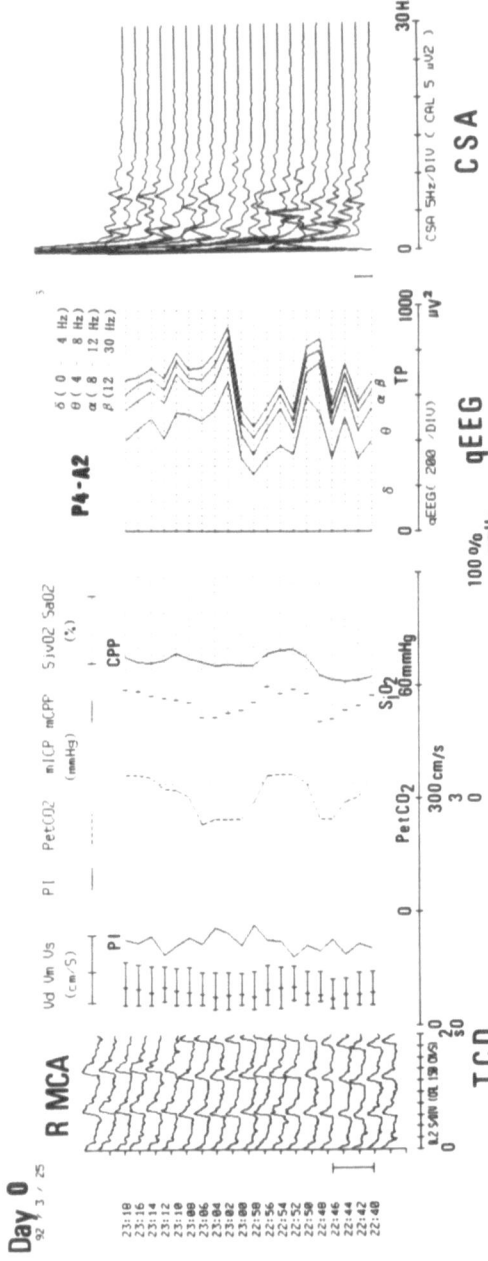

FIG. 1. Continuous monitoring on the day of head injury (day 0) during a cerebrovascular CO_2 reactivity test induced by hyperventilation of a 72-year-old patient with intracerebral hematoma in the right basal ganglionic region. Sequential changes recorded every 2 min are listed from *bottom* to *top*. From *left* to *right*: transcranial Doppler (*TCD*) waveforms in right middle cerebral artery (*RMCA*); parameters of TCD (end-diastolic velocity, *Vd*; mean velocity, *Vm*; peak systolic velocity, *Vs*; pulsatility index, *PI*); end-tidal CO_2 partial pressure (*PetCO$_2$*); mean intracranial pressure (*ICP*) and cerebral perfusion pressure (*CPP*); SjO_2 (*SjO$_2$*); arterial oxygen saturation measured by pulse oximeter, SpO_2 (*SaO$_2$*); absolute power spectral bands of quantitative EEG (*qEEG*) and compressed spectral arrays (*CSA*) at right parietal scalp (P4-A2 montage). $PetCO_2$ decreased by hyperventilation coincided with decreased SjO_2 below 50%, followed by increased δ and θ power bands, and slightly decreased α band to increased total power (*TP*) of qEEG

TABLE 1. Basic factors in the three groups based on minimal jugular bulb venous oxygen saturation (SjO$_2$) during hyperventilation[a]

	Ischemic	Normal	Hyperemic	P Values[b]
		Group		
n	13	13	12	
SjO$_2$ (%)	<55	55–70	≤70	
Age	41 ± 23	38 ± 20	37 ± 15	ns
GCS	5 ± 1.5	4 ± 1.5	4 ± 1.6	ns
Type of injury				ns
Focal	10	6	6	
Diffuse	3	7	6	
Barbiturate therapy	6	8	7	ns
GOS				ns
GR/MD	1	4	2	
SD/VS	10	8	8	
Dead	2	1	2	

GCS, Glasgow coma scale score; GOS, Glasgow outcome scale at 1 month after injury; GR, good recovery; MD, moderate disability; SD, severe disability; VS, vegetative state.
[a] Mean ± SD.
[b] ANOVA, Kruskal–Wallis test; ns, not significant ($P > .05$).

TABLE 2. Comparison of PetCO$_2$ and CO$_2$ reactivity, intracranial-pressure (ICP) and cerebral perfusion pressure (CPP) in the three groups during hyperventilation[a]

	Ischemic	Normal	Hyperemic	P Values[b]
		Group		
n	13	13	12	
SjO$_2$ (%)	<55	55–70	≥70	
PetCO$_2$ (mmHg)				
Minimal	23 ± 2.5	22 ± 2.0	24 ± 2.8	ns
Maximal	33 ± 2.5	32 ± 4.1	34 ± 2.8	ns
ΔCO$_2$ (mmHg)	10 ± 2.6	9.9 ± 3.0	11 ± 3.2	ns
Mean ICP (mmHg)	16 ± 5.5	14 ± 5.5	17 ± 13	ns
Mean CPP (mmHg)	65 ± 16	77 ± 16	63 ± 16	ns
ΔICP (mmHg)	7 ± 2.7	14 ± 13	8 ± 5.9	ns
ΔCPP (mmHg)	12 ± 6.3	19 ± 13	12 ± 5.1	ns
ΔVm/ΔCO$_2$	4.0 ± 1.9	3.8 ± 2.8	3.4 ± 2.0	ns
ΔSjO$_2$/ΔCO$_2$	1.9 ± 1.0	1.3 ± 0.8	0.8 ± 0.8	<.05

PetCO$_2$, end-tidal CO$_2$ partial pressure; Vm, mean velocity in middle cerebral artery.
[a] Mean ± SD.
[b] ANOVA; ns, not significant ($P > .05$).

d. Correlation with qEEG changes (increased TP and decreased α power) frequently was observed in the ischemic group (Figs. 1 and 2). qEEG changes of TP and α power were, to some degree, identified in all three groups (Fig. 2).

TABLE 3. Correlation coefficients of transcranial Doppler (TCD) parameters, ICP, and CPP with SjO_2[a]

| | Group | | | P Values[b] |
	Ischemic	Normal	Hyperemic	
n	13	13	12	
SjO_2 (%)	<55	55–70	≤70	
Vm (cm/s)	0.62 ± 0.37	0.27 ± 0.35	0.18 ± 0.40	<.05
CVR	−0.59 ± 0.28	−0.28 ± 0.29	−0.14 ± 0.40	<.01
PI	−0.47 ± 0.27	−0.18 ± 0.30	−0.18 ± 0.37	<.05
ICP (mmHg)	0.49 ± 0.49	0.34 ± 0.37	0.02 ± 0.49	ns
CPP (mmHg)	0.11 ± 0.50	−0.01 ± 0.46	−0.07 ± 0.42	ns

CVR = CPP/Vm.
[a] Mean ± SD.
[b] ANOVA; ns, not significant ($P > .05$).

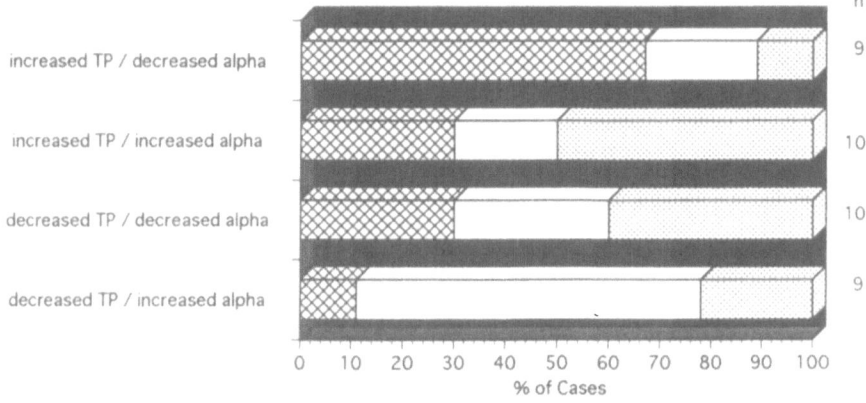

FIG. 2. Correlation between EEG and SjO_2 during a CO_2 reactivity test. TP, total power of qEEG. *Hatched bars*, ischemic ($SjO_2 < 55\%$); *white bars*, normal (SjO_2, 55%–70%); *dotted bars*, hyperemic ($SjO_2 > 70\%$)

Discussion

HV used to control ICP and to ameliorate cerebral acidosis in the management of acute severe head injury can result in reduction of CBF, which may produce brain ischemia [2]. The usefulness of SjO_2 monitoring, which can be evaluated by coupling CBF with cerebral metabolic rate of oxygen ($CMRO_2$), has been emphasized in the early detection of global ischemia during HV [1]. Our results confirmed a strong correlation of cerebral ischemia during HV detected by SjO_2 with decreased CBF and increased CVR [7,8], which is demonstrated by decreased Vm and increased PI. The importance of decreased CBF and increased CVR has been pointed out in the experimental development of ischemic brain damage after head injury [9]. Increased pulsatility of the Doppler velocity waveform reflects increased downstream vascular resistance during HV [10] or decreased intracranial compliance in relation to CPP [11] below an autoregulatory breakpoint of 70 mmHg [12]. In our ischemic and normal groups, there was a close correlation of SjO$_2$ with PI, but not with CPP. This discrepancy might result from relatively constant CPP values during HV above or around the threshold of the CPP breakpoint. The combined use of TCD and SjO$_2$ monitoring appears to be extremely useful in detecting early ischemic brain damage that cannot be evaluated by ICP or CPP alone, and in clarifying the underlying patho-physiology in severe head injury.

In our study, qEEG changes were observed during HV, especially increased TP and decreased α power in the ischemic group, which indicated CMRO$_2$ may change and affect SjO$_2$ values. This qEEG pattern has been pointed out in focal ischemia caused by chronic cerebrovascular accidents [13]. The slowing of EEG during active HV is thought to be the result of cerebral hypoxia as evidenced by decreased SjO$_2$ or jugular venous oxygen tension [14]. Generally, it is considered that CMRO$_2$ does not change during HV [15]. In our study, changes in total power and α power of qEEG were observed in almost all CO$_2$ reactivity tests during HV. These qEEG changes do suggest, however, that the possibility of increased CMRO$_2$ [4,7] or a relationship with anaerobic metabolism [16,17] should be taken into con-sideration, especially in cases of severe head injury.

Cerebrovascular CO$_2$ reactivity has a direct relationship with reduction of CBF and ICP [3]. In our study, despite an apparent decrease in CO$_2$ reactivity, based on SjO$_2$ (ΔSjO$_2$/ΔCO$_2$) in the order of ischemic group to normal and hyperemic groups, there was no significant difference among the three groups in preserved CO$_2$ reactivity based on TCD (ΔVm/ΔCO$_2$). This preserved CO$_2$ reactivity may indicate an inverse steal phenomenon [2] because there was a relatively large number of patients with focal injury. Increased CO$_2$ reactivity in hyperemic patients has been known and asso-ciated with increased ICP [18]. In our study, however, preserved CO$_2$ reactivity and decreased ICP during HV was observed in the hyperemic group, but was not always associated with intracranial hypertension. Our results support the preserved effectiveness of HV in hyperemic patients.

It has been suggested, based on a CBF study involving intravenous administration of xenon-133, that cerebrovascular CO$_2$ reactivity has a close relationship with prognosis of patients with severe head injury [4,5]. Jugular venous desaturation after severe head injury also contributes to a poor neurological outcome [19]. In the small series of our study, however, on the basis of SjO$_2$ monitoring during HV there were no apparent differences among the three groups. This difference may result from the timing of GOS assessment (1 month or 3 months after injury), the lower cutoff value of SjO$_2$ (50% or 55%), or the duration of desaturation. On the basis of TCD findings, disturbed CO$_2$ reactivity also did not predict an unfavorable outcome [20].

Therefore, there are risks of false prediction in which different modalities or methods of evaluation of CO_2 reactivity may result in different prognostic significances of patients with severe head injuries.

Conclusions

Cerebral ischemia during HV is closely related to cerebrovascular CO_2 reactivity, evaluated by SjO_2 monitoring, caused by decreased cerebral circulation and increased CVR, less frequently related to ICP and EEG changes, and scarcely related to CPP. Contributions to prediction of neurological outcome by CO_2 reactivity based on SjO_2 monitoring, however, are not obvious in patients with severe head injuries.

Acknowledgments. This work was supported by the Tokyo Institute of Medical Science, Japan.

References

1. Cruz J, Miner ME (1986) Modulating cerebral oxygen delivery and extraction in acute traumatic coma. In: Miner ME, Wagner KA (eds) Neurotrauma. Treatment, rehabilitation, and related issues. Butterworths, Boston, pp 55–72
2. Patel PM (1993) Hyperventilation as a therapeutic intervention: do the potential benefits outweigh the known risks? J Neurosurg Anesthesiol 5:62–65
3. Marmarou A, Bandoh K, Yoshihara M, Tsuji O (1993) Measurement of vascular reactivity in head-injured patients. Acta Neurochir 59(Suppl):18–21
4. Nordström CH, Messeter K, Sundbärg G, Schalén W, Werner M, Ryding E (1988) Cerebral blood flow, vasoreactivity, and oxygen consumption during barbiturate therapy in severe traumatic brain lesions. J Neurosurg 68:424–431
5. Schalén W, Messeter K, Nordström CH (1991) Cerebral vasoreactivity and the prediction of outcome in severe traumatic brain lesions. Acta Anaesthesiol Scand 35:113–122
6. Shiogai T, Sato E, Fujii Y, Takeuchi K, Saito I (1993) Continuous monitoring of transcranial Doppler, jugular venous oxygen saturation, and quantitative EEG in severe head injury. In: Nakamura N, Hashimoto T, Yasue M (eds) Recent advances in neurotraumatology. Springer, Berlin Heidelberg New York Tokyo, pp 297–300
7. Kety SS, Schmidt CF (1946) The effects of active and passive hyperventilation on cerebral blood flow, cerebral oxygen consumption, cardiac output, and blood pressure of normal young men. J Clin Invest 25:107–119
8. Pierce EC, Lambertsen CJ, Deutsch S, Chase PE, Linde HW, Dripps RD, Price HL (1962) Cerebral circulation and metabolism during thiopental anesthesia and hyperventilation in man. J Clin Invest 41:1664–1671
9. Pfenninger EG, Reith A, Breitig D, Grünert A, Ahnefeld FW (1989) Early changes of intracranial pressure, perfusion pressure, and blood flow after acute head injury: Part 1. An experimental study of the underlying pathophysiology. J Neurosurg 70:774–779

10. Beasley MG, Blau JN, Gosling RG (1979) Changes in internal carotid artery flow velocities with cerebral vasodilation and constriction. Stroke 10:331–335

11. Nelson RJ, Czosnyka M, Pickard JD, Maksymowics W, Perry S, Martin JL, Lovick AHJ (1992). Experimental aspects of cerebrospinal hemodynamics: the relationship between blood flow velocity waveform and cerebral autoregulation. Neurosurgery 31:705–710

12. Chan KH, Miller JD, Dearden NM, Andrews PJD, Midgley S (1992) The effect of changes in cerebral perfusion pressure upon middle cerebral artery blood flow velocity and jugular bulb venous oxygen saturation after severe brain injury. J Neurosurg 77:55–61

13. Slug I (1984) Quantitative EEG as a measure of brain dysfunction. In: Pfurtscheller G, Jonkman EJ, Lopes da Silva FH (eds) Brain ischemia: quantitative EEG and imaging techniques. Progress in brain research, vol 62. Elsevier, Amsterdam, pp 65–84

14. Gotoh F, Meyer JS (1965) Cerebral effects of hyperventilation in man. Arch Neurol 12:410–423

15. Alexander SC, Cohen PJ, Wollman H, Smith TC, Reivich M, Molen RAV (1965) Cerebral carbohydrate metabolism during hypocarbia in man: studies during nitrous oxide anesthesia. Anesthesiology 26:624–632

16. Alexander SC, Smith TC, Strobel G, Stephen GW, Wollman H (1968) Cerebral carbohydrate metabolism of man during respiratory and metabolic alkalosis. J Appl Physiol 24:66–72

17. Michenfelder JD, Sundt TM (1973) The effect of PaCO$_2$ on the metabolism of ischemic brain in squirrel monkeys. Anesthesiology 38:445–453

18. Obrist WD, Lagfitt TW, Jaggi JL, Cruz J, Gennarelli TA (1984) Cerebral blood flow and metabolism in comatose patients with acute head injury. J Neurosurg 61:241–253

19. Robertson C (1993) Desaturation episodes after severe head injury: influence on outcome. Acta Neurochir 59(Suppl):98–101

20. Steiger H-J, Aaslid R, Stoos R, Seiler RW (1994) Transcranial Doppler monitoring in head injury: relations between type of injury, flow velocities, vasoreactivity, and outcome. Neurosurgery 34:79–86

Continuous Monitoring of Jugular Bulb Oxygen Saturation in the Management of Patients with Severe Closed Head Injury

Yasufumi Mizutani[1], Tsuyoshi Katabami[1], Masahiko Udzura[1], Takeki Ogawa[1], Hiroaki Sekino[3], Yoshio Taguchi[3], and Ikuo Yamanaka[2]

Introduction

Continuous monitoring of intracranial pressure (ICP) is essential in the management of the patients with severe head injury, and various methods to decrease ICP have been utilized [1]. Hyperventilation, however, may occasionally cause inadequate cerebral perfusion, resulting in secondary brain damage in patients with increased ICP [2]. We have performed experimental and clinical studies using simultaneous monitoring of ICP and jugular bulb oxygen saturation (SjO_2) with a fiberoptic catheter to evaluate dynamic changes in cerebral perfusion and cerebral metabolic rate, with the aim of finding an appropriate treatment strategy for patients with severe head injury [3]. On the basis of our previous data [3] and a review of the literature [4,5], it was considered that a value for SjO_2 less than 50% indicated hypoperfusion and a value more than 80% suggested hyperemia. We present herein our early experience of the management of severely head-injured patients by using simultaneous monitoring of ICP and SjO_2 and discuss the treatment protocol we have developed.

Material and Methods

Patient Selection

This series consisted of 15 comatose patients with severe head injury in whom a simultaneous measurement of ICP and SjO_2 was made continuously. Immediately after each patient's arrival, resuscitative treatment and neuro-

[1] Department of Neurosurgery and [2] Department of Critical Care Medicine, Yokohama City Seibu Hospital, St. Marianna University School of Medicine, and [3] Division of Neurosurgery, The Second Department of Surgery, St. Marianna University School of Medicine, 1197-1 Yasashi-cho, Asahi-ku, Yokohama, Japan

logical assessment were made. The patients were examined by a computed tomography (CT) scan as soon as possible and assessed using the CT criteria advocated by Marshall et al. [6]. In patients with diffuse brain injury type II and III, continuous monitoring of SjO_2 and ICP was employed. When a large extraparenchymatous hematoma was found, the mass was evacuated before employing this monitoring. The following patients were precluded: patients in whom the monitoring systems did not work properly for various reasons, and patients who had pulmonary injury or severe systemic injury, shown by abnormal laboratory data such as hypoxia or severe blood loss.

Measurements of SjO_2 and ICP

A fiberoptic 4 Fr catheter system (Opticath and Oximetric III, Abbott Laboratories, Abbott Park, IL, USA) was used for continuous measurement of SjO_2. This catheter tip was placed in the right jugular bulb at the level between the skull and the top of the C-2 vertebra; placement was confirmed with a plain X-ray film. The system was calibrated in vivo using blood slowly withdrawn from the catheter. During continuous monitoring of SjO_2, the system was recalibrated every 8 h. The saturation of the systemic arterial blood (SaO_2) was monitored by pulse oximetry at the patient's finger.

ICP was measured with a subdural pressure monitoring system (Camino kit, digital pressure monitor model 420, Camino Laboratories, San Diego, CA, USA) inserted through a burrhole made on the frontal convexity in most patients. In the patients from whom masses had been evacuated, this pressure monitoring system was placed through the craniotomy. Increased ICP was defined as more than 20 torr.

In a few patients, local cerebral blood flow (LCBF) and brain temperature were monitored simultaneously by using a laser Doppler flowmeter in addition to continuous monitoring of SjO_2 and ICP.

Illustrative Case Presentations

Case 1

A 22-year-old man had a road traffic accident and was transferred to our hospital immediately after the injury. The initial Glasgow Coma Scale score (GCS) was 8 (E1, V2, M5). A CT scan showed a high-density spot in the posterior part of the corpus callosum, but no signs suggesting increased ICP. Laboratory examination including a complete blood count and a blood gas analysis showed no abnormalities. He was treated conservatively under the simultaneous monitoring of ICP and SjO_2 (Fig. 1). The initial values were within normal range. However, 14 h later, SjO_2 decreased to less than 50%, although ICP remained normal and other vital signs were stable. These data were highly suggestive of dehydration. Soon after administration of physiological saline, the SjO_2 returned to normal. The patient recovered uneventfully and returned to his previous life-style.

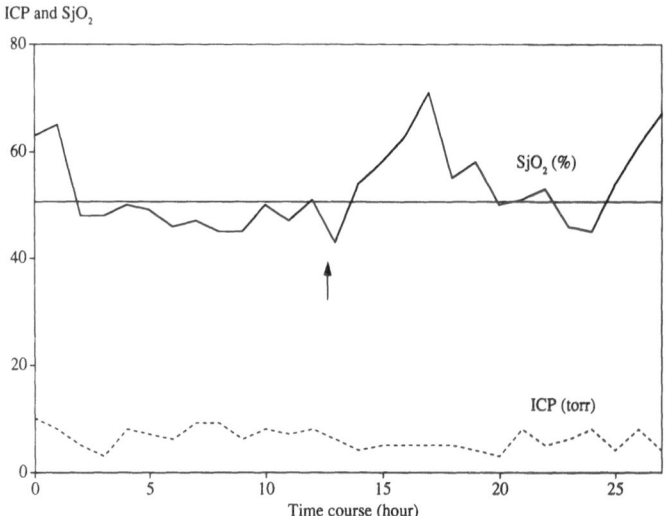

FIG. 1. Case 1: 22-year-old man with a diffuse brain injury, type II [6]. Fourteen hours after starting the continuous monitoring, jugular bulb oxygen saturation (SjO$_2$) decreased to less than 50%, although intracranial pressure (ICP) remained normal. The administration of physiological saline (*arrow*) was able to normalize the value for SjO$_2$

Case 2

A 46-year-old man was struck by a car while he was riding a bicycle. His GCS on admission was 8 (E2, V1, M5). A CT scan showed a massive subdural hematoma associated with cerebral contusion, and an evacuation of the hematoma was made as soon as feasible. Immediately after the operation, his ICP showed more than 70 torr and the SjO$_2$ value was about 30% (Fig. 2). Because administration of mannitol alone failed to control ICP, barbiturate coma therapy was introduced. This brought gradual changes in both ICP and SjO$_2$ in a symmetrical fashion, presumably because of decreased cerebral metabolic rate. Although the SjO$_2$ value was maintained normally over the following several hours, it decreased again with the increase of ICP. This suggested an uncontrollable brain swelling, and the patient eventually deteriorated into brain death.

Case 3

A 26-year-old man suffered a traffic accident while riding a motorcycle. His admission GCS score was 5 (E1, V1, M3). He was intubated. A CT scan revealed thin subarachnoid hemorrhage in the interhemispheric and basal cisterns, but no intraparenchymatous abnormalities except for a mild brain swelling. Multiple monitoring for SjO$_2$, ICP, LCBF, brain temperature, and end-tidal CO$_2$ was made continuously (Fig. 3). Because of mechanical ventilation, arterial oxygen saturation (SaO$_2$) indicated 100% during the

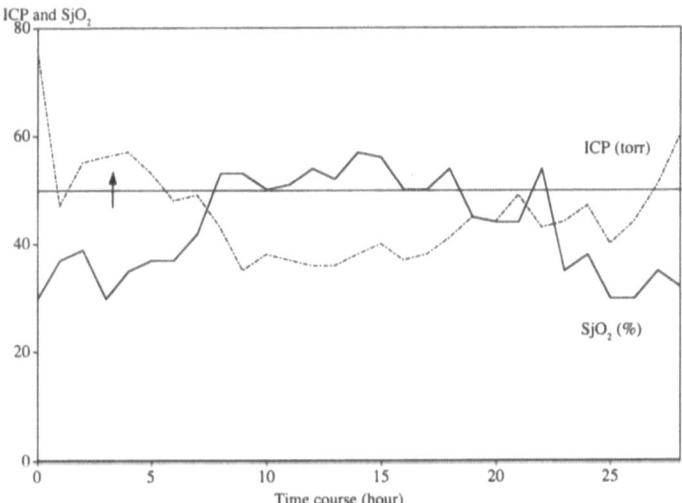

FIG. 2. Case 2: 46-year-old man with a massive subdural hematoma associated with cerebral contusion. The induction of barbiturate coma therapy (*arrow*) reduced ICP and increased SjO_2 considerably during the following several hours. However, this therapy eventually failed to control both ICP and SjO_2

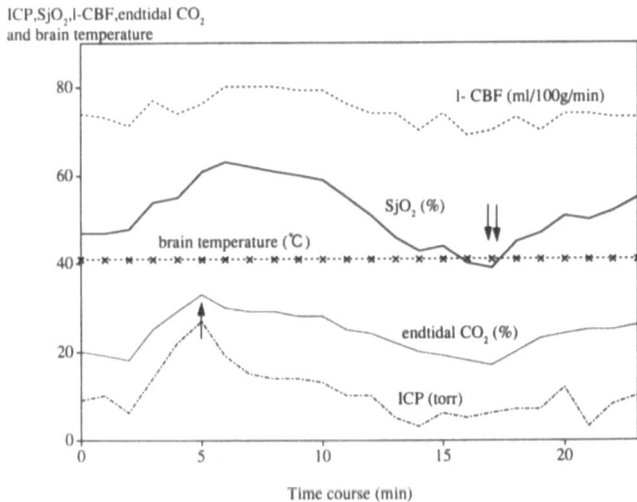

FIG. 3. Case 3: 26-year-old man with a diffuse brain injury, type III [6]. Multiple monitoring for SjO_2, ICP, local cerebral blood flow (LCBF), brain temperature, and end-tidal CO_2 was made continuously. On the third day of hospitalization, ICP increased to 28 torr, so that hyperventilation was applied (*single arrow*). This normalized ICP, but resulted in a decrease of SjO_2 below the normal limit. After cessation of hyperventilation (*double arrows*), the SjO_2 as well as ICP returned to normal values

following treatment period and was not shown. On his third day in hospital, ICP increased to 28 torr, and hyperventilation was applied. This caused SjO_2 to decrease below the normal limit, although ICP became normal. Along with the changes of end-tidal CO_2, LCBF decreased gradually. This change of LCBF was quite similar to that of SjO_2. When the artificial ventilation was returned to the previous setting, SjO_2 as well as LCBF returned to normal values. One month later, the patient became able to obey verbal commands, but remained bedridden because of a right femur fracture.

Discussion

Knowing cerebral blood flow (CBF) and the cerebral metabolic rate of oxygen ($CMRO_2$) as well as ICP is undoubtedly the most important factor in the management of the patients with severe head injury because cerebral ischemia is a common mechanism of secondary brain injury [7]. Robertson et al. [8] measured $CMRO_2$ and the cerebral metabolic rate of lactate, as well as CBF at the bedside, and reported that those measurements could indicate the presence of an evolving ischemic infarct after head injury. However, those measurements may involve technical difficulty and complexity. On the other hand, recent advances in fiberoptic technology are able to provide continuous measurement of SjO_2 with a simple procedure, and SjO_2 has been proven to reflect global cerebral hyperemia or ischemia sensitively [9]. The value for SjO_2 in normal individuals was reportedly 65%; values greater than 50% were considered to be acceptable [4]. When SjO_2 dropped to less than 50% (desaturation), global cerebral ischemia was indicated in most cases.

Cruz et al. [10] found a significant difference in outcome between patients with episodes of systemic hypoxemia and those without these episodes, and concluded that continuous monitoring was useful because it gave an outline assessment of oxygen delivery, established causal relationship for desaturation, and allowed for shorter response times to remedy hypoxemia once it was detected. However, several technical errors or systemic physiological abnormalities will produce a decreased value for SjO_2. Hence, desaturation may not always indicate decreased CBF. After confirming calibration of the catheter, the catheter position, SaO_2, and hemoglobin concentration should be checked before starting treatment for reduced CBF [5].

In our case 1, the cause of desaturation was thought to be merely dehydration, and the administration of physiological saline normalized a reduced value for SjO_2 immediately. We have encountered such episodes in several patients. In a similar situation in which the value for SjO_2 is reduced to less than 50% and ICP remains normal, an initial stage of vasospasm should be kept in mind. No matter what the cause, a circulatory volume expansion would be the initial treatment in this situation.

When increased ICP and desaturation are present at the same time, as in case 2, a cerebral ischemia is highly suggested. We have experienced this type of abnormality in 9 of 15 patients. In this case, control of ICP seems to be essential and mannitol should be given first. If the value for SjO_2 tends to increase and maintain its normal range after hyperventilation, this remedy can be justified. However, our experience revealed that hyperventilation caused a further decrease of the SjO_2 value in most patients who showed increased ICP and desaturation simultaneously. Therefore, hyperventilation would not be the treatment of choice in the situation just described.

We believe this strategy prevents secondary brain damage caused by inadequate cerebral perfusion. If increased ICP is refractory to the administration of mannitol, barbiturate coma therapy will be used. Theoretically, barbiturate can provide a decrease of cerebral metabolic rate [11] offering a decrease of ICP and consequently an increase in the SjO_2 value. Although the initial response to barbiturate was considerable in the majority of our patients who were induced to barbiturate coma, both ICP and SjO_2 eventually became uncontrollable, as seen in case 2. Recently, mild hypothermia treatment has been revived, and there have been several reports of the clinical application of mild hypothermia for patients with severe head injury [12]. This strategy may open the door for the treatment of uncontrollable ICP, but will need multiple continuous monitoring as we did in case 3 for safe management.

When ICP is high and SjO_2 is more than 80%, there must be hyperemia or arteriovenous shunt. In head-injured patients, this type of abnormality seemed to be related to brain swelling, in other words, increased cerebral blood volume [13]. Although we have experienced only two such cases, hyperventilation would be the treatment of choice.

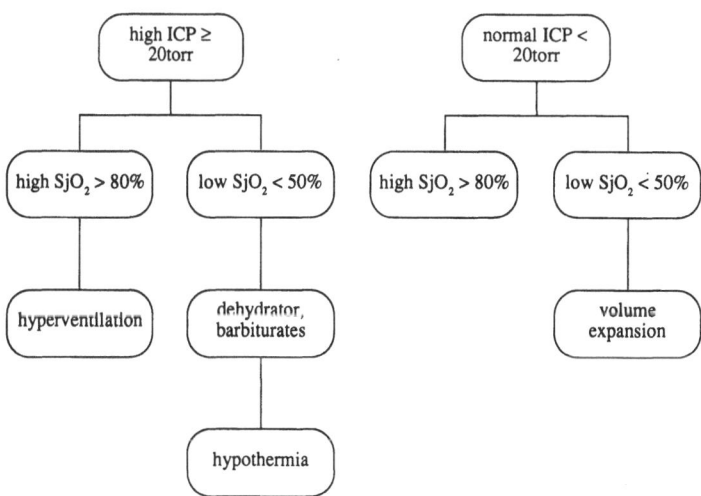

FIG. 4. A treatment protocol we have developed for patients with severe head injury uses continuous monitoring of ICP and SjO_2 simultaneously

Conclusions

Based on the foregoing considerations, we have developed a treatment protocol for patients with severe head injury by using a continuous monitoring of ICP and SjO_2 simultaneously (Fig. 4). Three of four types of abnormality have been discussed. The fourth type of abnormality consisted of normal ICP and increased SjO_2. Theoretically, this is a possibility but we have never experienced this type of abnormality.

Our experience is still limited, but we can conclude that simultaneous monitoring of SjO_2 and ICP is useful for the evaluation of the intracranial environment, offering an appropriate treatment strategy for patients with severe head injury.

References

1. Taguchi Y, Ogawa T, Sekino H (1988) Brain injury and intracranial pressure. Clin Neurosci 6:1118–1120
2. Obrist WD, Langfitt TW, Jaggi JL, Cruz J, Gennarelli TA (1984) Cerebral blood flow and metabolism in comatose patients with acute head injury. Relationship to intracranial hypertension. J Neurosurg 61:241–253
3. Katabami T (1993) The relationship between cerebral venous oxygen saturation and cerebral blood flow in focal brain injury: an experimental study. St Marianna Med J 21:725–736
4. Gibbs EL, Lennox WG, Nims LF, Gibbs FA (1942) Arterial and cerebral venous blood. Arterial-venous differences in man. J Biol Chem 144:325–332
5. Sheinberg M, Kanter MJ, Robertson CS, Contant CF, Narayan RJ, Grossman RG (1992) Continuous monitoring of jugular venous oxygen saturation in head-injured patients. J Neurosurg 76:212–217
6. Marshall LF, Marshall SB, Klauber MR, Clark MVB, Eisenberg HM, Jane JA, Luerssen TG, Marmarou A, Foulkes MA (1991) A new classification of head injury based on computerized tomography. J Neurosurg 75:S14–S20
7. Graham DI, Adams JH (1971) Ischemic brain damage in fatal head injuries. Lancet 1:265–266
8. Robertson CS, Grossman RG, Goodman JC, Narayan RK (1987) The predictive value of cerebral anaerobic metabolism with cerebral infarction after head injury. J Neurosurg 67:361–368
9. Andrews PJD, Dearden NM (1990) Validation of the Oximetrix III for continuous monitoring of jugular bulb oxygen saturation: comparison with IL 282 in vitro co-oximeter (abstrt). Br J Anaesth 64:393–394
10. Cruz J, Miner ME, Allen SJ, Alves WM, Gennarelli TA (1990) Continuous monitoring of cerebral oxygenation in acute brain injury: injection of mannitol during hyperventilation. J Neurosurg 73:725–730
11. Astrup J, Sorensen PM, Sorensen HR (1981) Inhibition of cerebral oxygen and glucose consumption in the dog by hypothermia, pentobarbital, and lidocaine. Anesthesiology 55:263–268
12. Shiozaki T, Sugimoto H, Taneda M, Yoshida H, Imai A, Yoshioka T, Sugimoto T (1993) Effect of mild hypothermia on uncontrollable intracranial hypertension after severe head injury. J Neurosurg 79:363–368

13. Langfitt TW, Gennarelli TA, Obrist WD, Bruce DA, Zimmerman RA (1982) Prospects for the future in the diagnosis and management of head injury: pathophysiology, brain imaging, and population-based studies. Clin Neurosurg 29:353–376

CO_2 Reactivity and Autoregulation in Severe Head Injury: Bedside Assessment by Relative Changes in Arteriojugular Differences of Oxygen

Juan Sahuquillo[1], Marcelino Báguena[2], Laura Campos[2], and Montserrat Olivé[3]

Introduction

It has been demonstrated both clinically and in experimental models that autoregulation and CO_2 reactivity can be impaired independently of each other in many brain insults, the so-called dissociated vasoparalysis [1]. The theoretical combination of preserved CO_2 reactivity and impaired or absent autoregulation can have many clinical implications in the overall daily management of brain-injured patients. To optimize their treatment, a bedside assessment of autoregulation and CO_2 reactivity is desirable. In spite of some unresolved and controversial methodological problems, monitoring hemodynamic parameters through a reverse catheter with its tip in the jugular bulb is an easy way of monitoring brain metabolism and cerebral blood flow (CBF) coupling and in some cases of estimating CBF [2–4]. When the cerebral metabolic rate of oxygen ($CMRO_2$) is constant, changes in arteriojugular differences of oxygen ($AVDO_2$) reflect changes in CBF [5]. In this situation, relative changes in $AVDO_2$ can be viewed as inverse changes in CBF and used as an evaluation method of CO_2 reactivity and autoregulation. Our aims in this chapter are to use relative changes in $AVDO_2$ after manipulations of mean arterial blood pressure and arterial pCO_2 to assess CO_2 reactivity and autoregulation in severe head injury patients.

Patients and Methods

In 48 consecutive severe head injury patients (postresuscitation, prehospital or admission Glasgow Coma Score (GCS) ≤ 8) with a mean age of 30 ± 18.4 years and a diffuse brain injury, cerebrovascular response to changes in

---

Department of Neurosurgery[1], Neurotraumatology Intensive Care Unit[2], and Anesthesiology Department[3], Vall d'Hebron University Hospital, Osona 6, 2-4, Barcelona 08023, Spain

pCO$_2$ was tested within the first 24 h after injury. Diffuse brain injury was considered in all the patients with no midline shift above 3 mm and no measured focal lesions above 25 ml. In 28 of these patients, autoregulation was also assessed. Immediately after admission a radial artery was canalized in each patient and a 14G catheter inserted percutaneously in the internal jugular bulb (IJ) using the technique described by Goetting and Preston [6]. The catheter was placed, whenever possible, in the right jugular bulb. X-Ray verification of the catheter position was obtained in all patients before obtaining jugular blood samples. Those cases with inappropriate situation of the reverse IJ catheter were excluded. Arterial and jugular blood samples were obtained at the same time, at least twice during the first 24 h after injury. AVDO$_2$ were calculated by the following equation: AVDO$_2$ = 1.34 × Hb(SaO$_2$ − SjO$_2$).

CO$_2$ Reativity Studies

To test CO$_2$ reactivity, and as a first step, arterial and jugular blood samples were extracted to establish baseline values for pCO$_2$ (pCO$_{2B}$), arterial pO$_2$, oxyhemoglobin saturation in the jugular bulb (SjO$_{2B}$), arterial oxyhemoglobin saturation (SaO$_2$), hemoglobin content (Hb), and basal arteriojugular differences of oxygen (AVDO$_2$B). Basal intracranial pressure (ICP$_B$) and mean arterial blood pressure (MABP) were also determined. These values were used as a reference for the following manipulations of arterial pCO$_2$. As a second step, manipulations in the ventilator settings were made to change the arterial pCO$_{2B}$. The goals in changing ventilator parameters were to increase or decrease arterial pCO$_2$ toward the "normoventilation range." To simplify these tests, and to avoid unnecessary ventilator manipulations, in those patients with a basal pCO$_2$ below 40 mmHg the ventilator settings were manipulated to increase the arterial pCO$_2$, while in those with pCO$_2$ above or equal to 40 mmHg the manipulations were directed to reduce arterial pCO$_2$. The mean absolute change in arterial pCO$_2$ in the entire group was 4.4 ± 2.3 mmHg (mean ± SD). After 10–15 min of the ventilator manipulations, AVDO$_2$ and all parameters were recalculated. Assuming a constant CMRO$_2$ during the test, changes in AVDO$_2$ reflect inverse changes in CBF. A relative CBF value (1/ADVO$_2$) was calculated from baseline AVDO$_2$ and was expressed as 100% [7]. Changes in 1/AVDO$_2$ after pCO$_2$ manipulation give a good estimate of changes in global CBF [7]. Two different indexes were calculated: (1) specific or absolute CO$_2$ reactivity (CO$_2$R$_{ABS}$) and (2) percentage reactivity (CO$_2$R%) [8]. Absolute reactivity refers to the absolute change of AVDO$_2$ per mmHg change in the arterial pCO$_2$ and was calculated as the change in AVDO$_2$ divided by the measured change in pCO$_2$: ΔAVDO$_2$/ΔpCO$_2$ [8]. The results were expressed as μmol/mmHg pCO$_2$. Percentage reactivity was calculated as the percent increase or decrease of estimated CBF (1/AVDO$_2$) per mmHg change in pCO$_2$. This index was calculated according to the following equation: ((1/AVDO$_2$H − 1/AVDO$_2$B)/1/AVDO$_2$B) × 100, where AVDO$_2$H is AVDO$_2$ after ventilator manipulations. The resulting percent change in estimated CBF was then divided by the ΔpCO_2 and the absolute value was considered. In this study, changes with hyper- and hypoventilation were grouped together. To avoid contamination of the results by hypoxemia-induced changes in CBF, patients with any pO_2 value less than 60 mmHg were excluded. Any patient with changes in MABP greater than 10 mmHg were also excluded to avoid superimposing changes in $AVDO_2$ provoked by autoregulatory mechanisms.

Testing Autoregulation

Changes in global CBF were estimated from repeated measurements of $1/AVDO_2$. To avoid oligemic insults, only $AVDO_2$ response to induced hypertension was studied in 28 patients. In all of them, CO_2 reactivity had been studied previously. In every patient, and to avoid influences of pCO_2 in the autoregulatory response, manipulations of the ventilator settings were done when necessary to obtain a baseline pCO_2 in the normoventilation range (35–45 mmHg). In each case, direct measurement of MABP was performed through a catheter introduced into the radial artery. In hemodynamically stable patients, phenylephrine was used to increase MABP by about 25%. Mean increase in blood pressure (BP) in the entire group was 25 ± 9 mmHg (mean ± SD). Arterial and jugular blood samples to calculate $AVDO_2$ were obtained before (baseline) and after a steady state of MABP was attained. All $AVDO_2$ values were corrected for changes in pCO_2 using CO_2R_{ABS} calculated in the previous study. Corrected changes were used in the calculations of the autoregulatory response. The percent change of $1/AVDO_2$ relative to the resting value was calculated according to the following equation: $\%AVDO_2 = ((1/AVDO_2B - 1/ADVDO_2H)/1/ABDO_2B) \times 100$. According to $\%AVDO_2$, and following the values seen in the following paragraphs, patients were classified as those with preserved autoregulation and those with impaired/absent cerebrovascular response to increased MABP.

Normal Range

The $CO_2R\%$ was used to separate patients with impaired/absent CO_2 reactivity from those with preserved CO_2 reactivity. From different published studies, the mean percent change of CBF per mmHg pCO_2 in normal awake hyperventilating volunteers ranged from 1.8 to 2.3 [9,10]. The calculated lower 2.5 percentile varied from different published studies because of the low number of cases studied. The lower 2.5 percentile in the McHenry study was 0.8 [11] and 1.2 in the Kety study [9]. Therefore, patients with $CO_2R\%$ greater than 1% were considered to be in the intact CO_2 reactivity group, and patients in whom $CO_2R\%$ was less than or equal to 1% were included in the impaired/absent CO_2 reactivity group.

If autoregulation is intact, no changes in CBF are expected when increasing MABP within the limits of autoregulatory curve. According to

Enevoldsen and Jensen's criteria [12], those patients with changes in $1/AVDO_2$ less than or equal to 20% were included in the intact autoregulation group. Patients with estimated CBF changes ($1/AVDO_2$) greater than 20% were classified as in the impaired/absent autoregulation group.

Results

The mean age of our series was 28 ± 16.7 years (mean $\pm$ SD) with a range from 14 to 85 years. Thirty-four of the patients were male (87%) and 5 were female (17%). Of the 39 patients, 31 (80%) had been injured in a road traffic accident. Analysis of the postresuscitation GCS recorded on admission showed that 18 patients (46%) scored equal to or below 6 points and 21 patients (54%) scored above 8 points. Basal cisterns were compressed in 12 cases (31%) and absent in 11 (28%). In 39 patients, CO_2 reactivity was tested within a mean of 18 ± 8 h after injury. Thirteen additional patients were tested but discarded from the study. Of these 13, 9 were excluded because alterations in MABP greater than 10 mmHg occurred when changing the ventilator settings. Four additional cases were also excluded because of unexpected and paradoxical changes in $AVDO_2$ with changes in pCO_2. Of the 39 cases, arterial pCO_2 was increased in 25 and decreased in 14. The mean absolute induced change in arterial pCO_2 was 4.6 ± 2.4 mmHg. In the entire group, the median of CO_2R_{ABS} was $0.1 \mu mol/mmHg$ pCO_2 with a lower 2.5 percentile of 0.001. The $CO_2R\%$ had a median of 4.4% with a lower 2.5 percentile of 0.06 and a higher 97.5 percentile of 29.3% change in estimated CBF per mmHg change in arterial pCO_2. According to the above mentioned criteria, only five patients (12.8%) presented an impaired/absent CO_2 reactivity (Fig. 1), and of these, four had a GCS less than 5 on admission. Three of these patients died, one was severely disabled, and one was in a persistent vegetative state 3 months after injury. The reduced number of cases ruled out statistical analysis of outcome.

In 35 of the 39 patients, autoregulation was also tested. Of the 35 cases studied, 5 were excluded because changes in pCO_2 during the autoregulation tests were above 2.5 mmHg and another 2 were excluded because of paradoxical decreases of mean BP with phenilefrine in hemodynamically unstable patients. The mean change in MABP in this subgroup of 28 cases was 26 ± 9.5 mmHg. In 12 patients (43%), changes in estimated CBF were below the 20% margin defined to consider autoregulation as intact. In the remaining 16 patients (57%), autoregulation was impaired. One patient with an induced decrease of 22% of estimated CBF when increasing MABP was included in the "intact" autoregulation group. In 15 of the 28 cases, ICP increased when increasing BP (Figs. 2, 3). Nevertheless, in all except 2 cases (10.7%), the net result was an increase of the cerebral perfusion pressure (CPP) (Fig. 2). The mean increase in CPP with the induced increase in MABP was 24.2 ± 11 mmHg (range, 1.30–44.6 mmHg). Of the 28 cases, CO_2 reactivity was impaired in 5. All patients with an impaired CO_2 reactivity also had impaired autoregulation.

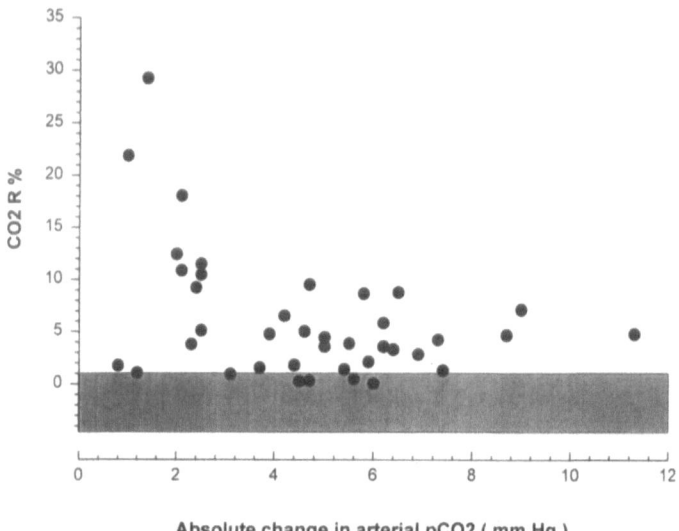

FIG. 1. Absolute change in arterial pCO_2 plotted against percentage reactivity of CO_2 ($CO_2R\%$). The *gray box* defines the zone of impaired/absent CO_2 reactivity. Observe the lack of correlation between the magnitude of change in pCO_2 during the test and CO_2 reactivity. Only five cases had an impaired autoregulation according to the established 1% limit

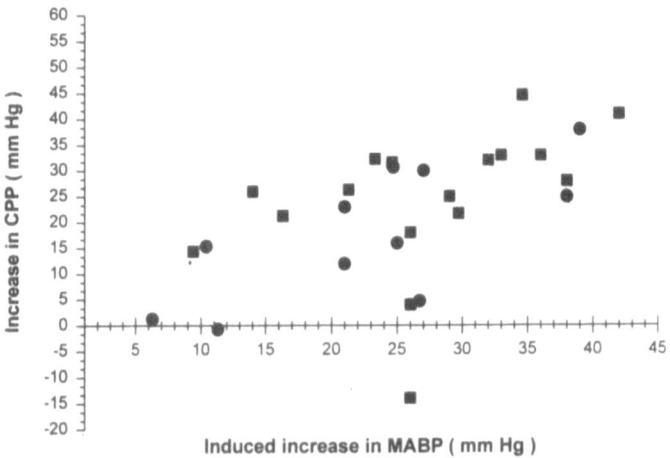

FIG. 2. Phenilephrine-induced increase in mean arterial blood pressure (MABP) plotted against increase in cerebral perfusion pressure (CPP) in patients with impaired autoregulation (*squares*) and preserved autoregulation (*circles*). In patients in whom CPP increased, a linear relationship between MABP and CPP was observed ($r = .65$)

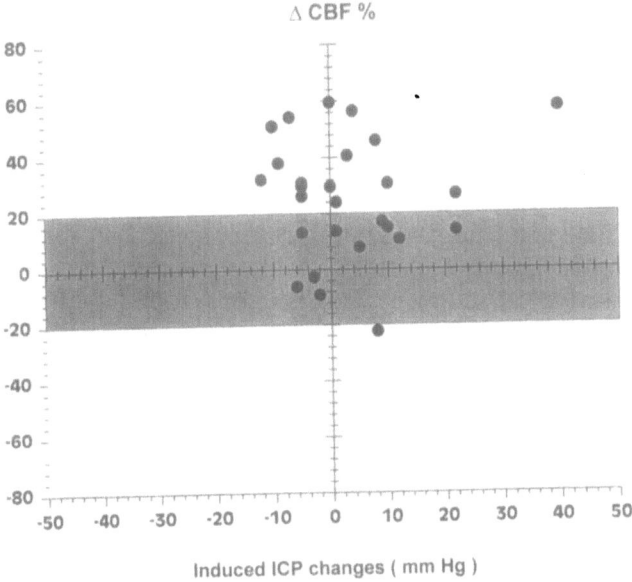

F$_{IG}$. 3. Induced intracranial pressure (ICP) changes plotted against increases in cerebral blood flow (CBF) during the autoregulation tests

Discussion

Impairment of autoregulatory mechanisms and CO$_2$ reactivity of the cerebrovascular bed are quite common in the acute phase of the severely head-injured patient and play an important role in the physiopathology of the increased cerebral blood volume (CBV) and high intracranial pressure (ICP) [13]. Manipulation of CBV through changes in pCO$_2$ is a widely used therapeutic measure to control high ICP in head-injured patients. However, hyperventilation may decrease CBF to the limit of ischemia in areas with preserved CO$_2$ reactivity and simultaneously increase CBF in areas with impaired or absent CO$_2$ reactivity (inverse steal phenomenon) [12]. Optimal blood presssure management in severe head-injured patients is still controversial [14,15]. While some authors advocate using vasoactive drugs to increase CPP or to control ICP in the acute phase, this management could be hazardous in patients with disturbed autoregulation. Increasing CPP in this subgroup would increase CBV and capillary pressure, therefore facilitating brain edema. About half the patients with a severe head injury have a variable degree of autoregulation impairment [16].

If we accept the fact that CMRO$_2$ is constant during the test, CBF is directly proportional to the reciprocal of AVDO$_2$. Therefore, it is possible to use AVDO$_2$ as a reliable estimate of CBF changes. This approach has been widely used by different authors and recently put forward as an accepted and reliable method to study the effects of drugs on autoregulation

[7]. $AVDO_2$ or CEO_2 (arterial minus jugular oxygen saturation) can be equally used to monitor CBF changes. Using $AVDO_2$ in testing CO_2 reactivity assumes that $CMRO_2$ is not altered by changes in arterial pCO_2. This point has been validated by many studies in awake and anesthesized humans with either hyper- or hypoventilation. [17,18]. According to our criteria, only 12.8% of the studied patients presented an impaired CO_2 reactivity in the first 24 h after injury. The median $CO_2R\%$ in our group (4.4%) was similar to the correction factor suggested by some authors to compare different groups of patients at different arterial pCO_2 levels [16]. However, the wide variability in $CO_2R\%$ in our study suggests that a better approach would be to use individualized $CO_2R\%$ to avoid unrealistic results. Some of our patients presented a $CO_2R\%$ greater than 10% and could be incorrectly classified as "hyperreactive." Nevertheless, the relationship between CBF and $AVDO_2$ follows an exponential pattern [19]. Because of this, patients with a low CBF can have relatively higher changes in $AVDO_2$ and be wrongly considered as hyperreactive. Thus, when studying CO_2 reactivity it is possible to state that reactivity is impaired or normal but unfeasible to say that it is above the normal range. Preserved CO_2 reactivity in head injury means that agressive hyperventilation should be avoided. If we hyperventilate patients with a normal CO_2 reactivity, it is possible to induce a shift to anaerobic metabolism. It has been demonstrated that moderate hyperventilation can induced a reduction of SjO_2 below the 50% threshold [20]. The continuous or intermittent monitoring of SjO_2, so-called optimized hyperventilation, allows us to monitor hyperventilation avoiding ischemic levels of arterial pCO_2.

When testing autoregulation, an important factor to consider is that between autoregulatory limits CBF is relatively, but not absolutely, constant [21]. Because of this, a ±20% limit was selected according to Enevoldsen's criteria [12]. Because autoregulation limits have not been clearly established, our results shoud be carefully analyzed. In some cases spontaneous changes in pCO_2 could be induced by changes in MABP when testing autoregulation. Therefore, correcting each patient's autoregulation results for changes in arterial pCO_2 with individual CO_2 reactivity is important to improve accuracy of data. Following Enevoldsen's criteria, 57% of our series had impaired/absent autoregulation. The patient with a 22% reduction of estimated CBF was included in the "intact" autoregulation group. In this case, the reduction in CBF could be the result of a hyperreactive vasoconstriction phenomena with intact autoregulatory mechanisms. An increase in brain tissue pressure and a secondary reduction of CBF in a nonautoregulating patient (false autoregulation), although possible, is less probable if we consider that in this case an increase of only 8 mmHg in ICP was observed.

Our data are in agreement with other studies in that autoregulation is a very vulnerable mechanism and that impaired autoregulation is highly prevalent in head injury [16]. As has been pointed out by Muizelaar et al. [22] autoregulation is not an all-or-nothing phenomenon and can be intact, slower than normal, intact with shifts in the pressure limits, or show smaller adjustements than normal. The 20% level in our study grossly distinguishes between intact and altered autoregulation. However, in the intact group, it is difficult to differentiate between patients with true normal autoregulation and those in whom lower or higher limits are abnormally shifted. Impaired autoregulation and preserved CO$_2$ reactivity was found in 43% of the cases, while preserved autoregulation and impaired CO$_2$ reactivity was not observed in any patient. Of the 28 cases in whom both autoregulation and CO$_2$ reactivity were studied, only 5 had a "complete vasoparalysis" (impaired autoregulation and CO$_2$ reactivity). Our data are in complete agreement in that this total vasoparalysis is infrequent and found only in the very damaged brain [1].

An interesting finding in our study was the observation that in spite of impaired autoregulation, increasing MABP induced a net increase of CPP in all except one patient. This finding supports the idea that to increase CPP by increasing MABP is not deleterious to patients with impaired autoregulation. However, no firm conclusions can be drawn about the effects of increasing capillary pressure and thus its facilitating effect on brain edema in nonautoregulating patients.

Conclusions

Monitoring relative changes in AVDO$_2$ permits the reliable study of CO$_2$ reactivity and autoregulation at the bedside. This can increase our knowledge of these parameters and their dynamic changes in the evolution of the head-injured patient. Introducing these variables on a day-to-day management basis should be considered in the treatment protocols. A consensus of the normal range for CO$_2$ reactivity and autoregulation would be desirable to standardize methods and to compare patients from different series.

Acknowledgment. Work was supported by grants 93/1257 and 94/0688 from the Fondo de Investigaciones Sanitarias de la Seguridad Social (FISS).

References

1. Paulson OB, Olesen J, Christensen MS (1972) Restoration of autoregulation of cerebral blood flow by hypocapnia (abstr). Neurology 22:286–293
2. Cruz J (1992) Jugular venous oxygen saturation monitoring (letter). J Neurosurg 77:162–163
3. Cruz J, Gennarelli TA, Alves WM (1992) Continuous monitoring of cerebral oxygenation in acute brain injury: multivariate assessment of severe intracranial "plateau" wave. Case report. J Trauma 32:401–403
4. Schmidt JF, Waldemar G, Vorstrup S, Andersen AR, Gjerris F, Paulson OB (1990) Computerized analysis of cerebral blood flow autoregulation in humans:

validation of a method for pharmacologic studies. J Cardiovasc Pharmacol 15:983–988

5. Robertson CS, Grossman RG, Goodman JC, Narayan RK (1987) The predictive value of cerebral anaerobic metabolism with cerebral infarction after head injury. J Neurosurg 67:361–368

6. Goetting MG, Preston G (1990) Jugular bulb catheterization: experience with 123 patients. Crit Care Med 18:1220–1223

7. Olsen KS, Videbaek C, Agerlin N, Kroll M, Bogerasmussen T, Paulson OB, Gjerris F (1993) The effect of tirilazad mesylate (u74006f) on cerebral oxygen consumption, and reactivity of cerebral blood flow to carbon dioxide in healthy volunteers. Anesthesiology 79:666–671

8. Davis SM, Ackerman RH, Correia JA, Alpert NM, Chang J, Buonanno F, Kelley RE, Rosner B, Taveras JM (1983) Cerebral blood flow and cerebrovascular CO_2 reactivity in stroke-age normal controls. Neurology 33:391–399

9. Kety SS, Schmidt CF (1948) The effects of active and passive hyperventilation on cerebral blood flow, cerebral oxygen consumption, cardiac output, and blood pressure of normal young men. J Clin Invest 25:107–119

10. Kety SS, Schmidt CF (1948) Effects of altered arterial tensions of carbon dioxide and oxygen on cerebral blood flow and cerebral oxygen consumption of normal young men. J Clin Invest 27:484–492

11. McHenry LC Jr, Slocum HC, Bivens HE, Mayes HA, Hayes CJ (1965) Hyperventilation in awake and anesthetized man. Effects on cerebral blood flow and cerebral metabolism. Arch Neurol 12:270–277

12. Enevoldsen EM, Jensen FT (1978) Autoregulation and CO_2 responses of cerebral blood flow in patients with acute severe head injury. J Neurosurg 689:698–703

13. Madsen FF (1990) Changes in regional cerebral blood flow after hyperventilation in the pig with an induced focal cerebral contusion. Acta Neurochir (Wien) 106:164–169

14. Muizelaar JP (1989) Induced arterial hypertension in the treatment of high ICP. In: Hoff JT (ed) Intracranial pressure VII. Springer-Verlag, Berlin Heidelberg, pp 508–510

15. Bouma GJ, Muizelaar JP (1990) Relationship between cardiac output and cerebral blood flow in patients with intact and with impaired autoregulation. J Neurosurg 73:368–374

16. Obrist WD, Langfitt TW, Jaggi JL, Cruz J, Gennarelli TA (1984) Cerebral blood flow and metabolism in comatose patients with acute head injury. Relationship to intracranial hypertension. J Neurosurg 61:241–253

17. Bloor BM (1975) Cerebral hemodynamics: the effect of hypoxia on autoregulation and CO_2 reactivity. In: Langfitt TW (ed) Cerebral circulation and metabolism. Springer-Verlag, Berlin Heidelberg, pp 55–58

18. Shapiro W, Wasserman AJ, Patterson JL Jr (1965) Human cerebrovascular response time to elevation of arterial carbon dioxide tension. Arch Neurol 13:130–138

19. Robertson CS, Narayan RK, Gokaslan ZL, Pahwa R, Grossman RG, Caram P, Allen E (1989) Cerebral arteriovenous oxygen difference as an estimate of cerebral blood flow in comatose patiens. J Neurosurg 70:222–230

20. Vonhelden A, Schneider GH, Unterberg A, Lanksch WR (1993) Monitoring of jugular venous oxygen saturation in comatose patients with subarachnoid haemorrhage and intracerebral haematomas. Acta Neurochir (Suppl) 59:102–106

21. Edvinsson L, MacKenzie ET, McCulloch J (1993) Disturbed cerebral autoregulation. In: Edvinsson L (ed) Cerebral blood flow and metabolism. Raven, New York, pp 599–609
22. Muizelaar JP, Becker DP, Lutz HA (1985) Present application and future promise of cerebral blood flow monitoring in head injury. In: Dacey RG (ed) Trauma of the central nervous system. Raven, New York, pp 91–102

Part 5

Characteristics of Near-Infrared Spectroscopy

Validation of a Noninvasive Measurement of Regional Hemoglobin Oxygen Saturation

VALERIE POLLARD[1], ERIC A. DeMELO[1], DONALD J. DEYO[1],
REBECCA DALMEIDA[1], R. WIDMAN[2], AND DONALD S. PROUGH[1]

Introduction

Near-infrared (NIR) spectroscopy may provide a continuous and noninvasive assessment of global brain hemoglobin oxygen saturation by measuring the differential absorption of infrared light [1–3]. As biological tissues are relatively transparent to infrared light at wavelengths between 400 and 1000 nm, infrared light may penetrate skin, subcutaneous tissue, bone, and dura to the brain [4–7], where it is absorbed by oxygenated hemoglobin, deoxygenated hemoglobin, and cytochrome aa₃. Thus, the attenuation of infrared light of specific wavelengths by these chromophores may be used to measure brain oxygenation [1,3,8–11]. The hemoglobin oxygen saturation measured by the cerebral oximeter receives contributions from arterial, venous, and capillary blood vessels, with a predominantly venous contribution [11,12], and may reflect the balance between cerebral oxygen consumption and delivery.

Clinical validation of the in vivo spectroscope has proven difficult as the saturation measured by the oximeter cannot be directly calibrated with a "gold standard" reference parameter because global hemoglobin oxygen saturation cannot be measured directly. Many studies have compared the spectroscopic signal to established methods that may assess cerebral function and perfusion, such as the electroencephalogram [13,14], nuclear magnetic resonance spectroscopy [15,16], and ^{133}Xe clearance techniques [17], with encouraging results. The most precise clinical reference parameter, however, remains the estimated global brain hemoglobin oxygen saturation ($CS_{comb}O_2$), which is calculated from arterial and jugular venous bulb oxygen saturations [13,18].

This chapter describes a validation study that evaluates a prototype cerebral oximeter in conscious volunteers breathing hypoxic gas mixtures, and details an algorithm to quantify brain hemoglobin oxygen saturation.

---
[1] Department of Anesthesiology, The University of Texas Medical Branch in Galveston, Suite 2A John Sealy Hospital, Galveston, Texas 77555-0591, USA
[2] Somanetics Corp., 1653 East Maple Road, Troy, Missouri 48083-4208, USA

Additional studies were performed to determine the effects of changes in position and carbon dioxide (CO_2) on the oximeter hemoglobin oxygen saturation signal (CS_fO_2), because the "gold standard" $CS_{comb}O_2$, is dependent on the assumption that the ratio of arterial to venous blood volume remains constant.

Methods

Description of the Cerebral Oximeter

A new prototype cerebral oximeter (Invos 3100, Somanetics Corporation, Troy, MO USA), measures the ratio of the concentration of oxyhemoglobin to that of deoxyhemoglobin and thus provides an index of global brain hemoglobin oxygen saturation. Infrared light is generated by an incandescent light source and is focused through a filter that separates the light into two wavelengths, 730 and 810 nm. Fiberoptic cables deliver the light to a miniature light-emitting diode in a self-adhesive sensor that attaches to the subject's forehead. The light then enters the underlying tissues, where it is scattered, causing the photons to travel in random paths through the brain. Computer simulations of the photon paths have shown them to follow an elliptical path between the emitter and detector [7,19]. A proportion of light is returned to the surface and is captured by two detectors on the sensor, which are placed at varying distances to control the length of the light path through the tissue. The more distant detector (D_2), placed 4 cm from the sensor, measures the hemoglobin oxygen saturation of all the tissues penetrated by the light beam, including skin, muscle tissue, skull, and brain. The closer detector (D_1), placed 3 cm from the sensor, measures the hemoglobin oxygen saturation from the superficial tissues. By subtracting D_1 from D_2, an approximate CS_fO_2 may be measured in the underlying brain. Monitoring cables deliver the detected light to photodetectors in the microcomputer, which then collects the spectroscopic measurements, averages them, and displays a sliding numerical average of the data points on the oximeter screen.

Description of the Cerebral Oximeter Algorithm:

The Beer–Lambert law describes the relationship between incident and received light of suitable wavelengths as follows:

$$I_w/I_{wo} = e^{-awCs}$$

where I_w is the intensity of transmitted light at wavelength w, I_{wo} is the intensity of incident light at wavelength w, a is the molar extinction coefficient of the chromophore, C is the concentration of chromophore molecules in the tissue, and s is the distance of the path length of light in the tissue. The extinction coefficients of oxy- and deoxyhemoglobin are known, and the transmitted light intensity is a measured parameter.

An algorithm based on the above equation is used to process the incoming intensity data as follows:

$$-\ln(I_w/I_{wo}) = \sum_{j=1}^{N} aw, jCjs$$

Absorption at a second wavelength, w', is then subtracted from the absorption at w to create the expression:

$$-\ln(I_w/I_{wo}) + \ln(I_{w'}/I_{w'o}) = \sum_{j=1}^{N} [a(w,j) - a(w',j)]Cjs$$

Repeated ($N + 1$) measurements are made to solve for C_{1s} for oxyhemoglobin and C_{2s} for reduced hemoglobin. Although these expressions do not represent the actual concentration of the molecules, they are proportional to them. The path length s, which varies with hemoglobin concentration, is assumed constant for all wavelengths over the range of measurement. Although the path length of photons has been measured with reasonably accuracy [5,20,21], the effects of unknown path lengths can be removed from the equation by calculating the ratio of the following expressions:

$$\frac{C_{2s}}{C_{1s}} = \frac{C_2}{C_1} = \frac{\text{concentration of deoxyhemoglobin}}{\text{concentration of oxyhemoglobin}}$$

Saturation of hemoglobin in the region of measurement is expressed as the ratio of oxyhemoglobin (HbO$_2$) to total hemoglobin (Hb):

$$CS_fO_2 = \frac{HbO_2}{HbO_2 + Hb} \times 100\%$$

Dividing the numerator and denominator of the fraction by HbO$_2$ yields the following:

$$CS_fO_2 = \frac{1}{(1 + Hb/HbO_2)} \times 100\% = \frac{1}{(1 + C_2/C_1)} \times 100\%$$

where C_2/C_1 is the parameter calculated by the processor based on measured intensities.

Volunteer Preparation

Healthy volunteers (age range, 19–49 years) were studied in three protocols that were approved by the institutional review board. A medical history was taken and examination performed, and informed consent was obtained, after which all volunteers underwent radial arterial catheterization and jugular venous bulb catheterization. Correct placement and positioning of the jugular venous bulb catheter were facilitated by use of a Doppler ultrasonic probe (DYMAX SiteRite, Pittsburgh, PA, USA) visualization of the vein.

Volunteers were continuously monitored using a pulse oximeter (Nellcor Model N 100C, Hayward, CA, USA), an end-tidal carbon dioxide monitor (DATEX Normocap 200, Helsinki, Finland), an electrocardiogram (Lifescope 6, Tokyo, Japan), and automated blood pressure monitor (Critikon Vital Signs Monitor 1846-X, Tampa, FL, USA). A self-adhesive probe containing a near-infrared light source and detector was also placed on each subject's right frontal forehead to continuously measure CS_fO_2. Subjects breathed randomly ordered hypoxic gas mixtures of nitrogen and oxygen through a tight-fitting mask and a closed circuit system. Each mixture was breathed until a stable pulse oximeter reading was obtained, at which time simultaneous arterial and jugular venous blood gases were slowly drawn. Heart rate, blood pressure, end-tidal CO_2, and pulse oximeter readings were documented at this time.

In the validation study, 12 subjects were initially studied (training group) to determine the association between CS_fO_2 and $CS_{comb}O_2$. The study was then validated in a second group of 10 volunteers (validation group). In a second study, 8 subjects breathed randomly ordered hypoxic gas mixtures in one of three randomized positions (supine, 20° Trendelenberg position, and 20° reverse Trendelenberg position) to determine the influence of position on CS_fO_2. Arterial and jugular venous blood gases were obtained in each position according to the initial study protocol.

Finally, to determine the influence of hypercapnia and hypocapnia on CS_fO_2, a third study was performed during which eight subjects were asked either to hyperventilate to an end-tidal CO_2 value less than 15 mmHg or to breathe a 7.3% CO_2 and air mixture through a tight-fitting continuous positive airway pressure (CPAP) mask during a 5-min period until the end-tidal CO_2 exceeded 55 mmHg. Simultaneous arterial and jugular venous blood gases were slowly drawn when end-tidal CO_2 measurements were stable. The influence of altered position during hypercapnia and hypocapnia on CS_fO_2, was also determined in this study.

In each study, subjects breathed the gas mixtures for at least 5 min before blood sampling, and were allowed a 5-min interval in which to recover between readings. In addition, 100% oxygen was inhaled after administration of a hypoxic gas mixture until baseline oxygen saturation was restored.

Statistics

All data sets were analyzed separately but in the same manner. Brain oxygen saturation ($CS_{comb}O_2$) was computed as

$$CS_{comb}O_2 = 0.25 \, SaO_2 + 0.75 \, SjO_2$$

where SaO_2 is arterial oxygen saturation and SjO_2 is jugular venous bulb oxygen saturation. Previous publications have indicated that the venous contribution to the cerebral blood content is 70%–80% [12,22]. The association between brain oxygen saturation and the in vivo spectroscope (CS_fO_2) was investigated, assuming a straight-line relationship:

$$CS_{comb}O_2 = (slope)\ CS_fO_2 + (intercept).$$

Pearson product-moment correlation coefficients between $CS_{comb}O_2$ and CS_fO_2 were computed for each subject to measure the intensity of the association. The data sets were also analyzed using the method described by Bland et al. for comparison of two measurements when the actual value is not known [23]. Finally, to determine the influence of position and CO_2 on $CS_{comb}O_2$ and CS_fO_2, an analysis of variance procedure was performed. Effects were assessed at the 0.05 level of significance.

Results

Validation Study

$CS_{comb}O_2$ and CS_fO_2 were highly correlated for each subject in both the training and validation data as $r^2 = .798$ to .987 for the training set and $r^2 = .794$ to .992 for the validation set (Table 1). The slopes ranged from 0.72 to 1.31 for the training data and from 0.49 to 1.11 for the validation data.

TABLE 1. Correlation coefficients, slopes, and intercepts for relationship between CS_fO_2 and $CS_{comb}O_2$

Group	Subject	Correlation coefficient	Slope	Intercept
Training	1	.951	0.8149	5.532
Training	2	.950	0.8139	9.0199
Training	3	.904	1.3064	−23.114
Training	4	.967	0.91168	6.9573
Training	5	.962	1.1409	−6.8769
Training	6	.798	0.71568	14.79
Training	7	.962	0.7267	18.543
Training	8	.967	0.75989	16.435
Training	9	.953	1.0972	−6.3078
Training	10	.875	0.78088	11.928
Training	11	.975	1.0536	4.6783
Training	12	.987	0.86384	14.008
Validation	1	.915	0.76183	7.8221
Validation	2	.982	1.1075	1.4236
Validation	3	.986	1.0419	−4.2881
Validation	4	.858	0.99429	2.3351
Validation	5	.979	1.0901	−2.6858
Validation	6	.909	1.0619	6.2437
Validation	7	.969	0.48723	30.061
Validation	8	.992	1.0012	4.8264
Validation	9	.927	0.76043	19.399
Validation	10	.794	0.89405	5.6883

CS_fO_2, oximeter hemoglobin oxygen saturation; $CS_{comb}O_2$, estimated global brain hemoglobin oxygen saturation.

Bland–Altman plots, which were obtained for each volunteer, demonstrated a close association between $CS_{comb}O_2$ and CS_fO_2 (Table 2 and Figs. 1–4).

The Influence of Position on CS_fO_2

$CS_{comb}O_2$ and CS_fO_2 were again closely correlated ($r^2 = .663$ to $.885$) (Table 3). The slopes ranged from 0.68 to 1.58 for the eight subjects studied. Bland–Altman plots for each subject also demonstrated a close association between $CS_{comb}O_2$ and CS_fO_2 (Table 4 and Figs. 5, 6).

$CS_{comb}O_2$ and CS_fO_2 increased significantly from baseline when the volunteers were placed in the 20° Trendelenberg position, but not in the 20° reverse Trendelenberg position.

The Influence of CO_2 on CS_fO_2

$CS_{comb}O_2$ and CS_fO_2 were variably correlated ($r^2 = .366$ to $.976$) (Table 5). The slopes ranged from 0.69 to 2.75. The limits of agreement were wide in the Bland–Altman plots, indicating that $CS_{comb}O_2$ and CS_fO_2 were not closely associated (Table 6 and Figs. 7, 8).

$CS_{comb}O_2$ increased significantly during hypercapnia and decreased significantly during hypocapnia from baseline values, as did SjO_2. CS_fO_2 increased significantly from baseline during hypercapnia but did not change

TABLE 2. Descriptive studies for differences between $CS_{comb}O_2$ and CS_fO_2

Group	Subject	n	Mean	SD	SE	Mean −2 SD	Mean +2 SD
Training	1	9	−4.74	2.12	0.71	−8.87	−0.61
Training	2	10	−1.69	3.11	0.99	−7.29	3.89
Training	3	8	−7.00	3.10	1.10	−12.79	−1.20
Training	4	10	2.24	1.80	0.57	−0.23	4.71
Training	5	10	4.00	2.85	0.86	−1.02	9.81
Training	6	9	0.95	2.46	0.82	−3.87	5.77
Training	7	10	−2.83	4.3	1.36	−11.98	6.32
Training	8	10	3.02	2.27	0.72	−1.83	7.88
Training	9	10	−0.35	2.05	0.65	−4.71	4.01
Training	10	10	−0.38	4.14	1.31	−8.34	7.58
Training	11	10	7.6	2.02	0.64	3.39	11.84
Training	12	10	6.43	1.97	0.62	2.3	10.57
Validation	1	9	−5.29	2.63	0.88	−10.55	−0.04
Validation	2	10	7.23	1.91	0.60	3.56	10.90
Validation	3	9	−2.01	0.89	0.30	−3.80	−0.23
Validation	4	9	2.07	3.75	1.25	−5.49	9.50
Validation	5	10	2.25	2.8	0.45	−0.57	5.07
Validation	6	10	9.84	2.75	0.87	4.35	15.33
Validation	7	10	−0.27	4.1	1.3	−7.92	8.48
Validation	8	8	4.9	1.09	0.39	2.72	7.07
Validation	9	9	5.78	2.96	0.99	−0.14	11.72
Validation	10	14	−1.38	3.34	0.89	−8.06	5.3

SD, standard deviation; SE, standard error; n, number of data points per subject.

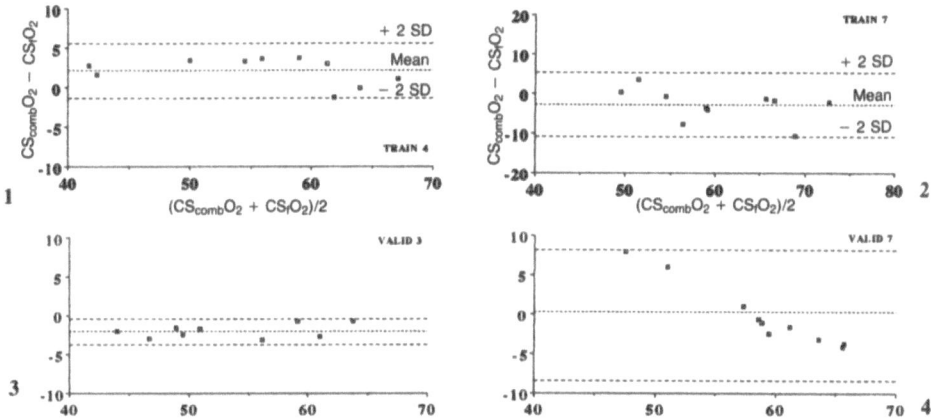

Figs. 1–4. Representative Bland–Altman plots for the training and validation groups demonstrate that oximeter hemoglobin oxygen saturation (CS_fO_2) and estimated global brain hemoglobin oxygen saturation oximeter ($CS_{comb}O_2$) are closely associated

TABLE 3. Correlation coefficients, slopes, and intercepts for different patient positions

Subject	Correlation coefficient	Slope	Intercept
1	.856	1.0669	−12.762
2	.799	1.2063	−14.659
3	.885	0.96457	3.5325
4	.740	0.68108	20.283
5	.723	1.5879	−25.773
6	.699	0.75586	15.289
7	.666	0.90235	8.2308
8	.663	0.69885	16.671

TABLE 4. Descriptive studies for differences between $CS_{comb}O_2$ and CS_fO_2 position influence

Subject	n	Mean	SD	SE	Mean −2 SD	Mean +2 SD
1	12	7.92	2.3	0.66	3.33	12.53
2	12	−2.75	4.52	1.31	−11.78	6.28
3	12	−0.33	3.21	0.93	−6.67	6.1
4	12	−0.93	4.95	1.43	−10.83	8.96
5	12	−4.85	5.89	1.7	−16.62	6.92
6	12	0.74	1.94	0.56	−3.13	4.63
7	12	−0.45	2.87	0.83	−6.19	5.27
8	12	4.16	2.88	0.83	−1.59	9.91

SD, standard deviation; SE, standard error; n, number of subjects studied.

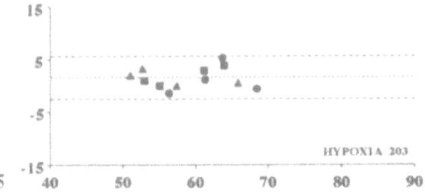 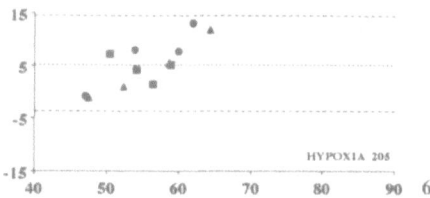

FIGS. 5, 6. Representative Bland–Altman plots for the hypoxia group also demonstrate that CS_fO_2 and $CS_{comb}O_2$ are closely associated. *Squares*, baseline; *triangles*, 20° Trendelenberg; *circles*, 20° reverse Trendelenberg

TABLE 5. Correlation coefficients, slopes, and intercepts for variation in blood CO_2 levels

Subject	Correlation coefficient	Slope	Intercept
1	.864	2.3414	−80.361
2	.976	2.75	−124.45
3	.601	0.68213	5.6472
4	.795	1.1043	−2.3365
5	.88	1.3555	−12.92
6	.915	1.9809	−60.555
7	.366	18.032	18.032
8	.656	1.2507	10.837

TABLE 6. Descriptive studies for differences between $CS_{comb}O_2$ and CS_fO_2 carbon dioxide influence

Subject	n	Mean	SD	SE	Mean −2 SD	Mean +2 SD
1	9	−0.48	9.62	3.21	−19.72	18.28
2	9	−0.59	9.27	3.09	−19.13	17.96
3	9	−2.89	8.40	2.80	−19.69	13.91
4	9	4.62	6.85	2.28	−9.08	18.32
5	9	8.02	5.99	2.00	−3.97	20.01
6	9	3.96	9.16	3.05	−14.36	22.29
7	9	−4.99	11.48	3.83	−27.95	17.97
8	9	6.01	8.21	2.74	−10.40	22.42

SD, standard deviation; SE, standard error; n, number of data points per subject.

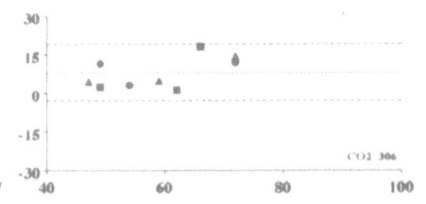 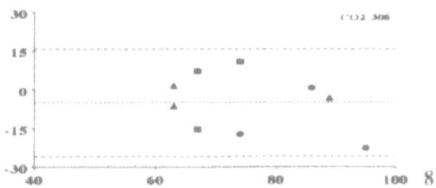

FIGS. 7, 8. Representative Bland–Altman plots for the CO_2 group demonstrate that CS_fO_2 and $CS_{comb}O_2$ are not closely associated as the limits of agreement are wide. *Squares*, baseline; *triangles*, 20° Trendelenberg; *circles*, 20° reverse Trendelenberg

during hypocapnia. These changes occurred irrespective of position. There were no significant differences within the CS$_{comb}$O$_2$ and CS$_f$O$_2$ groups when volunteers were placed either in a 20° Trendelenberg or 20° reverse Trendelenberg position.

Discussion

The concept of a simple, noninvasive, and continuous bedside monitor capable of detecting early cerebral ischemic events is certainly desirable, because irreversible cerebral damage may occur before changes in neurological status become apparent. Continuous monitoring of jugular venous bulb hemoglobin oxygen saturation has become increasingly popular in the management of the patient with severe head injury [24,25]. Monitoring SjO$_2$, however, requires frequent repositioning of the patient, and catheter recalibration, which is technically demanding. Although insertion of the catheter is relatively simple, it is nonetheless an invasive procedure.

Validation of the cerebral oximeter requires a "gold standard" against which CS$_f$O$_2$ may be calibrated. Because regional saturation underneath the probe cannot be measured directly, estimations of SjO$_2$ and SaO$_2$ must be made. We demonstrated a close correlation between CS$_f$O$_2$ and CS$_{comb}$O$_2$, which verifies the sensitivity of the cerebral oximeter.

Position changes may influence venous pressure, and may alter the proportion of arterial to venous blood in the cerebral vasculature [26], changing the ratio of SaO$_2$ and SjO$_2$ used to estimate CS$_{comb}$O$_2$, which might be expected to alter the correlation between CS$_f$O$_2$ and CS$_{comb}$O$_2$. Instead, we found that a close correlation was maintained, despite changes in position. Bland–Altman plots verified this association.

Local tissue metabolism may also influence cerebral vascular diameter [12,27,28], and thereby change the ratio of arterial to venous volume, which could alter the CS$_{comb}$O$_2$ calculation. This change may explain the variability in the correlation coefficients during hyper- and hypocapnia, as well as the lack of association between CS$_f$O$_2$ and CS$_{comb}$O$_2$ in the Bland–Altman plots. Of more concern, however, is the failure of CS$_f$O$_2$j1 to reflect a decrease in cerebral hemoglobin oxygen saturation during hypocapnia, despite a significant decrease in CS$_{comb}$O$_2$. This failure may limit the use of cerebral oximetry in head-injured patients where hyperventilation is a common therapeutic intervention.

Another possible variable is probe dioptode distance. Only one study has shown this to be a problem [29]. Most of the literature suggests that the probe dioptode distances of 1 and 2.7 cm, used in previous studies, are indeed satisfactory [1,11]. Nevertheless, probe dioptode distances of 3 and 4 cm were used in this study to allow further separation of the superficial and deep tissue contributions.

One final limitation of in vivo spectroscopy is that it measures regional oxygen distribution and may not reflect focal ischemic events. Thus, NIR spectroscopy should not be substituted for other established techniques, but should rather be used in conjunction with them to provide an early warning of a cerebral hypoxic-ischemic event. In conclusion, therefore, cerebral oximetry may prove a useful adjunct in monitoring patients at risk for cerebral ischemia. The influence of hyper- and hypocapnia on the spectroscopic signal merits further investigation, however, and the algorithm may require further adjustment in patients with relevant underlying pathology.

References

1. McCormick PW, Stewart M, Ray P, Lewis G, Dujovny M, Ausman JI (1991) Measurement of regional cerebrovascular hemoglobin oxygen saturation in cats using optical spectroscopy. Neurol Res 13:65–70
2. Chance B, Nioka S, Kent J, McCully K, Fountain M, Greenfeld R, Holtom G (1988) Time-resolved spectroscopy of hemoglobin and myoglobin in resting and ischemic muscle. Anal Biochem 174:698–707
3. Jöbsis-Vandervleit FF, Fox E, Sugioka K (1987) Monitoring of cerebral oxygenation and cytochrome aa_3 redox state. Int Anesthesiol Clin 25:209–230
4. Jöbsis FF (1977) Noninvasive, infrared monitoring of cerebral and myocardial oxygen sufficiency and circulatory parameters. Science 198:1264–1267
5. Delpy DT, Cope M, van der Zee P, Arridge S, Wray S, Wyatt J (1988) Estimation of optical path length through tissue from direct time of flight measurement. Phys Med Biol 33:1433–1442
6. Chance B, Leigh JS, Miyake H, Smith DS, Nioka S, Greenfeld R, Finander M, Kaufmann K, Levy W, Young M, Cohen P, Yoshioka H, Boretsky R (1988) Comparison of time-resolved and -unresolved measurements of deoxyhemoglobin in brain. Proc Natl Acad Sci USA 85:4971–4975
7. McCormick PW, Stewart M, Goetting M, Dujovny M, Lewis G, Ausman JI (1991) Noninvasive cerebral optical spectroscopy for monitoring cerebral oxygen delivery and hemodynamics. Crit Care Med 19:89–97
8. Wray S, Cope M, Delpy DT, Wyatt J, Reynolds EOR (1988) Characterization of the near infrared absorption spectra of cytochrome aa_3 and hemoglobin for the noninvasive monitoring of cerebral oxygenation. Biochim Biophys Acta 933:184–192
9. Keizer HH, Jöbsis-Vander Vliet FF, Lucas SS, Piantadosi CA, Sylvia AL (1985) The near-infrared (NIR) absorption band of cytochrome aa_3 in purified enzyme, isolated mitochondria and in the intact brain in situ. Adv Exp Med Biol 191: 823–832
10. Kariman K, Hempel FG, Jöbsis FF, Burns SR, Saltzman HA (1981) In vivo comparison of cerebral tissue PO_2 and cytochrome aa_3 reduction-oxidation state in cats during hemorrhagic shock. J Clin Invest 68:21–27
11. McCormick PW, Stewart M, Lewis G, Dujovny M, Ausman JI (1992) Intracerebral penetration of infrared light. J Neurosurg 76:315–318
12. Mchedlishvili G (1986) Arterial behavior and blood circulation in the brain. Plenum, New York, pp 55–60
13. McCormick PW, Stewart M, Goetting M, Balakrishnan G (1991) Regional cerebrovascular oxygen saturation measured by optical spectroscopy in humans. Stroke 22:596–602

14. Smith DS, Levy W, Maris M, Chance B (1990) Reperfusion hyperoxia in brain after circulatory arrest in humans. Anesthesiology 73:12–19

15. Delpy DT, Cope M, Cady EB, Wyatt JS, Hamilton PA, Hope PL, Wray S, Reynolds EOR (1987) Cerebral monitoring in newborn infants by magnetic resonance and near infrared spectroscopy. Scand J Clin Lab Invest 188:9–17

16. Tamura M, Hazeki O, Nioka S, Chance B, Smith DS (1988) The simultaneous measurements of tissue oxygen concentration and energy state by near-infrared and nuclear magnetic resonance spectroscopy. Adv Exp Med Biol 222:359–363

17. Colacino JM, Grubb B, Jöbsis FF (1981) Infra-red technique for cerebral blood flow: comparison with ^{133}Xenon clearance. Neurol Res 3:17–31

18. Pollard V, DeMelo E, Deyo DJ, Stoddard H, Hoffmann DJ, Prough DS (1994) Generation and validation of an algorithm for brain oxygen monitoring. Anesth Analg 78:S343

19. Van der Zee P, Delpy T (1987) Simulation of the point spread function for light in tissue by a Monte Carlo Model. Adv Exp Med Biol 215:179–191

20. Wyatt JS, Cope M, Delpy DT, Van der Zee P, Arridge S, Edwards AD, Reynolds EOR (1990) Measurement of optical path length for cerebral near infrared spectroscopy in newborn infants. Dev Neurosci 12:140–144

21. Van der Zee P, Cope M, Arridge SR, Essenpreis M, Potter LA, Edwards AD, Wyatt JS, McCormick DC, Roth SC, Reynolds EOR, Delpy DT (1992) Experimentally measured optical path lengths for the adult head, calf, and forearm, and the head of the newborn infant as a function of interoptode spacing. Adv Exp Med Biol 316:143–153

22. Portnoy HD, Chopp M, Branch C (1983) Hydraulic model of myogenic autoregulation and the cerebrovascular bed: the effects of altering systemic arterial pressure. Neurosurgery 13:482–498

23. Bland JM, Altman DG (1986) Statistical methods for assessing agreement between two methods of clinical measurement. Lancet 1:307–310

24. Cruz J (1993) Combined continuous monitoring of systemic and cerebral oxygenation in acute brain injury: preliminary observations. Crit Care Med 21:1225–1232

25. Sheinberg M, Kanter MJ, Robertson CS, Contant CF, Narayan RK, Grossman RG (1992) Continuous monitoring of jugular venous oxygen saturation in head-injured patients. J Neurosurg 76:212–217

26. Shenkin HA, Scheuerman WG, Spitz EB, Groff RA (1949) Effect of change of position upon the cerebral circulation of man. J Appl Physiol 2:317–326

27. Mueller SM, Heistad DD, Marcus ML (1977) Total and regional cerebral blood flow during hypotension, hypertension and hypocapnia. Effect of sympathetic denervation in dogs. Circ Res 41:350–356

28. Kontos HA (1981) Regulation of the cerebral circulation. Annu Rev Physiol 43:397–407

29. Harris DNF, Bailey SM (1993) Near-infrared spectroscopy in adults. Anaesthesia 48:694–696

Validation of Monitoring of Cerebral Oxygenation by Near-Infrared Spectroscopy in Comatose Patients

A. Unterberg, A. Rosenthal, G.H. Schneider, K. Kiening, and W.R. Lanksch

Introduction

Secondary ischemic brain damage is a common event in patients with severe brain injuries, and is often verified at autopsy, for example, following severe head injury. It is widely accepted that secondary brain ischemia contributes to morbidity and mortality of comatose patients. Until recently, monitoring of comatose patients focused on measurements of intracranial pressure (ICP) and cerebral perfusion pressure (CPP). The major limitation of the approach to manage ICP and CPP is the lack of metabolic information. Thus, monitoring of cerebral oxygenation was introduced.

Various techniques are currently available for monitoring. Jugular venous oximetry monitors the global oxygen saturation within the jugular bulb ($SjVO_2$) and represents an invasive technique. Direct measurements of cerebral tissue PO_2 are still more or less experimental. Some years ago, near-infrared spectroscopy (NIRS) was proposed to monitor cerebral tissue oxygenation focally. The great advantage of this technique is its noninvasiveness. So far, this technology has been validated only in special clinical conditions, as in newborn infants, healthy adult humans, and intraoperatively [1–6].

To date, there are no reports on the significance of cerebral oxygenation monitoring by NIRS in intensive care. Also, there is no information on the comparison of $SjVO_2$ and of NIRS-monitored cerebral oxygenation on a long-term basis. The aim of this investigation was thus to compare these different technologies, in the hope that NIRS-monitored cerebral oxygenation might supersede the invasive technique of jugular venous oximetry, which is prone to numerous artifacts.

Department of Neurosurgery, Rudolf Virchow Medical Center, Free University of Berlin, Augustenburger Platz 1, 13353 Berlin, Germany

Materials and Methods

In 15 patients comatose as the result of severe head injury (with a Glasgow Coma Score of 7 or less on admission), cerebral oxygenation was simultaneously monitored by NIRS and $SjVO_2$. Jugular bulb oxygen saturation was monitored by the Oximetrics 3 System (Abbott, Wiesbaden, Germany). Details of this technique are given elsewhere [7]. Regional frontal tissue oxygenation was measured by the INVOS 3100 Cerebral Oximeter (SOMANETICS, Troy, Michigan, USA). All probes were placed above the right frontal region. Two generations of NIRS probes were used in the study. In the second generation of probes, the geometry of the optodes had been changed to reduce the significance of an extracerebral blood "contamination" of scalp and skull.

ICP was simultaneously monitored by a Camino ® intraparenchymal device (Camino Laboratories, San Diego, USA). Arterial blood pressure was monitored invasively; cerebral perfusion pressure was calculated on line. Additionally, end-tidal CO_2 and the arterial oxygen saturation were monitored. Data were sampled via Hewlett-Packard ICU-monitor equipment (Model 685) and analyzed retrospectively.

Results and Discussion

General Technical Aspects of NIRS Monitoring

In most cases, tissue oxygenation ranged between 60% and 80% following positioning of the NIRS probes (frontally, right side). Placement of the probes above the temporal, parietal, or occipital region was also tested in some cases, but often failed to yield saturation data.

With the measurements ongoing, the NIRS system had frequent breakdowns and often stopped reporting oxygen saturation data. In some instances these errors could be solved by replacement of the sensor, firmer fixation of the probes, or by restarting the system. Altogether, however, NIRS monitoring had to be stopped because of a dysfunction of the system in about 60% of the cases. Figure 1 gives the duration of measurements of ten consecutive patients. It becomes obvious that there were a couple of periods in which there was no report of saturation values at all. Monitoring of more than 48 h was possible in three patients only. Moreover, the second generation of probes appeared to be even more sensitive to disturbances and errors than the first generation.

Our limited experience with the NIRS system thus calls for technological refinements to reduce artifacts and disturbances.

Comparison of NIRS and $SjVO_2$ Data

Figures 2–4 represent original tracings comparing cerebral oxygen saturation as measured focally by NIRS, or globally in the jugular bulb, together with

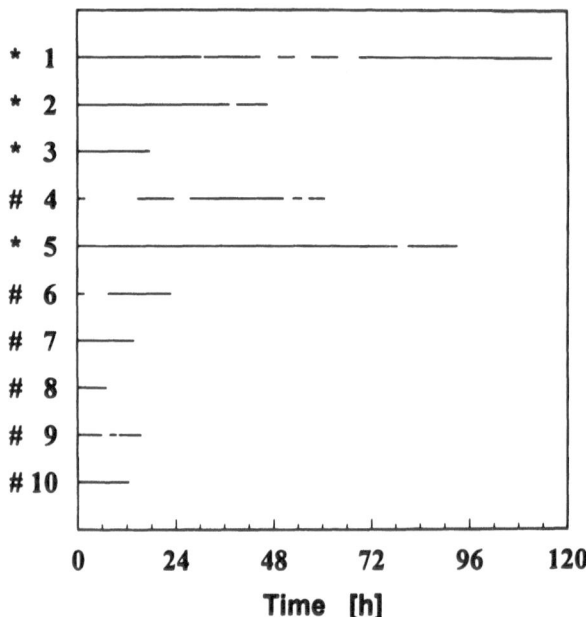

FIG. 1. Duration of monitoring of cerebral oxygenation by near-infrared spectros-copy (NIRS) in ten consecutive comatose patients. In most patients, monitoring was ended because of signal disturbances. The *solid lines* indicate that the system reported oxygen saturation values; *broken lines* indicate periods of signal distur-bances. *, first generation probe; #, second generation probe. Monitoring was even more prone to errors with the second generation of probes

monitoring of ICP and CPP. These figures illustrate that under "normal" conditions, that is, $SjVO_2$ between 60% and 80%, tissue oxygenation saturation (RSO_2) as measured by NIRS is running more or less parallel to the jugular bulb oxygen saturation. In most cases, RSO_2 was approximately 5–10% higher than $SjVO_2$ (Figs. 2 and 4). Closer analysis of the tracings indicated that increases of jugular bulb oxygen saturation were reflected by NIRS while decreases in $SjVO_2$ were mirrored less well, or not at all, by NIRS (Figs. 2–4).

Thus, the sensitivity of NIRS measurements to reflect increases or decreases in $SjVO_2$ was systematically analyzed (Figs. 5, 6). If $SjVO_2$ increased by more than 10% (22 episodes), RSO_2 increased in 82% (18 episodes) also. Thus, increases in global cerebral oxygenation were mirrored by increases of tissue oxygenation, although to a lesser extent. While $SjVO_2$ increased from 58% to 70%, RSO_2 rose from 64% to 69% (mean values). Decreases of $SjVO_2$ of more than 10% of the actual value, on the other hand, were insufficiently mirrored by NIRS. Of 31 episodes of marked $SjVO_2$ decreases, only 6 episodes (19%) of NIRS data reflected a drop. Most of these episodes were caused by increased ICP and a corresponding decrease in CPP (see Fig. 6). This phenomenon considerably limits the

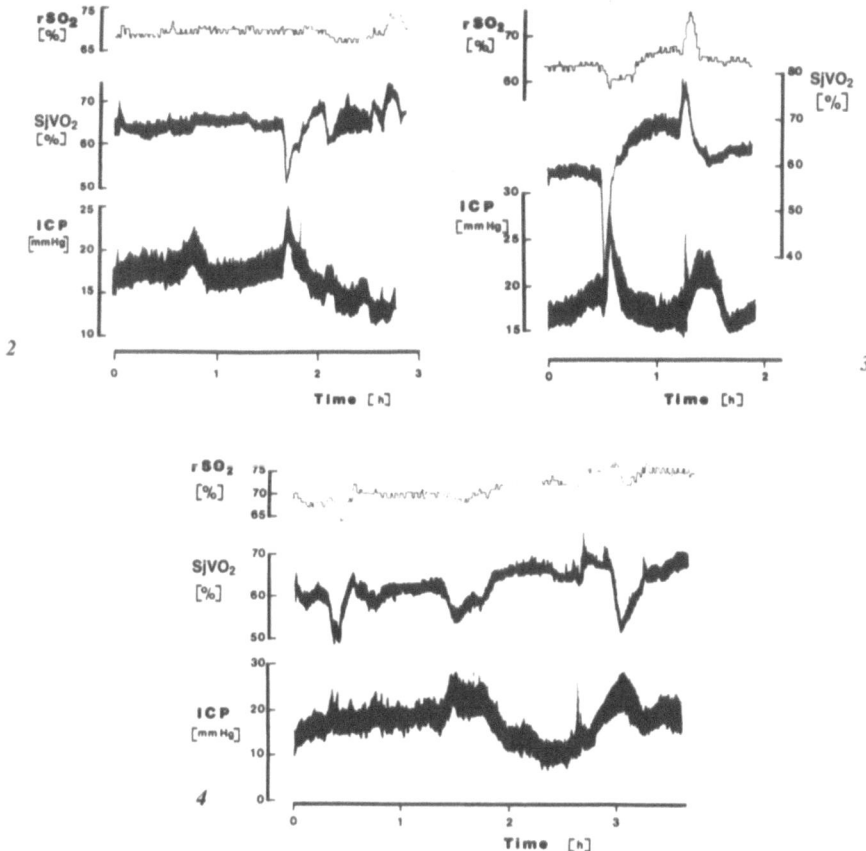

FIG. 2. Cerebral tissue oxygenation (RSO_2) as measured by NIRS, jugular venous oxygen saturation ($SjVO_2$), and intracranial pressure (ICP) in a severely head-injured patient with moderately elevated ICP. RSO_2 and $SjVO_2$ were parallel until an episode of intracranial hypertension when decrease of $SjVO_2$ occurred. This event is not seen on NIRS

FIG. 3. RSO_2 as measured by NIRS, $SjVO_2$, and ICP in a severely head-injured patient. In this case, the rapid and short-lasting jugular venous oxygen desaturation associated with intracranial hypertension is mirrored by a moderate decrease of RSO_2 while the following significant increase in $SjVO_2$ is mirrored more closely by NIRS

FIG. 4. RSO_2 as measured by NIRS, $SjVO_2$, and ICP in a severely head-injured patient. RSO_2 and $SjVO_2$ differ by about 10%. Increases and decreases in oxygen saturation are seen by NIRS, although to a much lesser extent. Moreover, the periods of severe jugular-venous desaturation (combined with intracranial hypertension) cannot be identified as critical episodes by NIRS monitoring

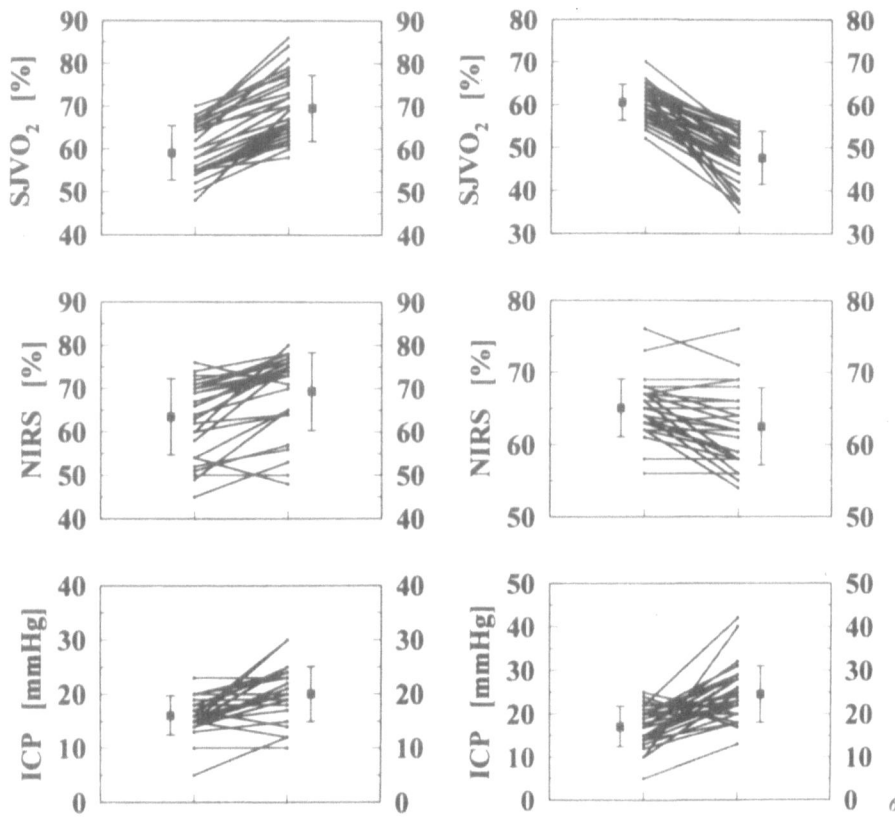

Fig. 5. Summary of episodes in which $SjVO_2$ markedly increased. In most instances, tissue oxygenation as monitored by NIRS also increased, although to a variable degree. ICP was not significantly affected

Fig. 6. Summary of episodes in which jugular venous oxygen saturation markedly decreased because of an episode of intracranial hypertension. Tissue oxygenation as measured by NIRS declined in only 20% of the episodes

significance of NIRS data to guide the therapy of comatose patients because episodes of reduced cerebral oxygenation cannot be recognized by NIRS monitoring.

Monitoring of Cerebral Oxygenation During Herniation and Cerebral Death

Monitoring of cerebral oxygenation during and following tentorial herniation with a following interruption of cerebral perfusion because of intracranial hypertension represents another issue of concern. Typically, $SjVO_2$ decreases during these instances from normal or reduced values to below 40% and then increases to above-normal ranges, because there is no longer any cerebral blood flow and the blood within the jugular bulb and vein represents "extracerebral contamination."

In the group of patients studied, there were two with tentorial herniation and cessation of cerebral blood flow. In both cases, RSO_2 indicated tissue oxygenation values of 60%–70% during the entire observation period of herniation. An example is given in Fig. 7. Again the typical episode of excessive desaturation was not picked up by NIRS. Moreover, placement of NIRS probes above the frontal brain of patients with a proven stagnation of flow in all cerebral arteries (brain death) yielded RSO_2 values in the normal range. The fact that changes in the inspired oxygen concentration were rapidly noticed by NIRS may indicate that the algorithm used by the NIRS monitor is still highly overestimating "extracerebral blood contamination."

Conclusions

The results of our experience with near-infrared spectroscopically monitored regional tissue oxygen saturation are ambiguous. Although there is correspondence between cerebral oxygenation as monitored by $SjVO_2$ and by NIRS in the "normal" range (60%–80%), episodes of global cerebral desaturation as picked up by jugular bulb oximetry were not mirrored by respective NIRS decreases.

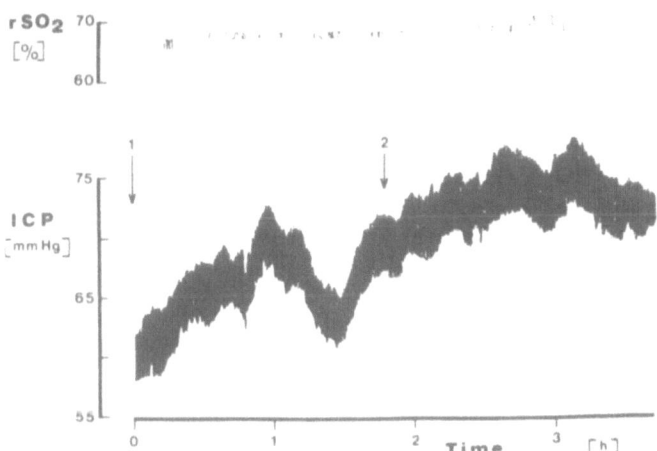

FIG. 7. RSO_2 and ICP in a severely head-injured patient who developed transtentorial herniation and cessation of cerebral blood flow. At the beginning of the tracing (1), the patient had a unilaterally dilated pupil indicating impeding herniation. Although ICP increased further, there was no change in RSO_2. Later (2), both pupils dilated and transcranial Doppler sonography revealed cessation of cerebral blood flow. There was no significant RSO_2 reaction during the entire event

It appears obvious that it is necessary to make significant technological refinements before this new technology enters into clinical routine for monitoring cerebral oxygenation. Additional validation studies are mandatory.

Acknowledgments. The excellent technical and secretarial assistance of Ms. R. Duisberg, C. Dürre, and A. Riede is highly appreciated.

References

1. Ausman JI, McCormick PW, Stewart M, Lewis G, Dujovny M, Balakrishnan G, Malik GM, Ghaly RF (1993) Cerebral oxygen metabolism during hypothermic circulatory arrest in humans. J Neurosurg 79:810–815
2. Brazy JE, Lewis DV, Mitnick MH, Jöbsis FF (1985) Noninvasive monitoring of cerebral oxygenation in preterm infants: preliminary observations. Pediatrics 75: 217–225
3. Jöbsis FF (1977) Noninvasive, infrared monitoring of cerebral and myocardial oxygen sufficiency and circulatory parameters. Science 198:1264–1267
4. McCormick PW, Stewart M, Goetting MG, Dujovny M (1991) Noninvasive cerebral optical spectroscopy for monitoring cerebral oxygen delivery and hemodynamics. Crit Care Med 19:89–97
5. McCormick PW, Stewart M, Goetting MG, Dujovny M (1991) Regional cerebrovascular oxygen saturation measured by optical spectroscopy in humans. Stroke 22:596–602
6. Smith DS, Levy W, Maris M, et al. (1990) Reperfusion hyperoxia in brain after circulatory arrest in humans. Anesthesiology 73:12–19
7. Unterberg AW, Schneider GH, Lanksch WR (eds) (1993) Monitoring of cerebral blood flow and metabolism in intensive care. Acta Neurochirurgica Suppl 59. Springer, Wien, New York

Near-Infrared Spectroscopy at the Sagittal Sinus Region: Comparison with Jugular Bulb Oxymetry

HIDEHIKO KUSHI, TADASHI SHIBUYA, MOTOAKI FUJII,
YOICHI KATAYAMA, AND TAKASHI TSUBOKAWA

Introduction

Since the first clinical application during the 1940s [1,2], infrared spectroscopy has become an important clinical technique through the development of a pulsed oxymeter [3]. More recently, near-infrared intracranial spectroscopy (NIS) has been introduced as a technique to monitor oxygenation of the brain noninvasively [4]. The NIS device is usually placed on the scalp of the forehead so that oxygenation of the frontal lobe at the depth of 2.5 cm is monitored [5–8]. Because the total blood volume of the brain consists of 75% venous blood, data from NIS can be regarded as reflecting the balance of oxygen supply and consumption [9,10]

Such a technique using the NIS has two disadvantages, however. First, because the data are also influenced by oxygen saturation of the arterial blood, this technique may not be sufficiently sensitive to detect early critical changes in oxygenation of the brain. Second, because the data reflect only the local condition of the frontal lobe, changes in oxygenation of other brain areas will escape detection. In contrast, jugular bulb oximetry sensitively provides information closely related to the balance between oxygen supply and consumption, although the technique is invasive. In this study, we examined whether similar information could be obtained noninvasively with NIS if the device was placed at the sagittal sinus region. The depth of the measurement is adjusted to 1.5 cm to detect oxygen saturation of the venous blood flowing through the sagittal sinus. The results were compared with data from jugular venous oximtery in the same patients.

Subjects and Methods

A total of 16 subjects were included in the present study (11 men and 5 women; age ranged from 16 to 70 years) (Table 1). Their best scores on the

Department of Neurological Surgery, Nihon University School of Medicine, 30-1 Oyaguchi-Kamimachi, Itabashi, 173 Tokyo, Japan

TABLE 1. Summary of patient characteristics

Case	Age	Sex	GCS	Diagnosis
1	36	M	5	DBI (moderate)
2	28	M	6	DBI (moderate)
3	34	F	6	DBI (moderate)
4	44	M	5	DBI (moderate)
5	22	F	7	DBI (moderate)
6	39	M	6	DBI (moderate)
7	54	M	5	DBI (severe)
8	18	M	4	DBI (severe)
9	25	M	5	DBI (severe)
10	30	M	5	DBI (severe)
11	16	F	4	Acute subdural hematoma
12	32	M	9	Acute subdural hematoma
13	19	M	9	Cerebral contusion
14	42	F	11	Cerebral contusion
15	70	F	3	Subarachnoid hemorrhage
16	65	M	3	Subarachnoid hemorrhage

GCS, Glasgow Coma Scale; DBI, diffuse brain injury.

Glasgow Coma Scale (GCS) during the initial 24 h ranged from 4 to 9 in 2 patients with acute subdural hematoma, from 9 to 11 in 2 patients with cerebral contusion, from 5 to 8 in 6 patients with a moderate form of diffuse brain injury, and from 4 to 5 in 4 patients with a severe form of diffuse brain injury. Three additional patients with severe subarachnoid hemorrhage were included who were resuscitated from cardiac arrest but remained at a score of 3 on the GCS. All the subjects underwent computed tomography (CT) scans immediately after admission, and magnetic resonance imaging (MRI) was done within 48 h. The 2 patients with acute subdural hematoma underwent craniotomy within 4 h after arrival.

Infrared rays generated by an incandescent light source were collected by a lens, relayed to a wavelength filter, and then led into a fiberoptic cable, where the infrared rays were continuously separated into near-infrared rays of different wavelengths (672, 726, 750, 803, and 840 nm). The timing of near-infrared ray distribution of each wavelength was controlled by a microcomputer built into the NIS mainframe system. This microcomputer enabled the selection of any one of the wavelengths listed to be applied to a patient's tissues for any desired period of time. Absorbance data of near-infrared rays were calculated by comparing the data with the reference wavelength, which was found to be 803 nm, or the point at which the absorbed wavelength of oxidized hemoglobin and that of reduced hemoglobin crossed. Concentrations of a specific substance were determined by the following Beer–Lambert equation on the basis of the absorbance values of the five wavelengths.

$$I(w) = I(w)o \times k \times aCs$$

where I(w) is a transmitted light at wavelength (w), I(w)o is an incident light at that wavelength, k is the absorption coefficient of a specific substance, a is an absorption coefficient, C is the concentration of the substance, and s is the length of optical route of the wavelength.

We placed the device over the superior sagittal sinus region. To detect oxygen saturation of the venous blood flowing through the superior sagittal sinus, near-infrared rays reflected from a depth of 1.5 cm were sampled by a sensor (light-intercepting part) that was located several centimeters away from the light source [4,6,7,9]. Because these infrared rays were mixed with signals from shallower regions, these mingling signals were removed by a second sensor [4,7]. This separation of signals from deeper and shallower regions of the brain was performed by a two-channel multiple wavelength tissue infrared spectrometer, INVOS Model 3100 (Somanetics, Troy, MI USA). Subjects whose scalp and skull were too thick to allow measurements were excluded from this study. Jugular bulb oximetry was performed with the technique previously described elsewhere [11].

Results

Oxygen saturation of the jugular bulb venous blood (SjO_2) monitored with jugular bulb oximetry and oxygen saturation of the sagittal sinus region (rSO_2) monitored with NIS of the 4 patients with severe diffuse brain injury were found to be always less than 60% on admission. Both SjO_2 and rSO_2 rose to more than 60% at 6–12 h after admission. In contrast, the 6 patients with moderate diffuse brain injury consistently showed values greater than 60%. The patient with acute subdural hematoma who scored 4 on GCS following surgical evacuation demonstrated a value less than 60%, whereas the patient with acute subdural hematoma who scored 9 and the 2 patients with cerebral contusion demonstrated values greater than 60%. These 14 patients exhibited high correlations between SjO_2 and rSO_2 (r = .512–.668; $P < .001$) during the initial 48 h after admission. However, the remaining 2 patients with subarachnoid hemorrhaging, who had sustained cardiac arrest at the time of arrival, did not show any significant correlation. Representative cases are presented in the following paragraphs.

Case 2

A 19-year-old man sustained injury in a traffic accident. He scored 4 on GCS and demonstrated a decerebrated posture. CT scans revealed evidence of diffuse brain injury. His SjO_2 and rSO_2 on admission were 55% and 52%, respectively, and returned to a level greater than 60% after approximately 12 h (Fig. 1).

Case 11

A 29-year-old man fell from height. CT scans disclosed an acute subdural hematoma in the right side. He underwent an emergency craniotomy, and

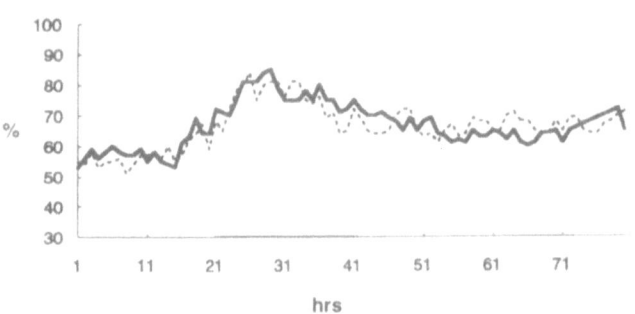

FIG. 1. Case 2: a 19-year-old man was injured in a traffic accident. He scored 4 on the Glasgow Coma Scale (GCS) and demonstrated a decerebrated posture. Computed tomography (CT) scans revealed evidence of diffuse brain injury. SjO_2, jugular bulb venous oxygen saturation (*dotted line*); NIS, near-infrared intracranial spectroscopy (*solid line*)

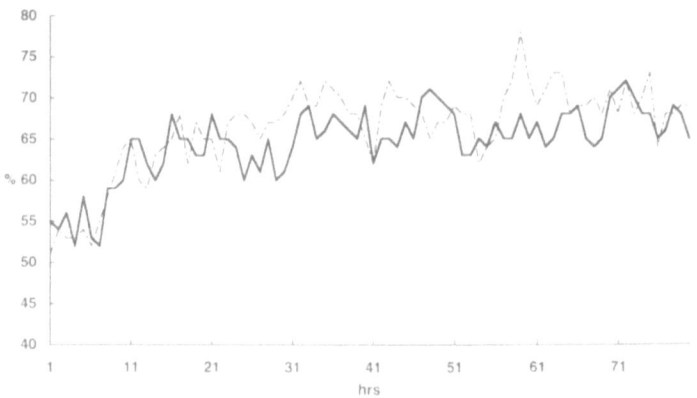

FIG. 2. Case 11: a 29-year-old man fell from height. CT scans disclosed an acute subdural hematoma on the right side. He underwent an emergency craniotomy and the hematoma was evacuated. SjO_2, *dotted line*; NIS, *solid line*

the hematoma was evacuated. SjO_2 and rSO_2 immediately after the surgery were 51% and 55%, respectively. Both SjO_2 and rSO_2 returned to a level greater than 60% at 7h after surgery (Fig. 2).

Case 16

A 65-year-old man suffered a sudden disturbance of consciousness at home and was brought to the emergency service of our hospital. He was in a state of cardiac and pulmonary arrest on arrival. His SjO_2 was 51% immediately after resuscitation but jumped to approximately 90% 1h later. In contrast, rSO_2 showed only gradual increase; it took 70h to reach 90% (Fig. 3). The condition of the patient was consistent with brain death.

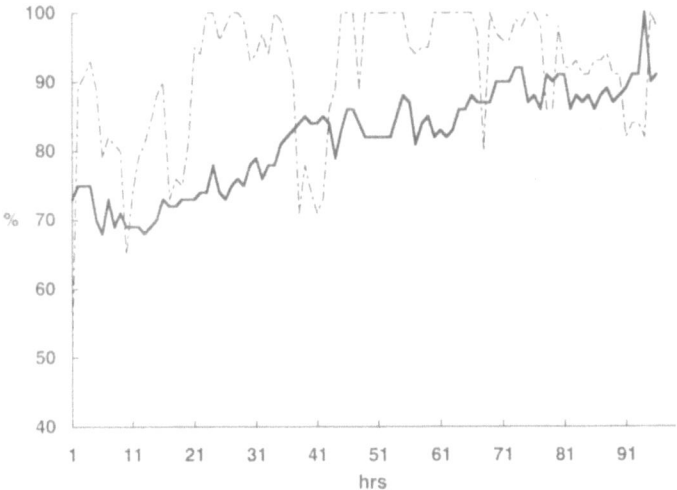

FIG. 3. Case 16: a 65-year-old man suffered a sudden disturbance of consciousness at home and was brought to the emergency service of our hospital. He was in a state of cardiac and pulmonary arrest on arrival. The condition of the patient was consistent with brain death. SjO$_2$, *dotted line*; NIS, *solid line*

Discussion

Near-infrared rays with a wavelength of 650–1000 nm are known to have unique characteristics. These rays penetrate human tissues to a depth of several centimeters [8,9,12,13]. Consequently, they pass through the skull to reach the brain tissues and return to the light-intercepting part of the device, providing a variety of information from the brain. More specifically, red rays that return from intracranial tissues provide information on the characteristics of the emission spectral group contained in the tissues that includes oxyhemoglobin, deoxyhemoglobin, and cytochrome aa_3 [14–16]. The measurement area and the sensor can be optically coupled so that the infrared rays can be projected onto any specific site in tissues to receive the reflecting rays. In other words, NIS is based on the same principle as that of pulsed oxymeters; therefore, it can directly measure the ratio of oxidized hemoglobin contained in the total hemoglobin, instead of continuously measuring the volume of oxidized or reduced hemoglobin separately. The NIS device enables noninvaisve, continuous, and direct measurement of oxygenation of the brain. There have been several reports on direct measurement of oxygenation of the human brain by means of near-infrared rays [17–19]. NIS recently has been employed to monitor oxygenation of the brain during carotid endarterectomy [5,7].

It has become increasingly clear that monitoring of SjO$_2$ provides critical information for the treatment of patients with severe traumatic brain injury [20–24]. The current study confirmed that patients with severe traumatic brain injury tended to show a level less than 60% on admission, suggesting a state in which oxygen supply does not meet oxygen consumption. Such a condition continues if the patient is not appropriately treated. This study also demonstrated that rSO_2 monitored at the sagittal sinus region exhibits a high correlation with SjO_2 in these patients. This implies that NIS may be useful to assess oxygenation of the brain similar to SjO_2. The monitoring of rSO_2 with NIS at the sagittal sinus region has the following advantages: (1) it permits simple and noninvasive measurement; (2) measurements are not affected by changes in the body or neck position of the patient, unlike jugular bulb oximetry; and (3) there is no need for calibration.

Good correlation was not found in the patients with subarachnoid hemorrhage after cardiac arrest and resuscitation. The discrepancy between SjO_2 and rSO_2 in such patients is most likely caused by the difference in the site of measurement. This finding may be interpreted as showing that the highly oxygenated venous blood at the jugular bulb does not reflect the actual status of oxygenation of the brain in patients with impending brain death. Thus, rSO_2 may provide information related more closely to oxygenation of the brain in such circumstances. NIS at the sagittal sinus region has, however, at least two disadvantages: (1) data may be unreliable when the scalp and skull of the patient are too thick, and (2) artifactual variation of data could be induced by patient perspiration, so that a sensor must be cleaned at least once a day. Despite these disadvantages, it is clear that use of NIS at the sagittal sinus region warrants further clinical study.

References

1. Jones RA (1985) Analytical application of vibrational spectroscopy: a historical review. In: Chemical, biological, and industrial application of infrared spectroscopy. New York, Wiley, pp 1–43
2. Dobriner K, Katzenellenbogen ER, Jones RN (1953) Infrared absorption spectra of sterid, vol 2. Interscience, New York
3. Takatani S, Cheung PW, Ernst EA (1980) A noninvasive tissue reflectance oximeter. Ann Biomed Eng 8:1–15
4. McCormic PW, Stewart M, Goetting MG (1991) Noninvasive cerebral optical spectroscopy for monitoring cerebral oxygen delivery and hemodynamics. Crit Care Med 19:89–97
5. James IA, Patric WM, Melville S, Gary L, Gurusway B, Ghaus MN, Ramsis FG (1993) Cerebral oxygen metabolism during hypothermic circulatory arrest in humans. J Neurosurg 79:810–815
6. McCormic PW, Stewart M, Goetting MG (1991) Regional cerebrovascular oxygen saturation measured by optical spectroscopy in humans. Stroke 22:596–602
7. McCormic PW, Stewart M, Lewis G (1991) Noninvasive measurement of regional cerebrovascular oxygen saturation in human using optical spectroscopy. In: Time-resolved spectroscopy and imaging of tissues. Proceedings of the International Society for Optical Engineering, vol 1431. pp 294–302
8. Delpy DT, Cope M, van der Zee P (1988) Estimation of optical pathlength through tissue from direct time flight measurement. Phys Med Biol 33:1433–1442

9. Smith DS, Levy W, Maris M (1990) Reperfusion hypoxia in brain after circulatory arrest in humans. Anesthesiology 73:12–19
10. Mchedlishvili G (1986) Cerebral arterial behavior providing constant blood flow pressure and volume. In: Bevan JA (ed) Arterial behavior and blood circulation in the brain. Plenum, New York, pp 42–95
11. Katayama Y, Tsubokawa T, Hirayama T, Himi K (1994) Continuous monitoring of jugular bulb oxygen saturation as a measure of the shunt flow of cerebral arteriovenous malformations. J Neurosurg 80:826–833
12. Wan S, Parrish JA, Anderson RR (1981) Transmittance of nonionizing radiation in human tissue. Photochem Photobiol 34:679–681
13. Chance B, Leigh JS, Miyake H (1988) Comparison of time-resolved and -unresolved measurements of deoxyhemoglobin in brain. Proc Natl Acad Sci USA 85:4971–4975
14. Hazeki O, Tamura M (1988) Quantitative analysis of hemoglobin oxygenation state of rat brain in situ by near-infrared spectrometry. J Appl Physiol 64:796–802
15. Seed JW, Cefalo RC, Proctor HJ (1984) The relationship of intracranial infrared light absorbance of fetal oxygenation: I. Methodology. Am J Obstet Gynecol 149:679–684
16. Willford DC, Hill EP, Moores WY (1986) Theoretical analysis of oxygen transport during hypothermia. J Clin Monit 2:30–43
17. Cope M, Delpy DT, Reynolds EOR (1988) Methods of quantitating cerebral near infrared spectroscopy data. Adv Exp Med Biol 222:183–189
18. Jobisis FF (1977) Noninvasive, infrared monitoring of cerebral and myocardial oxygen sufficiency and circulatory parameters. Science 198:1264–1267
19. Wiernsperger N, Sylvia AL, Jobsis FF (1981) Incomplete transient ischemia: a non-destructive evaluation of in vivo cerebral metabolism and hemodynamics in rat brain. Stroke 12:864–868
20. Bouma GJ, Muizelaar JP, Choi SC, Newlon PG, Yong HF (1991) Cerebral circulation and metabolism after severe traumatic brain injury: the elusive role of ischemia. J Neurosurg 75:685–693
21. Cruz J, Miner ME, Allen SJ, Alves WM, Gennarelli TA (1991) Continuous monitoring of cerebral oxygenation in acute brain injury: assessment of cerebral hemodynamic reserve. Neurosurgery 29:743–749
22. Sheinberg M, Kanter MJ, Robertson CG, Contant CF, Narayan RK, Grossman RG (1992) Continuous monitoring of jugular venous saturation in head-injured patients. J Neurosurg 76:212–217
23. Robertson CG, Contat CF, Narayan RK, Grossman RG (1992) Cerebral blood flow, AVDO$_2$, and neurologic outcome in head-injured patients. J Neurotrauma 9(Suppl I):349–358
24. Tsubokawa T, Katayama Y (1992) Continuous monitoring of jugular venous oxygen saturation in the management of severe head injury. Crit Rev Neurosurg 2:210 219

Bilateral Simultaneous Monitoring of Regional Cerebrovascular Oxygen Saturation Using Near-Infrared Spectroscopy

Issei Nara, Toshiyuki Shiogai, Nahoko Tanaka, Manabu Tokitsu, and Isamu Saito

Introduction

Near-infrared spectroscopy recently has come to be utilized in neurointensive care settings for continuous, noninvasive, and bedside evaluation of regional oxygen metabolism and hemodynamics [1–3]. Using near-infrared spectroscopy, regional cerebrovascular oxygen saturation (rSO_2) can be calculated [2,4] on the basis of measured oxyhemoglobin and deoxyhemoglobin. Normal control values of rSO_2 in multiple cerebral regions, however, have not been fully established by means of near-infrared spectroscopy. Furthermore, the correlation of rSO_2 with other modalities utilized in neurointensive care, such as intracranial pressure (ICP) [5] and jugular bulb venous oxygen saturation (SjO_2) [6], has been attempted experimentally or in intraoperative monitoring but these results have not been conclusive.

The aim of this study, using near-infrared spectroscopy, was to establish normal control values of rSO_2 in the bifrontal lobes and to evaluate the relationships of bilateral rSO_2 with SjO_2, mean velocity in the middle cerebral artery (Vm) by means of transcranial Doppler ultrasound, and ICP during a CO_2 reactivity test induced by hyperventilation in patients with severe brain damage.

Subjects and Methods

Measurement of rSO_2 in both frontal lobes was performed with two cerebral oximeter probes (INVOS 3100, Somanetics, Troy, MI, USA) attached to the bilateral forehead. Twenty normal healthy adult employees of Kyorin University Hospital (10 men and 10 women aged 23–61 years [mean, 38]) served as controls. Bifrontal rSO_2 values were monitored for 20–48 min (mean, 29 min) at rest in a prone position. Maximum, mean, and minimum

Department of Neurosurgery, Kyorin University School of Medicine, 6-20-2 Shinkawa, Mitaka, Tokyo 181, Japan

rSO_2 monitored values, divided into three age groups (20–30 years, $n = 7$; 31–40 years, $n = 7$; 41–60 years, $n = 6$), were analyzed.

Two comatose patients with severe brain damage (a 56-year-old patient with acute subdural hematoma and a 50-year-old patient with intracerebral hemorrhage) were subjected to CO_2 reactivity tests induced by hyperventilation (9–10 mmHg changes of end-tidal CO_2 partial pressure, $PetCO_2$), and data were collected every 2 min for 40 min (total, 20 data points). These data were compared with those of age-matched controls and correlated with other modalities such as ICP, systemic blood pressure (BP), SjO_2 and arterial oxygen staturation measured by pulse oximeter (SpO_2), and Vm. Bifrontal rSO_2 was correlated with SjO_2 and SpO_2, Vm, and ICP or BP during CO_2 reactivity tests.

In statistical analyses, differences in means were tested using the paired t test or one-way analysis of variance (ANOVA).

Results

Normal Control Subjects

No significant differences between left (L) and right (R) frontal lobes in mean (L = 70.1% ± 5.5%, R = 69.7% ± 3.6%), maximum, or minimum rSO_2 values were observed in any subjects ($n = 20$). Significant increases in mean, minimum, and maximum rSO_2 ($P < .01$, ANOVA) were identified in the oldest age group (40–60 years). In this group, all three rSO_2 values tended to increase in the right side rather than the left side. There were, however, no significant differences between lobes among the three age groups (Table 1).

Case Reports of Severe Brain Damage

In case 1 (a 56-year-old with left acute subdural hematoma), the patient's Glasgow Coma Score at admission was 8. Decompressive craniectomy and evacuation of the hematoma were performed on the day of admission. Computed tomography (CT) scans at admission and 2 days after injury are shown in Fig. 1. A CO_2 reactivity test induced by hyperventilation was carried out 4 days after injury (Fig. 2). During the test, decreased rSO_2 was observed in both sides, in comparison with age-matched control data. rSO_2 values were higher in the craniectomized left frontal lobe than in the non-craniectomized right side. Correlation of $PetCO_2$ changes with ICP, SjO_2, and Vm were apparent, but was not obvious with rSO_2 in either side.

In case 2 (a 50-year-old with right intracerebral hematoma), the patient's Glasgow Coma Score was 7 at admission. Decompressive craniectomy and evacuation of the hematoma were performed on the day of admission. CT scans at admission and 3 days after onset are shown in Fig. 3. Three days after onset, a CO_2 reactivity test induced by hyperventilation was carried out (Fig. 4). During the test, rSO_2 values in both sides remained within the

TABLE 1. Maximum, mean, and minimum regional oxygen saturation (rSO_2) in three normal control age groups

Age	n	Maximum rSO_2			Mean rSO_2			Minimum rSO_2		
		L	R	P value[a]	L	R	P value[a]	L	R	P value[a]
20–30	7	75.7 ± 3.5	74.0 ± 2.8	NS	69.8 ± 3.6	69.1 ± 4.8	NS	63.7 ± 6.9	63.9 ± 7.6	NS
31–40	7	69.1 ± 3.3	69.6 ± 5.3	NS	67.1 ± 2.5	66.9 ± 4.3	NS	65.0 ± 2.0	64.0 ± 3.9	NS
41–60	6	75.8 ± 4.2	76.8 ± 5.5	NS	72.5 ± 3.7	75.0 ± 4.0	NS	69.0 ± 4.4	72.7 ± 3.7	NS
P values[b]		<.01	<.01		<.01	<.01		<.01	<.01	

[a] mean ± SD; paired t test; ns = not significant, $P > .05$.
[b] ANOVA.

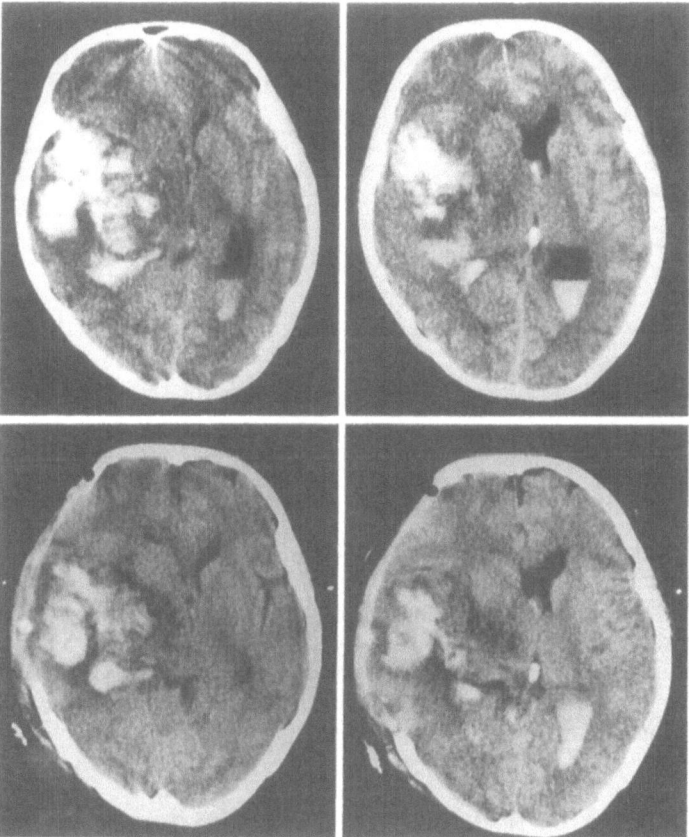

FIG. 1. Case 1: preoperative and postoperative computed tomography (CT) scans were obtained on admission day (*upper row*) and 2 days after injury (*lower row*). Left acute subdural hematoma was evacuated and craniotomized bone removed for external decompression (*lower*)

normal range (mean $\pm$ 2 SD) in comparison with age-matched controls. rSO_2 values were higher in the craniectomized right frontal lobe than in the noncraniectomized left side. Correlation of $PetCO_2$ changes with SjO_2 and Vm were apparent, but was not obvious with rSO_2 in either side.

Discussion

Transcranial measurement of regional cerebrovascular oxygen saturation using near-infrared spectroscopy was first introduced by Jöbsis in 1977 [7] and has since been utilized clinically for both neonates [3] and adults [2]. To date, there has been no clear establishment of normal rSO_2 values in both frontal lobes as obtained by near-infrared spectroscopy. On the basis of

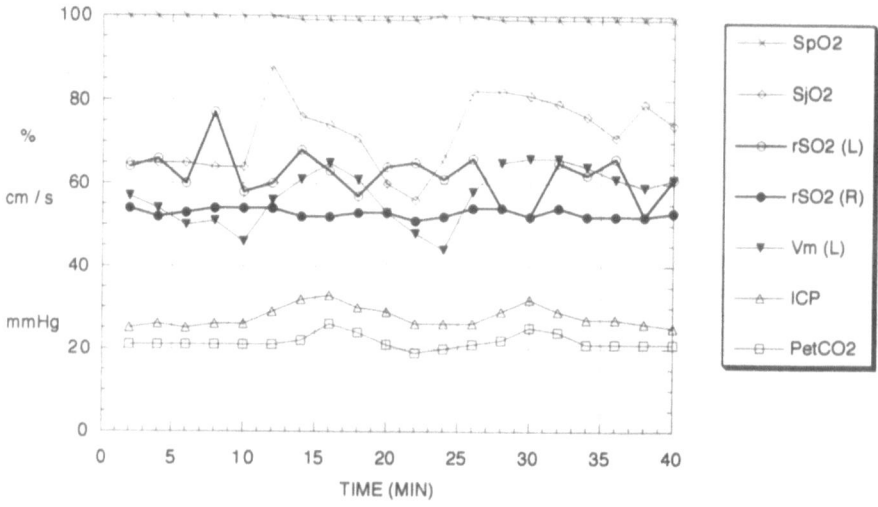

FIG. 2. Case 1: serial changes in pulse oximetric arterial oxygen saturation (SpO_2) and jugular bulb venous oxygen saturation (SjO_2), regional cerebrovascular oxygen saturation (rSO_2) on both sides, mean velocity in the left middle cerebral artery (Vm) , intracranial pressure (ICP), and end-tidal CO_2 partial pressure ($PetCO_2$) were measured during a CO_2 reactivity test. rSO_2 values in the craniectomized left frontal lobe were higher than in the noncraniectomized right side. Correlation of $PetCO_2$ changes with ICP, SjO_2, and Vm were apparent, but was not obvious with rSO_2 on either side

measured arterial oxygen saturation (SaO_2) and SjO_2, normal rSO_2 values in adults were estimated by the following equation: $rSO_2 = x(SaO_2) + (1 - x)$ (SjO_2), with x being the percentage of regional cerebral blood volume [2,4]. If the reported normal SaO_2 value of 98% and SjO_2 values of 54%–70% (mean $\pm$ 2 SD) [8] and x values of 0.18 or 0.28 were substituted in this equation, the normal rSO_2 range would be estimated as follows: 62%–75% ($x = 0.18$) and 66%–77% ($x = 0.28$), respectively. In our study, the range of measured rSO_2 values (mean $\pm$ 2 SD), 59%–81% in the left side and 62%–78% in the right side, approximated the estimated values.

In relation to age, the progressive reduction with advancing age of regional cerebral blood flow (rCBF) or the regional cerebral metabolic rate of oxygen (rCMRO$_2$), especially in the frontal lobe [9,10], has been pointed out using the N$_2$O technique [11], the ^{133}Xe inhalation method [12,13], and positron emission tomography [9,10]. In our study of the oldest age group, rSO_2 values were significantly as compared with the younger age groups. This result probably indicates that decreased rCMRO$_2$ is more apparent than rCBF, particularly in the frontal lobe [10]. With respect to side difference, decreased rCMRO$_2$ [10] or rCBF [14] in the left hemisphere has been reported. In our study, there was no significant side difference, but in the oldest age group the left side rSO_2 tended to be lower than right rSO_2,

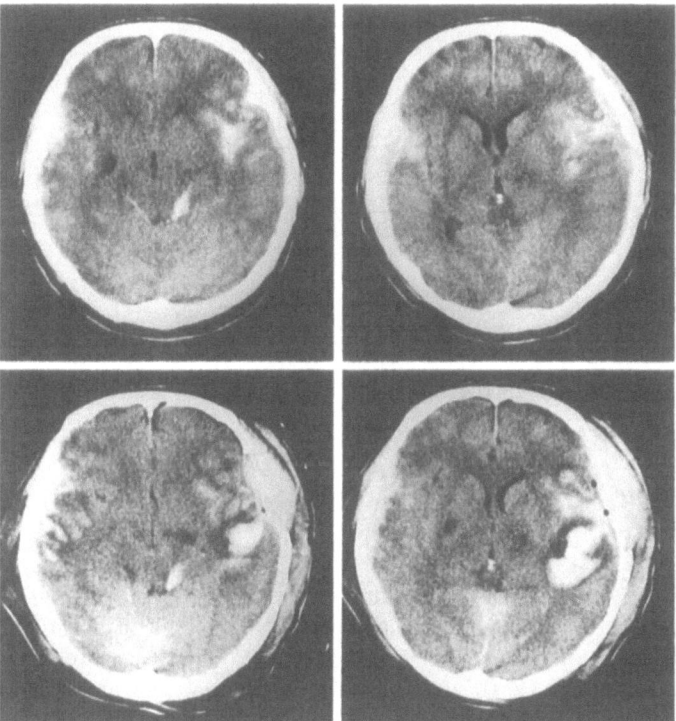

FIG. 3. Case 2: preoperative and postoperative CT scans were obtained on admission day (*upper row*) and 3 days after onset (*lower row*). Right intracerebral hematoma was evacuated and craniotomized bone removed for external decompression (*lower*)

suggesting that decreased rCBF is more apparent than $rCMRO_2$ in the left frontal lobe in this age group.

With respect to correlation between rSO_2 and other parameters during CO_2 reactivity tests induced by hyperventilation, there was no apparent correlation with rSO_2 on either side despite close correlations of $PetCO_2$ with SjO_2, Vm, and ICP. It will not be possible to determine the cause of discrepancies on the basis of these preliminary data. However, focal disturbance of CO_2 reactivity, correlation between rSO_2 and $rCMRO_2$, and systemic errors [6,15] should be taken into consideration. Further study is required for clarification in this regard.

Conclusion

Simultaneous bilateral monitoring of regional cerebrovascular oxygen saturation usisng near-infrared spectroscopy appears to be useful for the noninvasive evaluation of serial and regional changes of cerebral oxygen

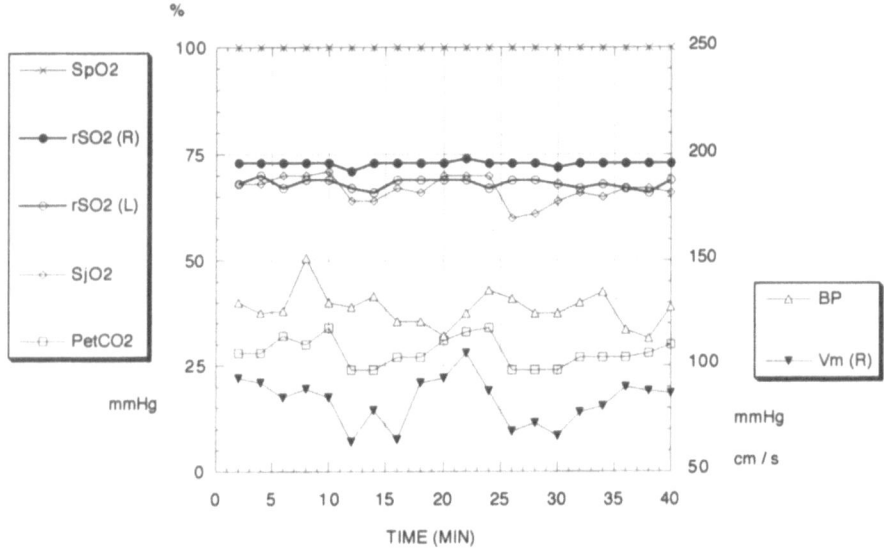

FIG. 4. Cases 2: serial changes in pulse oximetric arterial oxygen saturation (SpO_2), regional cerebrovascular oxygen saturation (rSO_2) on both sides, jugular bulb venous oxygen saturation (SjO_2), systemic blood pressure (BP), means velocity in right middle cerebral artery (Vm), and end-tidal CO_2 partial pressure ($PetCO_2$) were measured during a CO_2 reactivity test. rSO_2 values were higher in the craniectomized right frontal lobe than in the noncraniectomized left frontal lobe. Correlation of $PetCO_2$ changes with SjO_2 and Vm was apparent, but was not obvious with rSO_2 on either side

metabolism and hemodynamics in normal subjects and in patients with various brain damage.

Acknowledgments. This work was supported by the Tokyo Institute of Medical Science Japan.

References

1. McCormick PW, Stewart M, Goetting MG, Dujovny M, Lewis G, Ausman JI (1991) Noninvasive cerebral optical spectroscopy for monitoring cerebral oxygen delivery and hemodynamics. Crit Care Med 19:89–97
2. McCormick PW, Stewart M, Goetting MG, Balakrishnan G (1991) Regional cerebrovascular oxygen saturation measured by optical spectroscopy in humans. Stroke 22:596–602
3. Brazy JE (1991) Cerebral oxygen monitoring with near-infrared spectroscopy: clinical application to neonates. J Clin Monit 7:325–334
4. McCormick PW, Stewart M, Ray P, Dujovny M, Ausman JI (1991) Measurement of regional cerebrovascular hemoglobin oxygen saturation in cats using optical spectroscopy. Neurol Res 13:65–70

5. Cairns CB, Fillipo D, Proctor HJ (1985) A nonivasive method for monitoring the effects of increased intracranial pressure with near-infrared spectrophotometry. Surg Gynecol Obstet 161:145–148

6. Brown R. Wright G, Royston D (1993) A comparison of two systems for assessing cerebral venous oxyhemoglobin saturation during cardiopulmonary bypass in humans. Anaesthesia 48:697–700

7. Jöbsis FF (1977) Non-invasive, infrared monitoring of cerebral and myocardial oxygen sufficiency and circulatory parameters. Science 198:1264–1267

8. Robertson CS (1993) Jugular venous oxygen saturation monitoring in head injured patients. In: Proceedings of the 4th biannual conference of cerebral venous oxygen saturation monitoring, December 18, 1993, Tokyo, pp 7–12

9. Pantano P, Baron J-C, Lebrun-Grandié P, Duquesnoy N, Bouser M-G, Comar D (1984) Regional cerebral blood flow and oxygen consumption in human aging. Stroke 15:635–641

10. Yamaguchi T, Kanno I, Uemura K, Shishido F, Inugumi A, Ogawa T, Murakami M, Suzuki K (1986) Reduction in regional cerebral metabolic rate of oxygen during human aging. Stroke 17:1220–1228

11. Kety SS (1956) Human cerebral blood flow and oxygen consumption as related to aging. J Chronic Dis 3:478–486

12. Naritomi H, Meyer JS, Sakai F, Yamaguchi F, Shaw T (1979) Effects of advancing age on regional cerebral blood flow: studies in normal subjects and subjects with risk factors for atherothrombotic stroke. Arch Neurol 36:410–416

13. Melamed E, Lavy S, Bentin S, Cooper G, Rinot Y (1980) Reduction in regional cerebral blood flow during normal aging in man. Stroke 11:31–35

14. Rodriguez G, Warkentin S, Risberg J, Rosadini G (1988) Sex differences in regional cerebral blood flow. J Cereb Blood Flow Metab 8:783–789

15. Kruth CD, Steven JM, Benaron D, Chance B (1993) Near-infrared monitoring of the cerebral circulation. J Clin Monit 9:163–170

Effects of Hyperventilation and CO_2 Inhalation on Cerebral Oxygen Metabolism of Moyamoya Disease Measured by Near-Infrared Spectroscopy

Kaoru Sakatani[1], Masafumi Ohtaki[1], Masataka Kashiwasake[2], and Kazuo Hashi[1]

Introduction

Near-infrared spectroscopy (NIR) can give continuous, direct information about cerebral oxygen metabolism not only in infants but also in adults by providing signals from oxyhemoglobin (oxy-Hb), deoxyhemoglobin (deoxy-Hb), and the redox state of cytochrome aa$_3$ (Cyt). Using NIR, we examined the cerebral oxygen metabolism of normal adults and patients with moyamoya disease.

Methods

We studied ten patients with moyamoya disease and nine normal adult volunteers using NIR. Table 1 summarizes the patients studied. The disease was diagnosed in all patients by angiography, which demonstrated stenosis or occlusion of bilateral internal carotid arteries with moyamoya vessels. Besides angiography, computed tomography (CT) scan or magnetic resonance imaging (MRI) were performed in all patients, and single photon emission CT was performed in seven patients. Extracranial-intracranial (EC-IC) bypass, such as superficial temporal artery–middle cerebral artery (STA–MCA) anastomosis, were performed in seven of ten patients.

We measured the relative changes in the concentrations of oxy-Hb, deoxy-Hb, and the redox state of Cyt using an NIR instrument (NIRO-500, Hamamatsu Photonics, Hamamatsu, Japan). For measurement of these parameters, the transmitting fiberoptic bundle pulsed six consecutive wavelengths of NIR light (780, 808, 828, 850, 870, and 904 nm), and reflected

[1] Department of Neurosurgery, Sapporo Medical University, S-1, W-16, Chuo-ku, Sapporo, 060 Japan
[2] Hamamatsu Photonics Tsukuba Laboratory, 5-9-4, Tsukuba city, Ibaraki, 300-26 Japan

light was collected in the receiving fiberoptic bundle and transmitted to a photomultiplier tube. We used the differential path length fraction of adult heads (5.93 ± 0.42, mean ± SD), which was determined by time-of-fight measurement of an ultrashort optical pulse through the tissues [1]. Using an algorithm developed by Wray et al. [2], concentrations of oxy-Hb, deoxy-Hb, and Cyt were continuously analyzed by means of a computer incorporated into the apparatus. The change in cerebral blood volume (CBV) was considered to be that of total hemoglobin (oxy-Hb + deoxy-Hb) [3].

Results

Effects of Hyperventilation

Hypervenilation decreased PaCO$_2$ and increased PaO$_2$ with respiratory alkalosis in both control and moyamoya groups. In both groups, hyperventilation caused an decrease of oxy-Hb with only a mild increase in deoxy-Hb, resulting in a decrease of total Hb (Fig. 1). These changes recovered to the control levels after hyperventilation.

Effects of CO$_2$ Inhalation

Inhalation of CO$_2$ increased PaCO$_2$ and PaO$_2$ with respiratory acidosis in both groups. In both normal adults and the patients with moyamoya disease, CO$_2$ inhalation caused an increase of oxy-Hb with a mild decrease in deoxy-Hb, resulting in an increase of total Hb. However, these changes were smaller in the moyamoya group than those in the control group. Figure 2 compares the changes of the NIR parameters taken before, during, and after CO$_2$ inhalation in normal adult and a patient with moyamoya diseases. Note that oxy-Hb rapidly increased with a mild decrease of deoxy-Hb in the normal adult immediately after the start of CO$_2$ inhalation, but these same changes were smaller in the patients with moyamoya disease than those in the normal adults.

Comparison of CO$_2$ Responses in Normal Adults and Patients with Moyamoya Disease

Figure 3 shows the correlation between the changes of arterial PCO$_2$ and oxy-Hb. In both normal adults and the patients with moyamoya disease, oxy-Hb increases linearly with increase of arterial PCO$_2$. However, these changes in moyamoya disease patients are slightly smaller than those in the normal adult. To clearly see the difference in CO$_2$ responses of control and moyamoya groups, we calculated the CO$_2$ response index as the changes in oxy-Hb, deoxy-Hb, and total Hb, while eliminating the effects of arterial PCO$_2$ change (Table 2). We excluded the cases without EC-IC bypass surgery. There is no significant difference in the CO^2 response index between

TABLE 1. Summary of the cases of moyamoya disease

Case	Age (years)	Sex	Onset (age)	CT/MRI	SPECT	Surgery	Interval (surgery–NIR)
1.	16	F	TIA (9 yr)	Normal	Right hemisphere CBF↓	Right, STA-MCA + EMS Left, omentum	6 yr
2.	38	F	TIA (7–12 yr)	Normal	Bitemporooccipital CBF↓	Right, left, STA-MCA + EMS	2 yr
3.	11	F	TIA (5 yr)	Normal	(−)	Right, STA-MCA + omentum	6 yr
4.	13	F	TIA (3 yr)	Lacunar infarction in right frontal lobe	Left parietooccipital CBF↓	Right, left, EMS	9 yr
5.	48	F	Hemorrhage (44 yr)	Old hematoma in left temporal lobe	Left temporal, right occipital CBF↓	Right, left, STA-MCA + EMS	4 yr
6.	40	F	Seizure (?)	Lacunar infarction in bifrontal lobe	(−)	Right, left, STA-MCA	7 yr
7.	56	M	Infarction (56 yr)	Watershed infarction in right temporooccipital lobe	Right hemisphere CBF↓	Right, STA-MCA + EMS	1 mo
8.	14	F	Seizure (13 yr)	Normal	(−)	(−)	
9.	37	F	Infarction (37 yr)	Infarction in right temporoparietal lobe	Right hemisphere CBF↓	(−)	
10.	24	F	TIA (10 yr)	Lacunar infarction in bifrontal lobe	Bifrontal CBF↓	(−)	

CT/MRI, computed tomography/magnetic resonance imaging; SPECT, single photon emission computed tomography; TIA, transient ischemic attack; STA, superficial temporal artery; MCA, middle cerebral artery; CBF, cerebral blood flow; EMS, encephalomyosynangiosis.

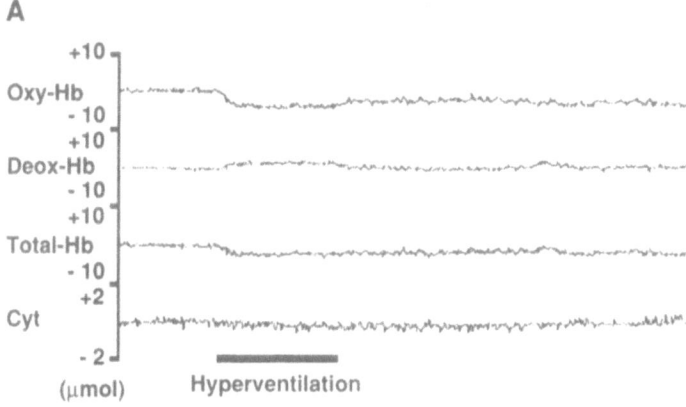

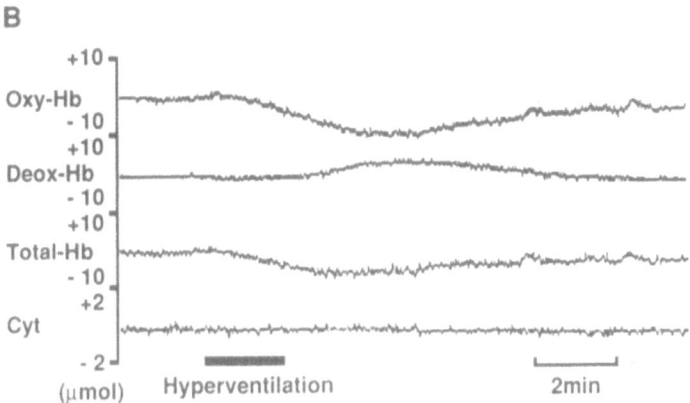

FIG. 1A,B. Effects of hyperventilation on cerebral oxygen metabolism in a normal adult (**A**) and a patient with moyamoya disease (**B**). Hyperventilation causes an decreases of oxyhemaglobin (*oxy-Hb*) with a mild increase in deoxyhemoglobin (*deoxy-Hb*), resulting in a decrease of total Hb in both groups. (*Cyt,*) These changes recovered to control levels after hyperventilation

control and moyamoya groups during hyperventilation. However, the increase of oxy-Hb in moyamoya disease during CO_2 inhalation is significantly smaller than that in normal adults ($P < .01$).

Changes in Cytochrome aa₃ During Hyperventilation

We observed reductions of Cyt in one case of moyamoya disease during hyperventilation (Fig. 4A). After hyperventilation, deoxy-Hb increases as oxy-Hb decreases without changes in total Hb, indicating a hypoxic change. The patient complained numbness of the extremities during this period. Cyt reduces with these changes. In another case of moyamoya

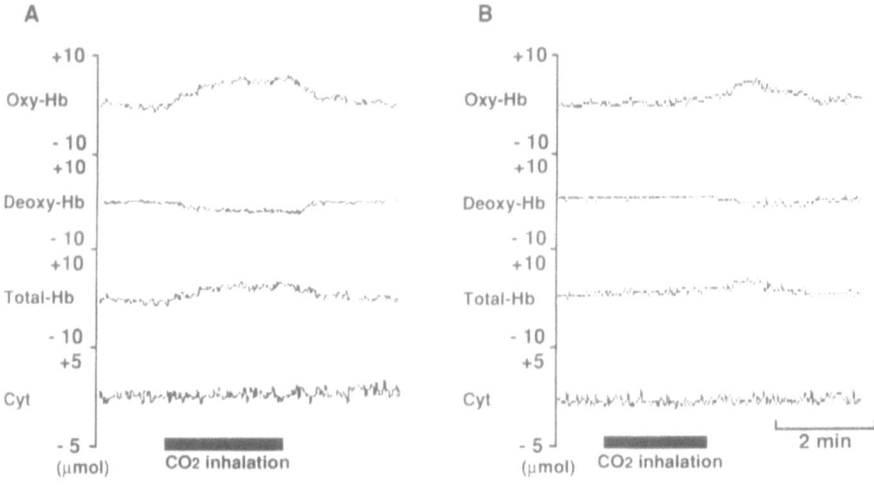

FIG. 2A,B. Effects of CO_2 inhalation on cerebral oxygen metabolism in a normal adult (**A**) and a patient with moyamoya disease (**B**). Note that changes in the near-infrared (NIR) parameters of moyamoya disease are smaller than those in the normal adult

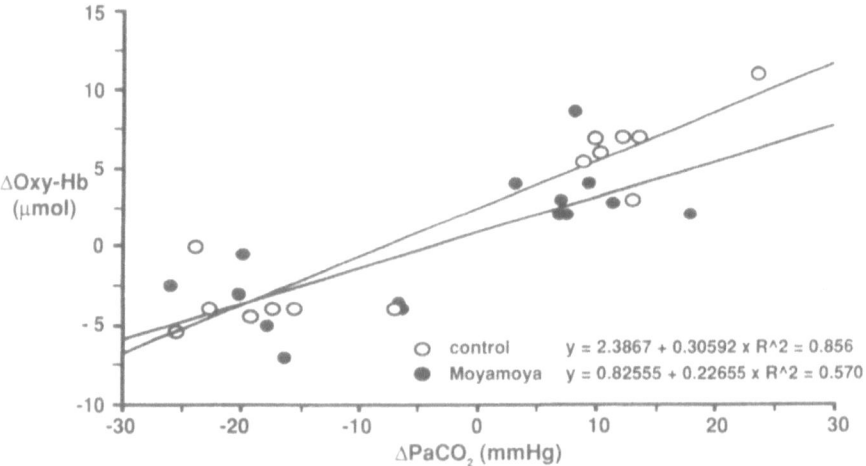

FIG. 3. The correlation between the changes of arterial $PaCO_2$ and oxy-Hb. In both normal adults and the patients with moyamoya disease, oxy-Hb increases linearly with increase of arterial PCO_2. Note that these changes are slightly smaller in moyamoya disease than those in the normal adult

disease, hyperventilation caused ischemic changes of the NIR parameters and transient hemiparesis without any changes in Cyt (Fig. 4B). EC-IC bypass surgery was not performed in either patient at the time of measurement.

TABLE 2. Changes in oxy-Hb, deoxy-Hb, and Total Hb after CO_2 inhalation and hyperventilation

Condition	ΔOxy-Hb/ΔPaCO$_2$	ΔDeoxy-Hb/ΔPaCO$_2$	ΔTotal Hb/ΔPaCO$_2$
CO_2 inhalation			
Contral ($n = 8$)	0.5 ± 0.1	0.0 ± 0.1	0.4 ± 0.1
Moyamoya ($n = 4$)	0.3 ± 0.1	0.0 ± 0.0	0.3 ± 0.1
Hyperventilation			
Control ($n = 6$)	0.3 ± 0.1	0.0 ± 0.0	0.2 ± 0.2
Moyamoya ($n = 4$)	0.4 ± 0.2	0.0 ± 0.1	0.4 ± 0.3

(For CO_2 inhalation Oxy-Hb values: $P < 0.01$)

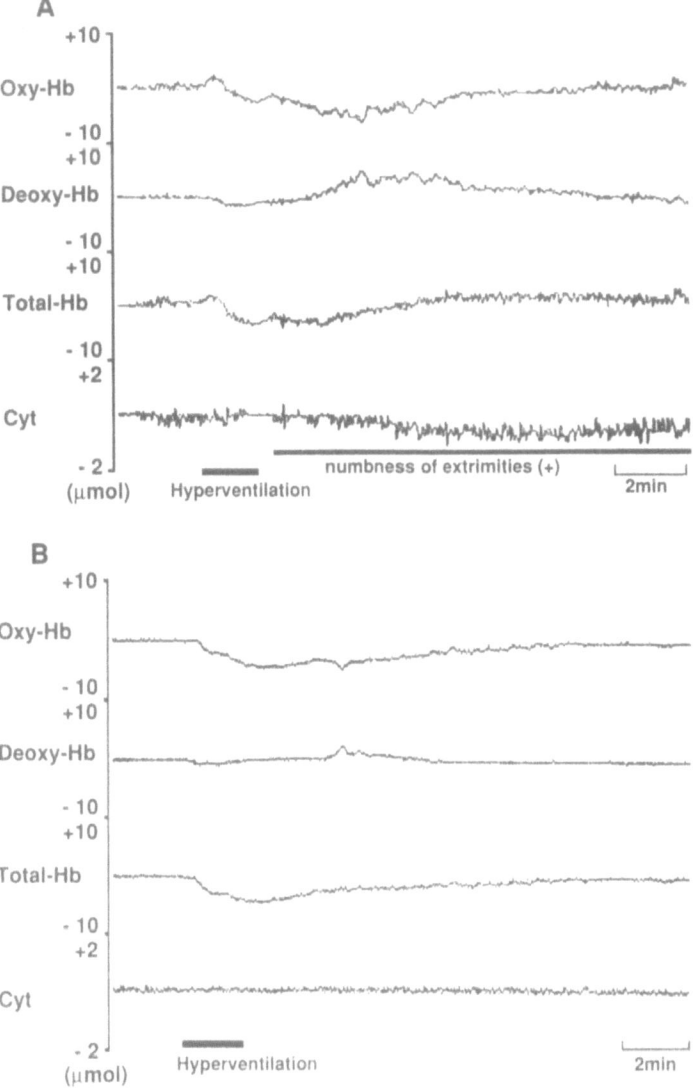

FIG. 4A,B. Changes in redox state of cytochrome aa$_3$ (Cyt) of Moyamoya disease during hyperventilation. Hyperventilation induced clinical symptoms in these patients with (**A**) and without (**B**) a reduction of Cyt

Dependence of Cerebral Oxygen Metabolism on Blood Flow of Extracranial Arteries After EC-IC Bypass

We also examined whether NIR can detect the dependence of cerebral oxygen metabolism on the blood flow of the extracranial arteries after EC-IC bypass. Figure 5 shows changes of the NIR parameters during compression of the superficial temporal artery (STA), which was anastomosed to the branch of the middle cerebral artery (MCA) 5 years previously. Compression of STA decreases oxy-Hb and total Hb with a mild increase of deoxy-Hb. These changes are similar to the changes in cerebral ischemia. These changes induced by STA compression were observed in four of seven operated cases.

Discussion

The changes of oxy-Hb, deoxy-Hb, and total Hb induced by hyperventilation were divided into three patterns. First, oxy-Hb decreases without changes in deoxy-Hb resulted in a decrease of total Hb, indicating ischemia from constriction of small arteries. Second, oxy-Hb decreases and deoxy-Hb increases of the same size resulting in no change of total Hb. This pattern indicates hypoxia. Third, oxy-Hb decreases with a mild increase in deoxy-Hb resulting in a decrease of total Hb, and suggesting hypoxic ischemia. We observed ischemic or hypoxic ischemic changes mainly during hyperventilation. Hypoxic change was observed only after hyperventilation. These

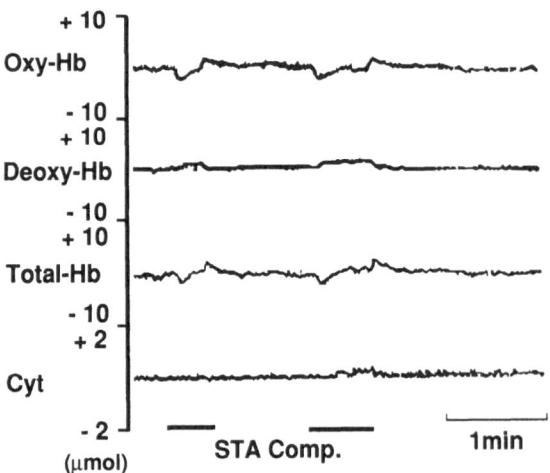

Fig. 5. Dependence of cerebral oxygen metabolism on blood flow of extracranial arteries after extracranial-intracranial (EC-IC) bypass. Compression of the superficial temporal artery decreases oxy-Hb and total Hb with a mild increase of deoxy-Hb, indicating ischemic changes. This patient underwent superficial temporal artery–middle cerebral artery (STA–MCA) anastomosis 5 years ago

observations suggest that CBV returned to the control level as arterial PCO$_2$ recovered to the baseline after hyperventilation, but systemic hypoxia developed after hyperventilation. Indeed, systemic arterial O$_2$ saturation measured by a pulse oxymeter decreased after hyperventilation in some cases (unpublished data). Such hypoxic change measured by NIR was similar to the rebuildup phenomena of the electroencephalograph (EEG), which is specific in moyamoya disease [4], but the hypoxic change was also observed in normal adults.

All patients who underwent EC-IC bypass surgery improved clinically. In addition, the cerebral vasodilatory capacity induced by hypercapnea was likely to be maintained (see Fig. 3). It has been reported that EC-IC bypass surgery improves cerebral blood flow in moyamoya disease. However, the increase of oxy-Hb with EC-IC bypass surgery during CO$_2$ inhalation in moyamoya disease was significantly smaller than that in a normal adult (see Table 2). These results suggest that EC-IC bypass surgery may increase cerebral blood flow but fail to improve the CO$_2$-induced vasomotor reactivity in patients with moyamoya disease. These results are inconsistent with the study of xenon-133 inhalation and single photon emission CT, which demonstrate an increase in the regional vasodilatory capacity induced by acetazolamide after EC-IC bypass surgery [5]. The conflicting results may be caused by the limitation of the monitored field of NIR or the difference in vasodilatory activity of CO$_2$ inhalation and acetazolamide.

The NIRO-500 allows us to measure changes of brain Cyt, which reflects oxidative metabolism at the cellular level. We observed reductions of Cyt in a case of moyamoya disease during hyperventilation (see Fig. 4A). Clinical symptoms were associated with the reduction of Cyt. We also observed a reduction of Cyt during a balloon Matas test with abolishment of somatosensory evoked response (unpublished data). However, in another case of moyamoya disease, hyperventilation caused ischemic changes in NIR parameters and clinical symptoms without any changes in Cyt (see Fig. 4B). This inconsistency of Cyt changes measured by NIR may result from the limitation of the monitored field of NIR because the case without changes of Cyt showed a reduced cerebral blood flow in areas that were far from the frontal lobes. Another possibility is that changes of oxy-Hb and deoxy-Hb may affect the measurement of Cyt. We injected saline into the internal carotid artery to decrease the concentration of hemoglobin (unpublished data). However, Cyt did not show any change during hemodilution, suggesting that the change of Cyt is not caused by the changes of oxy-and deoxy-Hb.

Compression of STA caused ischemic changes in the patients who underwent EC-IC bypass surgery. These results suggest that NIR can monitor the patency of EC-IC bypass noninvasively. However, we do not know whether the blood flow of the skin affects the parameters measured by NIR. To clarify this point, we tested the effect of STA compression and the effect of saline injection into the external carotid artery on NIR parameters during angiography of the cases without EC-IC bypass (unpublished data).

These effects were small but not negligible in these cases, indicating that blood flow of skin can affect the NIR parameters. Thus, we may not be able to use the STA compression technique in the case of a single anastomosis.

Finally, we conclude that the NIR technique is clinically very useful for detecting changes of cerebral oxygen metabolism. However, there are also limitations and problems with this technique.

References

1. Van der Zee P, Cope M, Arridge SR, et al (1991) Experimentally measured optical pathlengths for the adult head, calf and forearm and the head of the newborn infants as a function of inter optode spacing. Adv Exp Med Biol 316:143–151
2. Wray S, Cope M, Delpy DT, et al (1988) Characterization of the near infrared absorption spectra of cytochrome aa$_3$ and haemoglobin for the noninvasive monitoring of cerebral oxygenation. Biochim Biophys Acta 933:184–192
3. Wayatt JS, Cope M, Delpy DT, et al (1986) Quantification of cerebral oxygenation and haemodynamics in sick newborn infants by near-infrared spectrophotometry. Lancet ii:1063–1066
4. Kodama N, Aoki Y, Hiraga H, Wada T, Suzuki J (1979) Electroencephalographic findings in children with Moyamoya disease. Arch Neurol 36:16–19
5. Vorstrup S, Brun B, Lassen NA (1986) Evaluation of the cerebral vasodilatory capacity by the acetazolamide test before EC-IC bypass suggery in patients with occlusion of the internal carotid artery. Stroke 17:1291–1298

Index

A

acetazolamide 233
acute subdural hematoma (SDH) 64,
   72, 100, 117, 120, 134, 135, 212,
   213, 219
aerobic metabolism 31, 117
afterdischarge (AD) 17, 43, 44, 46
amino acid 65, 79, 82
2-amino-5-phosphonovalerate (APV)
   17, 43, 43, 46
AMPA receptor 31, 49
anaerobic metabolism 81, 169,
   186
anemia 88, 94, 123, 125
anesthesia 94, 127, 128, 132, 140
anoxia 3, 6, 13, 14, 15
anoxic depolarization 16, 17, 18
arterial oxygen saturation (Sao$_2$) 106,
   117, 164, 165, 173, 174, 181,
   196, 201, 205, 222
arteriojugular venous lactate content
   difference (AJDL) 88
arteriovenous malformation (AVM)
   146, 148, 149
arteriojugular venous oxygen
   content difference (AJDO$_2$,
   AVDO$_2$) 65, 66, 68, 88, 106,
   109, 180, 181, 182, 183, 185,
   186
aspartate 38, 54, 55, 60, 61, 65, 66,
   80, 81
astrocyte 29, 31, 70, 71, 81
autoragiogram 7, 28, 31, 36
autoradiography 27, 31, 34, 35
autoregulation 109, 110, 180, 181,
   183, 185, 186, 187

B

balloon Matas test 233
barbiturate therapy 80, 113, 117, 134,
   135, 137, 138, 139, 165, 174, 177
bilateral catheterization 154
bilateral jugular bulb 112
blood flow velocity 105, 107, 164,
   165, 168, 169, 218
brain compliance 110
brain damage 47, 49, 120, 218, 219
brain death 102, 121, 174, 214, 216
brain edema 39, 185, 187
brain energy metabolism 61
brain injury 59, 81, 88, 94, 99, 105,
   106, 110, 204, 215, 216
brain ischemia 105, 168
brain oxygen metabolism 120
brain swelling 70, 117, 121, 125, 137,
   174, 177
brain temperature 173, 174
brain trauma 64, 87, 93, 94
brain tumor 72

C

^{45}Ca accumulation 35, 36, 38, 39
^{45}Ca autoradiography 5, 36, 39
Ca^{2+} 5, 12, 13, 14, 15, 17, 18, 46
Ca^{2+} dependent 14, 15, 76
calcium 32, 34, 54, 55
calcium antagonist 135
CA1 pyrmidal cell 17, 42, 46
carbon dioxide reactivity 107, 108,
   110
cardiopulmonary bypass (CPB) 127,
   132, 140, 141, 142, 143, 144

carotid endarterectomy   215
cell death   26, 32
cellular membrane   3, 4, 6, 8, 9, 10, 11, 12, 13, 18, 76
cellular swelling   4, 6, 7, 8, 9, 10, 11, 15
central nervous system (CNS)   3, 4, 11, 72
cerebral acidosis   164, 168
cerebral blood flow (CBF)   49, 50, 51, 52, 53, 54, 60, 68, 81, 87, 88, 90, 98, 100, 101, 102, 103, 109, 110, 120, 123, 124, 125, 134, 138, 139, 153, 156, 158, 160, 162, 164, 168, 169, 173, 174, 176, 180, 181, 182, 183, 185, 186, 209, 222, 223, 233
cerebral blood volume (CBV)   110, 177, 185, 222, 227, 233
cerebral contusion   64, 66, 72, 79, 80, 100, 120, 122, 174, 212, 213
cerebral damage   64, 132
cerebral extraction ratio (CEO$_2$)   88, 186
cerebral function   127, 159, 193
cerebral hemorrhage   101, 134
cerebral hyperemia   106
cerebral hypoperfusion   93, 94, 95
cerebral infarction   61
cerebral ischemia   3, 6, 7, 8, 11, 12, 13, 14, 15, 16, 17, 31, 32, 42, 87, 88, 90, 101, 103, 105, 106, 112, 122, 125, 126, 127, 132, 158, 176, 201, 202
cerebral metabolic rate of oxygen consumption (CMRO$_2$)   61, 88, 109, 110, 134, 139, 168, 169, 176, 180, 181, 185, 222, 223
cerebral oxygenation   127, 204, 205, 206, 207, 208, 209
cerebral oxygen extraction (CEO$_2$)   64, 68, 69
cerebral oxygen metabolism   98, 102, 103, 164, 228, 232, 234
cerebral oximeter   193, 194, 201
cerebral perfusion pressure (CPP)   61, 66, 68, 70, 79, 87, 93, 94, 105, 106, 107, 108, 109, 110, 113, 156, 164, 165, 169, 183, 185, 187, 204, 205, 206

cerebral swelling   100, 135
cerebral trauma   12
cerebral tissue oxygenation (RSO$_2$)   206, 209
cerebral vascular reactivity   107
cerebrovascular disease   98, 99, 101, 103
cerebrovascular disorder   120
cerebrovascular permeability   10
cerebrovascular resistance (CVR)   165, 168
cerebrovascular response   180
choline   6, 9
CI-977   13, 47, 49, 50, 52, 53, 54, 55
Cl$^-$ 15
^{14}C-labeled sucrose   6, 7, 8, 9, 10, 11
^{14}C-labeled deoxyglucose autoradiography   12, 15
Co^{2+} 13, 14
compressed spectral array (CSA)   165
computed tomography (CT)   61, 70, 72, 106, 135, 137, 147, 154, 161, 173, 174, 212, 213, 219, 226
CT stereotactic operation   135, 137
contused brain tissue   72, 76
contusion   70, 78
CO$_2$ reactivity   164, 165, 169, 170, 180, 181, 182, 183, 185, 186, 187, 218, 219, 223
CO$_2$ response   227
cortical spreading depression   6, 14, 16
cytochrome aa$_3$ (Cyt)   193, 215, 226, 228, 233
cytoplasm   26, 55
cytosol   76

D
delayed neuronal damage   34
deoxyhemoglobin (deoxy-Hb)   193, 194, 215, 218, 226, 227, 229, 232
desaturation   101, 120, 121, 122, 123, 124, 125, 126, 156, 157, 176, 177, 209
dialysis probe   4, 6
diffuse brain injury   62, 66, 98, 99, 173, 180, 181, 212, 213
dopamine   36, 38, 40, 94, 109

E

electroencephalography (EEG)   127, 128, 129, 132, 133, 165, 169, 193, 233

EEG power spectrum   128, 132, 133

electron microscopic study   27

embolization procedure   146, 149

endoarterectomy   128

end-tidal carbon dioxide concentration (ETCO$_2$)   106, 107

end-tidal CO$_2$ pressure (Pet CO$_2$)   164, 165, 174, 176, 196, 205, 219, 221, 223

energy depletion   76

epidural hematoma   64, 79

EPSP slope   43

excitatory amino acid (EAA)   11, 13, 14, 15, 17, 34, 38, 47, 54, 59, 60, 61, 64, 66, 68, 69, 70, 71, 72, 78, 80, 81

EAA antagonist   12, 14, 15, 16, 18, 64, 70

excitatory postsynaptic potential (EPSP)   42, 43

excitotoxic effects   31, 34

excitotoxicity   60, 72, 76, 81

external jugular vein   101, 102

extracellular fluid (ECF)   59, 61, 62, 66, 69, 70, 71

extracellular EAA   76, 81

extracellular glutamate concentration   26, 31, 38, 47, 54, 55, 61, 76

extracellular space (ECS)   3, 4, 6, 7, 8, 10, 11, 12, 18, 26, 76, 78

ECS concentration   7, 9, 10, 13, 72

ECS shrinkage   6

ECS volume   8

extracerebral contamination   209

F

femorofemoral venoarterial bypass (F-F bypass)   128, 129, 130, 132

fentanyl   140, 144

fiberoptic catheter   93, 95, 98, 99, 113, 127, 128, 134, 147, 149, 160, 172

Fick's principle   88, 109, 141

fluid-percussion brain injury   10, 12, 13, 14, 15, 17, 69

free fatty acid   9, 17, 18

G

gamma-amino butyric acid (GABA)   81

giant cerebral aneurysm   128

Glasgow Coma Score (GCS)   80, 94, 98, 100, 106, 134, 137, 153, 156, 164, 165, 173, 174, 180, 183, 205, 212, 213, 219

Glasgow Outcome Scale (GOS)   61, 80, 94, 101, 165, 169

glial volume   81

global brain oxygen saturation (CS$_{comb}$O$_2$)   193, 194, 196, 197, 198, 201

glucose   16, 49, 50, 54, 59, 60, 61, 62, 113

glucose utilization   12, 15

glutamate   13, 26, 27, 28, 29, 30, 31, 34, 36, 38, 40, 47, 52, 53, 54, 55, 60, 61, 62, 64, 65, 66, 70, 72, 73, 74, 76, 80

glutamate antagonist   26, 28, 31, 62

glutamate neurotoxicity   26, 30, 31, 32, 62

glutamate uptake   31, 32

glycine   80, 81

glycolysis   60

H

head injury   26, 49, 59, 64, 70, 78, 81, 98, 99, 101, 103, 109, 113, 120, 134, 145, 153, 155, 157, 164, 168, 169, 170, 172, 176, 178, 180, 185, 186, 201, 205

head trauma   79, 81, 123

hematocrit   90

hemoglobin   88, 90, 92, 103, 106, 122, 156, 176, 195, 215, 227, 233

hemoglobin oxygen saturation (CS$_f$O$_2$)   194, 196, 197, 198, 201

high-performance liquid chromatography (HPLC)   36, 60, 66, 72, 79

hippocampal pyramidal cell   12, 18, 42

hippocampus   14, 42

^{3}H-labeled inulin   9

hypercapnia   196, 198, 201, 202

hyperemia   117, 146, 165, 172, 176, 177

hypertensive rat   34, 39, 40
hyperventilation (HV)   94, 99, 125,
   164, 168, 169, 172, 176, 177,
   186, 196, 218, 219, 223, 227,
   229, 230, 232, 233, 201
hyperventilation therapy   100, 101,
   121, 122, 125
hypocapnia   122, 123, 156, 196, 198,
   201, 202, 233
hypoperfusion   88, 172
hypotension   68, 87, 105, 156
hypothermia   103, 113, 128, 129, 132,
   133, 145, 177
hypoventilation   186
hypoxanthine   59, 60, 62
hypoxia   60, 68, 94, 105, 153, 155,
   158, 160, 169, 173, 232, 233

I
induced hypertension   108, 109, 110
infrared light   193, 194
intensive care   39, 60, 61, 62, 81, 82,
   87, 94, 103, 134, 135, 137, 156,
   204
internal carotid endarterectomy   128
internal jugular vein   88, 89, 93, 99,
   103, 106, 112, 134, 154, 155, 158
intracellular space (ICS)   3, 9, 10, 11
intracerebral hematoma (ICH)   79,
   112, 116, 161, 219
intracranial hematoma   87, 88, 93,
   134, 135, 160, 161, 162
intracranial hypertension   60, 112,
   117, 123, 156, 169, 208
intracranial pressure (ICP)   60, 61, 65,
   68, 70, 78, 79, 80, 81, 87, 89, 90,
   99, 100, 101, 103, 105, 106, 107,
   109, 110, 117, 122, 123, 125,
   135, 137, 138, 154, 156, 158,
   162, 164, 165, 168, 169, 172,
   173, 174, 176, 177, 178, 181,
   185, 204, 205, 206, 218, 219, 223
ion channel   13, 15, 16, 17, 42, 46
ionic concentration   32
ionic fluxes   3, 13, 15
ionic homeostasis   15, 70
ionic shift   4, 8, 14, 15, 17
ion permeability   11
ion pump   13, 15, 16, 17

ion-sensitive microelectrode   71
ischemia   9, 11, 12, 15, 17, 26, 30, 34,
   50, 52, 53, 54, 59, 60, 61, 76, 87,
   95, 116, 119, 120, 121, 122, 123,
   126, 127, 132, 133, 138, 146,
   153, 156, 160, 165, 169, 176,
   185, 232
ischemic brain injury   3, 4, 8, 37, 47,
   59, 81
ischemic insult   37, 76, 87, 90, 116,
   132
ischemic neuronal damage   18, 26, 30,
   72, 87, 128, 164, 169
ischemic neuronal death   13, 34

J
jugular bulb   87, 88, 89, 90, 98, 99,
   106, 113, 138, 139, 147, 149,
   154, 160, 180, 181, 216
jugular bulb pressure   91
jugular bulb oximetry   90, 209, 211,
   213, 216
jugular bulb saturation   90, 98, 102
jugular bulb temperature   92
jugular vein   92, 158
jugular vein oxygen saturation
   (JSATO$_2$)   66, 68
jugular venous desaturation   80, 94,
   153, 169
jugular venous flow   119

K
K^+ 5, 6, 7, 8, 11, 12, 13, 14, 15, 69,
   70, 71
K^+-free   5, 6
K^+-sensitive electrode   8
kynurenic acid (KYN)   14, 15, 16, 17,
   18

L
lactate   11, 16, 17, 18, 59, 60, 61, 79,
   80, 81, 82, 88, 141, 142, 143,
   144, 176
lactic acidosis   59, 78
laser Doppler   100, 173
LOI   88, 94, 95
long-term potentiation   17

M

magnetic resonnce (MR)   61, 73, 130, 212, 226
mannitol   103, 121, 123, 137, 174, 177
Mg^{2+} 13, 14
membrane function   11, 76
metabolic monitoring   59
MK-801   28, 30, 31, 35, 36, 37
molecular size   9
moyamoya disease   101, 226, 227, 229, 233

N

Na^+ 5, 69, 71
NBQX   28, 30
neuroactive amino acid   59, 60
neurochemical change   3, 6, 11, 12
neurochemical environment   3, 11, 12
neurochemical process   3
neuron   31
neuronal damage   38, 40, 55
neuronal depolarization   38
neuronal vacuplation   49
neuronal swelling   49
neuroprotective effect   26, 64
neuroprotective drug   47, 49, 54
neurotoxic effect   59
neurotransmission   76
neurotransmitter   13, 17, 18, 34, 38, 40
N-methyl-D-aspartate (NMDA) antagonist   43, 47, 49
NMDA receptor   31, 38, 42, 43, 46, 47, 80, 81
NMDA receptor antagonist   37
nuclear magnetic resonance spectroscopy   193

O

opioid agonist   47
opioid receptor   55
oxidative metabolism   233
oxygen consumption (VO_2)   134, 135, 137, 138, 139, 140, 142, 143, 144, 145, 153, 193, 211, 216
oxygen delivery (DO_2)   88, 105, 109, 110, 142, 144, 153, 176, 193

oxygen demand   102, 105, 110, 127, 132, 140, 145
oxygen extraction ratio   145
oxygen-glucose index (OGI)   117
oxygen saturation   120, 193, 196, 211, 213, 218
oxygen saturation catheter   153, 154
oxygen saturation of the perfusion flow ($SjPO_2$)   147, 149
oxygen saturation of the shunt flow ($SjSO_2$)   147
oxygen saturation of the systemic arterial blood (SaO_2)   88, 107, 147, 155
oxygen supply   102, 105, 127, 132, 140, 145, 211, 216
oxyhemoglobin (oxy-Hb)   193, 194, 195, 212, 215, 218, 226, 227, 229, 232, 233
oxymetrix continuous oxygen saturation monitoring system   66

P

$PaCO_2$ 99, 100, 107, 117, 121, 180, 181, 182, 183, 185, 186, 227
PaO_2 88, 107, 181, 182, 227
pathological condition   6, 31
pathological process   18
pathophysiological event   80, 81
pH   16, 107, 145
phenylephrine   107, 110, 182
phenylephrine test   107
phospholipase A2   17
phospholipase C   17
population spike (PS)   42
positive end-expiratory pressure (PEEP)   156
positron emission tomography (PET)   60, 61, 81, 138, 222
postischemia   43, 44, 46
postischemic potentiation (PIP)   17, 42, 43, 46
postresuscitation   112, 116, 183
potassium   64, 65, 66
prolonged seizure   26
pulsatility index (PI)   165, 168, 169
purine   60
pyknosis   29

pyruvate   59, 60, 79

Q

quantitive electroencephalogram
    (qEEG)   164, 165, 167, 169
Queckenstedt's test   99

R

recovery rate   8, 9, 65
regional cerebral oxygen saturatyion
    (rSO$_2$)   127, 128, 129, 132, 133
reperfusion   46
repetitive stimulation   43, 44, 46
respiratory quotient (RQ)   117
resuscitation   125, 216

S

Schaffer collateral   42, 43
secondary brain damage   64, 76, 78,
    120, 172, 177, 204
secondary brain injury   59, 81, 176
secondary insult   70, 160
secondary ischemia   59
secondary ischemic injury   68
selective death   12, 18, 42
serine   54, 66
shock   123, 125
single photon emission CT   226, 233
sodium   64, 65, 66
somatosensory evoked response   233
space-occupying lesion (SOL)   113,
    114, 123
striatum   28, 34, 36, 37, 38, 39, 40

subarachnoid hemorrhage (SAH)   26,
    59, 61, 62, 88, 93, 94, 101, 112,
    134, 135, 174, 212, 213, 216
subdural hematoma   79, 174
sucrose   7, 10
synaptic response   43, 44

T

taurine   80, 81
temperature   11
tentorial herniation   68, 208, 209
tetraethylammonium   6
tetraethyltrismethylammonium   6
thalamus   37, 39
thoracic aortic aneurysm (TAA)   128,
    129
threonine   66
thrombosis   90, 158
transcranial doppler (TCD)   61, 105,
    106, 164, 165, 169
traumatic brain injury (TBI)   3, 4, 8,
    10, 11, 12, 15, 17, 18, 59, 70, 71,
    72, 105, 122
trimethylammonium   9

V

vaculation   29
vasoconstriction   110
vasoparalysis   180, 187
vasospasm   87, 94, 101, 105, 156, 176

X

xenon-133 (^{133}Xe)   169, 193, 222, 233

.